Promoting Biodiversity in Food Systems

Promoting Biodiversity in Food Systems

Edited by
Irana W. Hawkins
PhD, MPH, RDN

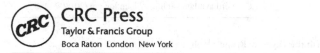

CRC Press
Taylor & Francis Group
Boca Raton London New York

CRC Press is an imprint of the
Taylor & Francis Group, an **informa** business

CRC Press
Taylor & Francis Group
6000 Broken Sound Parkway NW, Suite 300
Boca Raton, FL 33487-2742

First issued in paperback 2020

© 2019 by Taylor & Francis Group, LLC
CRC Press is an imprint of Taylor & Francis Group, an Informa business

No claim to original U.S. Government works

ISBN-13: 978-1-138-62697-3 (hbk)
ISBN-13: 978-0-367-73297-4 (pbk)

Library of Congress Cataloging-in-Publication Data

Names: Hawkins, Irana W., editor.
Title: Promoting biodiversity in food systems / edited by Irana W. Hawkins.
Description: Boca Raton, Florida : CRC Press, Taylor & Francis, [2018] |
Includes bibliographical references and index.
Identifiers: LCCN 2018023405| ISBN 9781138626973 (hardback : alk. paper) |
ISBN 9781315212647 (e-book)
Subjects: LCSH: Agrobiodiversity. | Food industry and trade--Environmental
aspects. | Food security. | Nutrition. | Functional foods. |
Lifestyles--Health aspects.
Classification: LCC S494.5.A43 P76 2018 | DDC 333.95--dc23
LC record available at https://lccn.loc.gov/2018023405

Visit the Taylor & Francis Web site at
http://www.taylorandfrancis.com

and the CRC Press Web site at
http://www.crcpress.com

Dedication

To My Father

Mr. Ira James Hawkins

1921–2013

A steadfast advocate for and student of the natural environment

Contents

SECTION I   Biodiversity Loss, Planetary Boundaries, Food Systems, and Human Health

SECTION II   Creating Biodiversity-Friendly, Sustainable Solutions

Preface

Registered Dietitian Nutritionists (RDNs) are the only credentialed healthcare providers solely trained in the application of food, nutrition, and dietetics. They are mandated by a Code of Ethics to protect public health, and are charged with recommending the healthiest foods for optimal well-being across the lifecycle. These foods should come from and contribute to healthy ecosystems.

This book culminated from the session I planned entitled, "Biodiversity: Achieving an Abundance of Wholesome Foods From Healthy Ecosystems," for the 2015 Academy of Nutrition and Dietetics Annual Food & Nutrition Conference & Exposition. It is thought to be the largest gathering of food and nutrition professionals in the world. My presentation was entitled "Promoting Biodiversity in Dietetics Practice." I was fortunate to co-present with Dr. Catherine Badgley of the University of Michigan who discussed "Biodiversity and Sustainable Agriculture."

Our session piqued the interest of Ms. Randy Brehm, Senior Editor of Agriculture and Nutrition at CRC Press. I am most grateful to Ms. Brehm and CRC Press for the opportunity to produce *Promoting Biodiversity in Food Systems* with a talented group of contributing authors who have an impressive breadth of expertise in food systems, environmental care, healthcare, and higher education. Each chapter offers a piece to the puzzle for creating healthy food systems that produce healthy foods that support healthy people on a healthy planet. Each author offers a unique perspective of understanding and applying the evidenced-based data to the multifaceted and complex issues at hand. I sincerely thank each author for their contribution, as well as CRC Press and Ms. Randy Brehm; Ms. Lara Spieker who prepared the manuscript for production; Mr. Andrew Corrigan, Project Manager; Ms. Shayna Murry, Design Artist; Ms. Laura Piedrahita, Editorial Assistant; Ms. Cynthia Klivecka, Production Editorial Manager; and Ms. Rachael Panthier, Production Editor.

Promoting Biodiversity in Food Systems recognizes that bolstering biodiversity is both an overarching necessity and a foundational solution. *Promoting Biodiversity in Food Systems* underscores that with an interdisciplinary approach, we can eat healthfully *and* support the living being and living systems of the natural environment upon which our lives depend.

Photo credits back cover:

Top left- ACOPAGRO organic agroforestry farmer Maria Adile Sangama Guerra. Photo credit Aurelio Loret de Mola and Stephanie Pellny. Courtesy of Ms. Jessica Jones-Hughes, Equal Exchange.

Top middle- Regenerative design with swales in Santa Cruz, California. Photo credit Ms. Lydia Neilsen, Rehydrate the Earth. Courtesy of Ms. Neilsen.

Top right- Morroccan Chickpea Sorghum Bowl. Photo credit: Ms. Sharon Palmer, The Plant-Powered Dietitian. Courtesy of Ms. Palmer.

Bottom left- Dalin Tzu Chi Hospital workers complimentary workplace bicycles. Photo credit Tzu Chi Medical Foundation, Hualien,Taiwan. Courtesy of Dr. Chin-Lon Lin, Tzu Chi Medical Foundation.

Bottom middle- Skyline Garden at Taipei Tzu Chi Hospital. Photo credit Tzu Chi Medical Foundation, Hualien, Taiwan. Courtesy of Dr. Chin-Lon Lin, Tzu Chi Medical Foundation.

Bottom right- Diversified farming system, Occidental Arts and Ecology Center, Sonoma County, California. Photo credit Dr. Catherine Badgley, University of Michigan. Courtesy of Dr. Badgley.

Editor

Dr. Irana W. Hawkins is a Registered Dietitian Nutritionist (RDN), a Native Plant Steward, and a Master Recycler-Composter. She teaches in the Doctoral Programs in Public Health at Walden University, Minneapolis, Minnesota (MN). Dr. Hawkins understands that the healthiest foods should come from and contribute to the healthiest ecosystems. While *Promoting Biodiversity in Food Systems* identifies the problems associated with the modern food system, the solutions offered are teaming with co-benefits. The contributing authors offer perspectives that place food, food systems, health, healthcare, and the natural environment together as they cannot be separated—with biodiversity front and center.

Contributors

Mildred L. Alvarado, Ph.D.
Independent Sustainable
   Agriculture Consultant
Amherst, MA

Catherine Badgley, PhD
University of Michigan
Ann Arbor, MI

Michael M. Bell, PhD
University of Wisconsin—Madison
Madison, WI

Michael Berger, PhD
Simmons College
Boston, MA

Tina H.T. Chiu, PhD, RDN
Tzu Chi Medical Foundation
New Taipei City, Taiwan

Stacia Clinton, BS, RDN
Health Care Without Harm
Reston, VA

Bonnie Farmer, MS, RDN
PlantWise Nutrition Consulting
Galesburg, MI

Anandi Gandhi, MA
Independent Researcher
Berkeley, CA

Dary Goodrich, BA
Equal Exchange [Chocolate]
West Bridgewater, MA

Alison H. Harmon, PhD, RDN
Montana State University
Bozeman, MT

Irana W. Hawkins, PhD, MPH, RDN
Walden University
Minneapolis, MN

Katrina Hoch, PhD, MS, RDN, CD
Seattle Children's Hospital
Seattle, WA

Kimberley Hodgson MURP, MS, AICP, RDN
Cultivating Healthy Places
Vancouver, British Columbia

Ravdeep Jaidka, MS
Equal Exchange [Produce]
West Bridgewater, MA

Jessica Jones-Hughes, MS, RDN
Equal Exchange [Fresh Produce]
West Bridgewater, MA

Carly Kadlec, BA
Equal Exchange [Coffee]
West Bridgewater, MA

Cristina Liberati, MALD
Equal Exchange [Grant Management
   & Chocolate]
West Bridgewater, MA

Chin-Lon Lin, MD, FACC
Tzu Chi Medical Foundation
Hualien City, Taiwan

Tobias Lunt, MS
University of Wisconsin—Madison
Madison, WI

Bill McDorman, BA
Rocky Mountain Seed Alliance
Ketchum, ID

Kayellen Edmonds-Umeakunne, MS, RDN
Morehouse School of Medicine
Atlanta, GA

Loyal A. Mehrhoff, PhD
Center for Biological Diversity
Honolulu, HI

Tara Moreau, PhD
University of British Columbia
  Botanical Garden
Vancouver, British Columbia

Lydia Neilsen, BA
Rehydrate the Earth
Santa Cruz, CA

Sharon Palmer, BS, RDN
The Plant-Powered Dietitian
Bradbury, CA

Rebecca Prince-Ruiz, BSc
Plastic Free July
South Fremantle, Western
  Australia

Leif Rawson-Ahern, MBA
Equal Exchange [Tea]
West Bridgewater, MA

Monique Richard, MS, RDN, LDN, RYT-200
East Tennessee State University
Johnson City, TN

Mona Seymour, PhD
Loyola Marymount University
Los Angeles, CA

Kumara Sidhartha, MD, MPH
Emerald Physicians/Cape Cod
  Healthcare
Cotuit, MA

Saray Stancic, MD
Stancic Health and Wellness
Ramsey, NJ

Jasia Steinmetz, PhD, RDN
University of Wisconsin—Stevens Point
Stevens Point, WI

Valerie J. Stull, PhD, MPH
University of Wisconsin—Madison
Madison, WI

Stewart Tai, Certified Engineer
Khoo Teck Puat Hospital
Singapore

Caroline Trapp, DNP, ANP, CDE
University of Michigan
Ann Arbor, MI

Angie Tagtow, MS, RDN
Minnesota Institute for Sustainable
  Agriculture
St. Paul, MN

Stephen Thomas, BA
Colorado State University
Fort Collins, CO

John Westerdahl, PhD, MPH, MA, RDN, CNS
LifeTalk Radio Network
Newbury Park, CA

Section I

Biodiversity Loss, Planetary Boundaries, Food Systems, and Human Health

1 The Intersection of Biodiversity, Food, and Health

Irana W. Hawkins

CONTENTS

1.1 INTRODUCTION

When Mr. Randy Bekendam of Amy's Organic Farm in Ontario, California, was asked for a donation of farm fresh produce for a free health clinic serving persons without health insurance in San Bernardino, California, he replied, "It wouldn't be a health event without offering healthy foods" (Hawkins 2017). He contributed a carload of organic pomegranates, butternut squash, and eggplant. Farmer Bekendam's sentiments align with the premise of this book: Food, food systems, health, and healthcare cannot be separated from each other or the natural environment.

As food comes from food systems—whether it be the complex, industrialized, mainstream food system or the food that we grow in our front- and backyards—attention to the value of *how* and *what* is produced and consumed has never been more important for biodiversity, health outcomes, and the delivery of healthcare. Biodiversity is comprised of the millions of living beings on the planet—whether they are plants, animals, or soil microbes—and along with their respective ecosystems help support humanity's well-being in the Earth system (Millennium Ecosystem Assessment 2005; Chivian and Bernstein 2010; Steffen et al. 2015).

Why place an emphasis upon biodiversity? Along with the overexploitation of resources, agriculture is a top driver of biodiversity loss (Butchart et al. 2010; Maxwell et al. 2016). Other drivers include but are not limited to urban development, invasion and disease, pollution, climate change, and energy production (Maxwell et al. 2016). Scientists affirm that we are in the midst of what is considered a biodiversity crisis or a "sixth mass extinction" (Ceballos 2015). Not only does biodiversity provide us with food, clothing, shelter, medicine, and enumerable ecosystem services such as water purification, soil fertility, carbon sequestration and storage, vector-borne disease control and pollination- but biodiversity is a key factor in regulating

3

the Earth system (Steffen et al. 2015). Biodiversity contributes to the stability of the Earth system, and increasingly diverse ecosystems become more resilient over time (Cardinale et al. 2012).

Why focus on health and healthcare? The Western diet produced by the industrialized food system contributes to the demise of human health. The Western diet and what we know in the U.S. as the Standard American Diet (SAD) has a far-reaching impact on human health as documented by the nutrition transitions around the world and a large body of evidence-based data (Popkin et al. 2012; World Health Organization 2017; The 2015 Global Burden of Disease Collaborators 2017). Highly processed convenience foods laden with added fats, sugar, and salt, and low in fiber are commonplace. As meals are now readily consumed outside the home, the astronomical use of single-use, disposable food and beverage packaging and food-serving implements are a routine lifestyle practice in the U.S and around the globe. What may be less obvious but extremely important is the negative impact disposable food-serving plastics impart on biodiversity and the natural environment.

Additionally, the U.S. healthcare system systematically fails to address the burden of chronic diet-related diseases despite spending the most monies on healthcare in the world (Woolf and Laudan 2013). The U.S. and other countries around the globe are facing epidemic rates of chronic diseases such as diabetes and obesity (United Nations Systems Standing Committee on Nutrition 2017; World Health Organization 2017; The 2015 Global Burden of Disease Collaborators 2017). In the U.S., it has been projected that one in three will have diabetes by 2050 (Boyle et al. 2010). The burden of diabetes is altogether immense and disproportionately impacts persons of color (Huang et al. 2009; Indian Health Service 2017). Likewise, the burdens of infectious diseases and the rise of chronic diseases in developing countries strains limited resources while imposing further undue suffering.

While humanity is using more natural resources than ever, we are also wasting these precious resources. Food waste has increased in the U.S. in recent years from 900 calories per person per day in 1974 to 1400 calories wasted per person per day in 2003 (Hall et al. 2009). This not only represents an extraordinary waste of natural resources, but contributes to food insecurity and simply makes no sense whatsoever, except to the person or business engaging in the waste. As the chef Hugh Fearnley-Whittingstall from the United Kingdom (U.K.) stated, "Watching twenty tons of freshly dug parsnips consigned to the rubbish heap in a Norfolk farmyard—purely because they didn't look pretty enough—is still one of the most shocking things I've ever seen" (BBC News July 27, 2016). Additionally, in 2015 the *Boise Weekly* reported that of the 53,000 tons of food sent to the Ada County Landfill per year, over 30% was considered edible food (Prentice 2015). As methane gas is produced when food enters landfills, (Hall 2009), a whole systems perspective is warranted and overdue.

While there are many forces that impact the production and distribution of food such as neoliberal policies and other social and economic injustices, we're at a critical junction where the entirety of stakeholders in the food system must address the anthropogenic maladies imposed on the natural environment. Additionally, in an era of unprecedented biodiversity loss and climate change, the foods grown for production and the nutrients they contain may change altogether.

Another consideration is that during extreme heat events, animals such as cows cannot withstand such conditions and will perish (U.S. Environmental Protection Agency 2016). How will regional food producers contend with such issues? How can we prevail through drought and water shortages? How can those concerned with improving regional food systems, offering wholesome foods, reversing chronic disease trends, and bolstering biodiversity create inroads?

This book examines not only the problems associated with the mainstream food system but offers solutions that can be incorporated into our respective professional practice every day whether it be in the production or procurement of food—in our delivery of healthcare—how we educate our students that will enter the workforce—the foods we recommend for good health—or by including youth in the healthy food systems we strive to achieve.

As delineated in this book, healthy foods should come from healthy ecosystems—and how foods are grown and what is produced should contribute to the health of ecosystems, bolster biodiversity, and contribute positively to human health. This chapter introduces these connections while offering a roadmap to this book that is framed by way of the planetary boundaries and through the lens of planetary health. Ultimately, we cannot speak of healthy ecosystems, healthy food systems, or healthy people without acknowledging the vital role of biodiversity and the inordinate number of ecosystem services that our lives depend upon. The next section offers a broad overview of how we got here with respect to resource utilization and its subsequent impact on the Earth system.

1.2 THE ANTHROPOCENE AND ECOLOGICAL OVERSHOOT

In an era of excessive anthropogenic resource utilization that has been labeled "The Anthropocene," scientists note that the accelerated use of resources seen in the Industrial Era (1800–1945) and subsequently during "The Great Acceleration" (1945–2010) contributed to unprecedented changes in the Earth system (Steffen et al. 2007, 2015). During the period of The Great Acceleration, scientists point to the sharp increase in the human population and urban populations, real GDP, foreign investment, energy use, fertilizer use, dams, water use, paper production, tourism, transportation, and telecommunications (Steffen et al. 2015). Subsequently, the Earth system was impacted through steep increases in greenhouse gas emissions such as carbon dioxide, nitrous oxide, and methane, as well as a decrease in the ozone layer. Increases in the Earth's surface temperatures, tropical forest loss, marine fish capture, aquaculture, nitrogen in coastal zones, land changes, terrestrial biosphere degradation, as well as the acidification of the ocean (Steffen et al. 2015) all effected the Earth system. Additional information on the Anthropocene is located in Chapter 7.

Additionally, data from the Global Footprint Network (Oakland, CA) demonstrates that humanity is using more resources that can naturally be replenished in one year, referred to as "ecological overshoot" or "Earth overshoot" (Global Footprint Network 2017). Hence, the Earth's natural resources cannot be replenished in a year's time and thus the regenerative capacity of the Earth is being outstripped by approximately 50% (Galli et al. 2014). Furthermore, the day that humanity utilizes a year's supply of natural resources has occurred earlier in each year since the 1970s, known as "Earth Overshoot Day" (Global Footprint Network 2017). However, scientists indicate that focusing on this date is not as effective as understanding the totality of and reversing the massive amount of resources that are being overused.

1.3 THE PLANETARY BOUNDARIES

The planetary boundaries framework offers a way to understand the integral and interconnected processes of the Earth system while examining how the anthropogenic processes of utilizing the Earth's resources detracts or contributes to the stability of the Earth system (Steffen et al. 2015). This framework and corresponding graphic in Figure 1.1 helps discern the integrated processes of the Earth system that impact what scientists consider our "safe operating space" on the planet, where biosphere integrity and climate change are considered core drivers (Steffen et al. 2015).

The nine planetary boundaries include climate change, biosphere integrity (which includes genetic diversity and functional diversity), land system change, freshwater use, biochemical flows that include phosphorus and nitrogen overuse, ocean acidification, atmospheric aerosol loading, stratospheric ozone depletion, and novel entities that entails persistent chemical pollution (Steffen et al. 2015). The question marks in Figure 1.1 indicate those boundaries that are in the process of being quantified (Steffen et al. 2015).

Four planetary boundaries have been breached and are directly linked to food systems—climate change, genetic diversity, land system changes, and biochemical

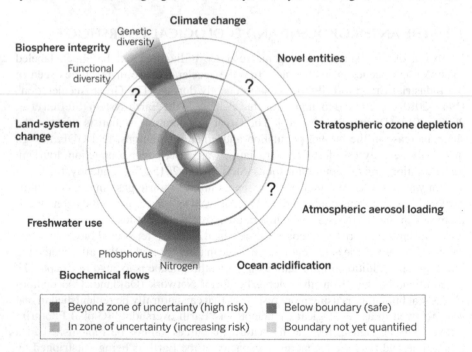

FIGURE 1.1 The status of the planetary boundaries. (From Steffen, W. et al., *Science*, 347, 1259855, 2015. With Permission.)

flows. Climate change and land system change denote an increased risk of uncertainty in maintaining our "safe operating space" while genetic diversity and biochemical flows indicate a high risk of uncertainty that may result in an increasingly inhospitable Earth system (Steffen et al. 2015). Hence, the importance of biodiversity loss cannot be overemphasized.

1.4 AN OVERVIEW OF THE CHAPTERS IN THIS BOOK

While agriculture and food systems have directly impacted the planetary boundaries that have been transgressed, they are also a solution in collectively reducing impact on the natural environment and improving human health in what we now call planetary health. Planetary health can be succinctly summarized as recognizing that both the health and well-being of humans and the natural environment must be considered together—as one cannot be separated from the other (Whitmee et al. 2015).

With some exceptions, the first half of *Promoting Biodiversity in Food Systems* primarily points to the problems associated with the industrial food system such as the loss of biodiversity and other burdens imposed on the natural environment; the burdens imposed on those producing food in the global food system; and the impact of the Western diet on human health. The second half of the book focuses on solutions to sustain biodiversity including: Regenerative agriculture; rehabilitating and rehydrating soils; a return to cooking, growing food and reclaiming local food systems; experiential learning; the importance of creating biodiversity-friendly healthcare infrastructure; institutionalizing prevention in healthcare practice; and shifting dietary patterns to increase the consumption of wholesome plant foods.

Promoting Biodiversity in Food Systems underscores that environmental care can be implemented in our respective professions—whether it be serving food, delivering healthcare, urban planning, growing food, or the dynamic processes of educating students and colleagues. From the outdoor teaching classrooms at Montana State University (MSU) and their student-run Towne's Harvest Garden (Community-Supported Agriculture)—or the global network of hospitals and healthcare facilities connected with Health Care Without Harm—food systems and healthcare systems can reverse the destructive processes forced upon the natural environment by creating new paths going forward where planetary health thrives.

In this first section, Dr. Loyal Mehrhoff expounds upon the innumerable benefits and consequences of biodiversity loss in Chapter 2. In Chapter 3, Dr. Kumara Siddhartha describes the physical aspects of food and energy, thereafter delineating the impact of the industrialized food system on biodiversity and the planetary boundaries.

In Chapter 4, Ms. Anandi Gandhi roots us in the soil, explaining the intricate pro cesses of "the biodiversity below our feet" as well as the state of our soils. Thereafter, in Chapter 5, Ms. Rebecca Prince-Ruiz focuses our attention on the rise and overall impact of disposable plastics—much of which is used to consume food and beverages. She also identifies excellent resources and the importance of working towards solutions. With over 5.25 trillion plastic particles in the ocean (Eriksen et al. 2014), the overall impact to biodiversity is both vast and dumbfounding.

In Chapter 6, Drs. Valerie Stull and Michael Bell explain how the food system that produces enough food to feed everyone leaves millions behind and they introduce the concepts of food justice and food sovereignty. They also highlight those working to end injustices by creating tangible solutions. Thereafter, Dr. Jasia Steinmetz expounds upon how food insecurity is characterized in the U.S. In Chapter 8, the industrialized food system's impact on public health is conveyed by Ms. Angie Tagtow that addresses not only chronic diseases but critical issues such as genetically modified organisms in the food supply. In Chapter 9, Ms. Jessica Jones-Hughes and colleagues (Dr. Mildred L. Alvarado, Ms. Dary Goodrich, Ms. Carly Kadlec, Ms. Cristina Liberati, Mr. Tobias Lunt, Ms. Ravdeep Jaidka, and Ms. Leif Rawson-Ahern) demonstrate how the global food system and biodiversity interface with commonly consumed foods and beverages: Bananas, cacao, coffee, sugar, palm oil, tea, and avocados. Solutions prominently emerge in this chapter as we transition to the second half of the book.

In Chapter 10, Dr. Catherine Badgley frames Section II in sustainable agriculture and offers additional insights to the common question, "How are we are going to feed the world?" Then, Dr. Mona Seymour introduces the concept of veganic agriculture. Designated by Civil Eats as what could be the next "plant-based movement" (Wall 2017), Dr. Seymour describes why it is becoming a growing trend. Mr. Bill McDorman and Mr. Stephen Thomas then focus on the power of saving seeds in Chapter 11, describing them as, "...self-replicating hard drives, allowing farmers to store newfound improvements and pass them on to future generations." In this chapter, Ms. Lydia Neilsen also discusses how creating swales can contribute to rejuvenating local water systems and offer places for biodiversity to live.

In Chapter 12, Ms. Kimberley Hodgson and Dr. Tara Moreau convey that while cities have contributed to biodiversity loss, they can also serve as a solution by bolstering biodiversity and strengthening local food systems. Dr. Alison Harmon then demonstrates in Chapter 13 how experiential learning not only contributes to local sustainable food systems—but can improve the processes of pedagogy altogether. Dr. Michael Berger follows with a vignette conveying the experience of designing an intensive, interdisciplinary course where students facilitated learning to create deliverables that solve global problems at the local level.

We then head into the kitchen with Ms. Sharon Palmer in Chapter 14, where she aptly conveys, "The Road to Good Health Goes Through the Kitchen." From there we shift to what to cook in the kitchen. Whole plant foods and their benefits are described by Ms. Monique Richard in Chapter 15. The vignettes in this chapter by Ms. Bonnie Farmer and Ms. Kayellen Edmonds-Umeakunne (1) Explain how centenarians of differing cultures and geographic locations share the common denominator of predominantly consuming whole plant foods, and (2) describe the processes of whole plant foods on the gut microbiome that convey positive benefits to human health.

From this understanding of the benefits of whole plant-based foods comes the charge from Dr. Saray Stancic that how we train medical doctors should focus on lifestyle medicine—as our healthcare system is ill-equipped to treat the epidemic of chronic diseases we see today. Dr. John Westerdahl then draws upon his experiences in planning plant-based meals at medical conferences—the very place where healthcare providers convene to discuss good health. Dr. Caroline Trapp then offers a unique and timely perspective from the nursing profession in Chapter 17: The rationale for de-prescribing medication in Type 2 Diabetes care while encouraging whole plant foods and healthy lifestyle behaviors.

In Chapter 18, we learn from Ms. Stacia Clinton how a growing global network of hospitals committed to improving planetary health offers transformative outcomes. When leveraging the purchasing power of healthcare institutions, thoughtful paths can direct how both health and regional food systems can be revolutionized. In Chapter 19, we see how a cutting edge, multi-hospital system, the Tzu Chi hospitals (Taiwan) and the Tzu Chi Medical Foundation incorporate reverence for biodiversity in all aspects of their operations. After discussing the harmful impact hospitals can have on the natural environment, Drs. Lin and Chiu discuss a number of impactful solutions implemented at their facilities. It may be the conservation efforts offered to individual patients such as collecting excess water from the shower that is then used to flush toilets, or the durable tableware set that is given to each employee for their personal use when eating meals in the workplace. The Tzu Chi hospitals' system-wide efforts include but are not limited to: an extensive greywater system; using renewable energy from solar panels; creating green spaces for biodiversity that also contribute to facilitating human healing; creating permeable surfaces for rainwater collection; exclusively serving vegetarian meals on resuable tableware; serving foods produced at the hospital's organic farm; and creating a non-profit subsidy that upcycles plastic waste—whether it be from dialysis tubing or the plastic bottles they collect in the community—that becomes items such as blankets that are used in their humanitarian operations around the world. In fact, when serving meals during a humanitarian crisis, those meals are served on reusable tableware. The Tzu Chi hospitals and subsidiaries demonstrate that with forethought and determination, care for both human health, biodiversity, and the natural environment can prevail. Additionally, Mr. Stewart Tai offers a case study of the extraordinary ecological accomplishments of Khoo Teck Puat Hospital in Singapore. Finally, in Chapter 20, Dr. Katrina Hoch conveys how children can thrive when being introduced to healthy foods systems.

As mentioned at the beginning of this chapter, we cannot remove food systems and the food it produces from human health or the health of the natural environment. What is conveyed throughout *Promoting Biodiversity in Food Systems* is that conserving and promoting biodiversity is of the utmost importance—with food systems being a critical component of this mission.

REFERENCES

Boyle, J., T. Thompson, and E. Gregg. 2010. Projection of the year 2050 burden of diabetes in the US adult population: Dynamic modeling of incidence, mortality, and prediabetes prevalence. *Population Health Metrics* 8: 29. http://www.pophealthmetrics.com/content/8/1/29.

Butchart, S.H.M., M. Walpole, B. Collen, A. van Strien, J.P.W. Scharlemann, R.E.A. Almond, J.E.M. Baillie, et al. 2010. Global biodiversity: Indicators of recent declines. *Science* 328: 1164–1168.

Cardinale, B., Duffy, J., Gonzalez A., et al. 2012. Biodiversity loss and its impact on humanity. *Nature* 486: 59–68. doi:10.1038/nature11148.

Ceballos G., Ehrlich P.R., Barnosky A.D., García A., Pringle R.M., Palmer T.M. 2015. *Sci Adv.* Jun 19; 1(5):e1400253. doi: 10.1126/sciadv.1400253. eCollection.

Chivian, E., and A. Bernstein. 2010. *How Our Health Depends on Biodiversity.* Boston, MA: Center for Health and the Global Environment, Harvard Medical School. http://www.chgeharvard.org/sites/default/files/resources/182945%20HMS%20Biodiversity%20booklet.pdf.

Eriksen, M., L.C.M. Lebreton, H.S. Carson, M. Thiel, C.J. Moore, J.C. Borerro, F. Galgani, P.T. Ryan, and J. Reisser. 2014. Plastic pollution in the World's oceans: More than 5 trillion plastic pieces weighing over 250,000 tons afloat at sea. *Plos One* 1–15, doi: 10.1371/journal.pone.0111913.

Fearnley-Whittingstall, H. October 28, 2015. Viewpoint: The rejected vegetables that aren't even wonky. *BBC News Magazine.* https://www.bbc.co.uk/news/magazine-34647454.

Galli, A., M. Wackernagel I. Katsunori, and E. Lazarus. 2014. Ecological footprint: Implications for biodiversity. *Biological Conservation* 173: 121–132.

Global Footprint Network. 2017. n.d. About earth overshoot day. https://www.overshootday.org/about-earth-overshoot-day/

Hall, K.K., J. Guo M. Dore, and C.C. Chow. 2009. The progressive increase of food waste in America and its environmental impact. *Plos One* 4(11): e7940.

Hawkins, I. 2017. *What a Difference Two Days Makes!* Center for Faculty Excellence Newsletter, December, volume 8, number 3, page 7, Walden University.

Huang, E., S. Brown N. Thakur, L. Carlisle, E. Foley, B. Ewigman, and D.O. Meltzer. 2009. Racial/ethnic differences in concerns about current and future medications among patients with type 2 diabetes. *Diabetes Care* 32(2): 311–316.

Indian Health Service. 2017. Indian health disparities. https://www.ihs.gov/newsroom/includes/themes/responsive2017/display_objects/documents/factsheets/Disparities.pdf. Accessed December 27, 2017.

Maxwell, S.L., R.A. Fuller, T.M. Brooks, and J.E.M. Watson. 2016. The ravages of guns, nets and bulldozers [comment]. *Nature* 536: 143–145.

Millennium Ecosystem Assessment. 2005. Overview of the millennium ecosystem assessment. http://www.millenniumassessment.org/en/About.html. Accessed December 14, 2015.

Popkin, B., L. Adair, and S. Ng. 2012. Now and then: The global nutrition transition: The pandemic of obesity in developing countries. *Nutrition Reviews* 70(1): 3–21. doi: 10.1111/j.1753-4887.2011.00456.x.

Prentice, G. January 21, 2015. What a waste: Analysis reveals a stunning amount of edible food and yard debris in Ada County landfill. *Boise Weekly.* http://www.boiseweekly.com/boise/what-a-waste/Content?oid=3388505.

Steffen, W., W. Broadgate L. Deutsch, O. Gaffney, and C. Cornelia Ludwig. 2015. The trajectory of the anthropocene: The great acceleration. *The Anthropocene Review* 2(1): 81–98.

Steffen, W., P. Crutzen, and J. McNeill. 2007. The anthropocene: Are humans now overwhelming the great forces of nature? *Ambio* 36(8): 614–621.

Steffen, W., K. Richardson, J. Rockström, S.E. Cornell, I. Fetzer, E.M. Bennett, R. Biggs, S.R. Carpenter, et al. 2015. Planetary boundaries: Guiding human development on a changing planet. *Science* 347(6223): 1259855, doi:10.1126/science.1259855.

The 2015 Global Burden of Disease Collaborators. 2017. Health effects of overweight and obesity in 195 countries over 25 Years. *The New England Journal of Medicine* 377(1): 13–27.

United Nations Systems Standing Committee on Nutrition. 2017. The UN decade of action on nutrition 2016–2025. https://www.unscn.org/en/topics/un-decade-of-action-on-nutrition. Accessed November 27, 2017.

United States (U.S.) Environmental Protection Agency. 2016. Climate impacts on agriculture and food supply. https://www.epa.gov/climate-impacts/climate-impacts-agriculture-and-food-supply. Accessed November 25, 2017.

Wall, A. 2017. Is vegan farming the next plant-based phenomenon? August 4. Civil Eats. https://civileats.com/2017/08/04/is-vegan-farming-the-next-plant-based- phenomenon/

Whitmee S., A. Haines C. Beyrer F. Boltz A.G. Capon B.F. de Souza Dias A. Ezeh H. Frumkin, et al. 2015. *Lancet* 386: 1973–2028.

Woolf, S.H., and A. Laudan, eds. 2013. *U.S. Health in International Perspective: Shorter Lives, Poorer Health*. Washington, DC: National Academy of Sciences and the Institute of Medicine. National Academy of Sciences. ISBN 978-0-309-38779-8, doi: 10.17226/13497.

World Health Organization. 2017. The top 10 causes of death: Top 10 causes of death worldwide. http://www.who.int/mediacentre/factsheets/fs310/en/. Accessed November 29, 2017.

2 Biological Diversity—Life on Earth

Loyal A. Mehrhoff

CONTENTS

2.1 INTRODUCTION

Biological diversity, or biodiversity for short, is a broad concept that encompasses the totality of life on Earth. Biodiversity includes all of the variation found in plants, animals, and the ecosystems they form. This includes their morphology (structural features), taxonomic uniqueness (e.g., a species, subspecies, or variety), genetics, abundance, and even behavior. Biodiversity also includes spatial and temporal elements of these factors. When we think of biodiversity we often imagine tigers, elephants, and polar bears, but biodiversity includes domesticated species as well. It is the different types of corn, apples, rice, and vegetables that we eat every day; our pets that provide companionship; and the plants that beautify our gardens. With this all-encompassing concept, we can understand that biodiversity is important to humanity. The oxygen we breathe, the food we eat, numerous economic activities, and many of our medicines all come from other living organisms—the Earth's biodiversity.

Because biodiversity is a complex concept involving multiple spatial and temporal scales, most discussions of biodiversity are simplified and focus one or a few aspects of diversity, such as the number and abundance of species present in an area, differences in species between areas, or the genetic structure of a particular species across space. One of the simplest measures is the number of species found in an area, though accurately quantifying even this on a global scale can be challenging. The well-known scientist Robert May noted that if an alien space-faring civilization showed up on our doorstep, one of their first questions would probably be to ask us how many species reside on Earth (May 2010). Unfortunately, we would not have a good answer. We have documented approximately 2.4 million species (Pimm et al. 2014), only a fraction of what we think resides on the planet. One estimate by Mora et al. (2011) is that there are about 8.7 million species, but other estimates range from around 3 million species to tens or hundreds of millions of species (May 2010; Locey and Lennon 2015).

2.2 WHERE IS EARTH'S BIODIVERSITY?

Biodiversity is everywhere because life is everywhere on this planet. From the depths of the oceans to the highest mountains and driest deserts, life exists. However, life and biodiversity are not uniformly distributed. There is a species diversity gradient that is highest near the equator and declines towards the poles. It is widely thought that tropical rainforests have the highest species diversity of terrestrial ecosystems, with coral reefs being the most biodiverse aquatic ecosystems. The factors that drive increases in species diversity are not universally agreed upon (Terborgh 2015; Brown 2014)—but areas with high species diversity frequently lack environmental extremes, have high productivity (high temperatures and moisture), and are on older landscapes (or waterscapes) (Figure 2.1).

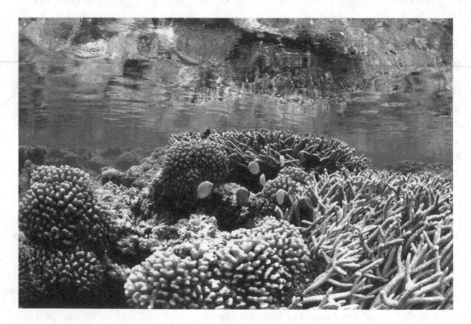

FIGURE 2.1 Coral reef at Rose Atoll National Wildlife Refuge American Samoa. (Photo by Jim Maragos, U.S. Fish & Wildlife Service.)

2.3 IS BIODIVERSITY DECLINING?

The total number of species on Earth is declining. In fact, it is declining very rap-idly because the rate of speciation (the formation of new species) is far less than the current rate of species extinctions (the loss of species). The extinction of spe-cies is occurring so fast that scientists are concerned that we may soon be enter-ing a worldwide mass extinction event or are already in one (Barnosky et al. 2011; McCallum 2015; Ceballos et al. 2017). There have been five previous mass extinction events in Earth's history. The last one occurred 65 million years ago at the close of the Cretaceous period, when 70% of the world's species went extinct including the dinosaurs (McCallum 2015). Today's global extinction rate is thought to be around 100 species per million species per year (Millennium Ecosystem Assessment 2005) with projections of an increase in the rate up to 1,500 species per million species per year by 2100 (Pimm et al. 2006). Since the background or natural rate of extinction is thought to be around one-tenth to one species per million species per year, these extinction rates are up to 1,500 times higher than normal.

But not all measures of biodiversity are declining. For example, at local or regional scales, the number of species is frequently stable or increasing due to increases in the number of non-native species introduced by humans (McGill et al. 2015). Even in places like the Hawaiian Islands, often referred to as the "extinction capital of the United States," the number of non-native species that have been introduced into the islands far exceeds the number of native species extinctions, so there has been an overall net increase in species diversity (Sax et al. 2002, 2003). So, what should we make of a situ-ation where some measures of biodiversity show a decline and others an increase? As with all scientific inquiries, it is important to understand how the different measures are calculated and how they differ, as well as understanding what the differences mean.

In the above example from Hawaii, we find that, indeed, the total number of species living in these islands has increased over the last 200 years. This is not, however, good news because the number of native Hawaiian species has declined due to extinctions. For example, 110 of the Hawaii's 1,216 endemic plants (those found only in Hawaii) have gone extinct, with another 238 species reduced to fewer than 50 wild individu-als, yet 1,367 plant species from other parts of the world have been introduced into the islands by humans (Wagner et al. 2005). So, if we are simply counting the number of all plant species, Hawaii has seen more than a two-fold increase of its local biodi-versity, even if all of the 238 plants on the brink of extinction are also lost. However, both endemic biodiversity and global biodiversity have actually declined because the endemic species lost from Hawaii are lost not just from Hawaii, but from all of the Earth. And while the human introduction of plants from Asia, South America, and other places into Hawaii has increased local biodiversity, it has not increased global diversity at the species level. Competing trends like these force us to think about what are the most important measures of biodiversity and at what scale.

2.4 CAUSES OF BIODIVERSITY LOSS

We humans have been very successful at surviving as there are now almost 7.5 billion of us (United Nations 2017). We are capable of maintaining large populations even in unfavorable climates by: (1) modifying naturally occurring ecosystems to better suit our needs; (2) exploiting ancient fossil fuel resources like coal and oil (stored solar energy from millions of years ago); (3) creating vast agricultural systems that allow us to produce large amounts of food and transport it to otherwise inhospitable areas; and (4) the development of medical and sanitary advancements that have greatly increased our survival rates. Humans inhabit every continent, where 25%–40% of the planet's total primary productivity ends up being coopted by humans (Krausmann et al. 2013; Viousek et al. 1986) and approximately 40%–50% of the Earth's land area has been altered to feed or support us (Vitousek et al. 1997)—with more recent estimates at 50% (Hooke et al. 2012). Man-made chemicals such as pesticides can be found even in the most remote areas (Vecchiato et al. 2015). Our use of fossil fuels has raised atmospheric carbon dioxide by 40% (IPCC 2013)—levels not seen in 800,000 years—threatening significant climate changes and rises in sea level.

Currently, humans are the primary cause of species extinction and biodiversity loss. We are also the only hope for stopping biodiversity loss. Most of our impacts are due to the combination of a large, rapidly increasing global population and a trend towards increasing per capita consumption of resources (Millennium Ecosystem Assessment 2005). As our population and consumption increases, so does our footprint on the natural world. Our ecological footprint measures our consumption of resources and generation of waste compared to Earth's ability to generate new resources and absorb our wastes (Wackernagel et al. 2002). Humanity's ecological footprint became unsustainable in the 1980s. In other words, that is when people began to annually consume more energy, plant productivity, and animal biomass than the Earth could naturally produce in a year as discussed in Chapter 1. We humans currently use 60% more than what the Earth annually produces (Global Footprint Network 2018), with the projection that by 2020 it may reach 175% of what the Earth can produce.

We have seen wild terrestrial vertebrates decline in abundance and range by 35%, marine vertebrates by 36%, and freshwater vertebrates by 81% (Ripple et al. 2017). The number (and biomass) of domestic vertebrate animals has continued to increase and is now 24 times larger than the total biomass of all wild vertebrates (Smil 2011).

Areas that can provide the food, commodities, and energy desired by humans are being altered to where they are no longer able to support the unique plants and animals that once lived there. With fossil fuel–driven climate change our actions will alter even the far reaches of the globe. We are clearly affecting all life on Earth and many species will be lost forever as a result.

2.5   THE MOST IMPORTANT THREATS TO BIODIVERSITY

This section discusses the most important threats to biodiversity: Changing land use; invasive species; overharvesting; climate change; pollution; and intentional persecution. But keep in mind that increases in human population and per capita resource consumption can be important drivers of these threats. In general, species with low population sizes and restricted ranges are at highest risk of extinction (Lawton 1995). But even extremely abundant species have been lost and it has happened more frequently than one would think. For example, three extremely abundant North

American species, the passenger pigeon (with 3 billion birds), the Rocky Mountain locust (with up to 12 trillion individuals), and the American bison (with tens of millions of animals) were driven to extinction or near extinction in the case of the bison. These examples will be discussed in the following sections.

2.5.1 CHANGING LAND USE

The loss of native habitat is the greatest cause of species extinctions. Worldwide, 25% of the globe has been converted to agricultural areas (Millennium Ecosystem Assessment 2005). In the last century, we have lost 40% of our forests and 50% of wetlands (Millennium Ecosystem Assessment 2005). As we convert native ecosystems to urban areas or agricultural systems to support our food, housing, and infrastructure needs, we reduce the amount of habitat available to sustain wild plants and animals. When the available habitat for a species declines to a certain point, the species may die out in the area and be lost from local biodiversity. If those species are endemic to that area, the species is also lost from global biodiversity. Deforestation in areas with high biodiversity and high endemism like tropical rainforests and coral reefs are of particular concern. For example, the conversion of a single forested ridge in Ecuador to cacao, coffee, and banana forced the extinction of a large proportion of the ridge's 90-plus endemic plant species (Dodson and Gentry 1991). The conversion of lowland forests in Hawaii for agriculture and cattle grazing likely caused the extinction of at least 16 endemic plant species (Beacham 1997).

The Rocky Mountain locust (*Melanoplus spretus*) was among the most abundant insects in North America with a single swarm estimated at 3.5 to 12.5 trillion individuals. After causing over $200 million dollars (USD) in agricultural damage in the 1870s (Garcia 2000), it was intentionally targeted for eradication. By 1902 they were eradicated (Hochkirch 2014), though the primary cause of extinction was through the conversion of its river valley habitat into farmland and not due to interventions solely targeting the Rocky Mountain locust (Lockwood 2001).

2.5.2 INVASIVE SPECIES

The anthropogenic movement of species from one area to another has altered many of the world's ecosystems. Introduced species cannot only alter basic habitats but may prey on endemic species to the point of extinction. Of particular note has been the introduction of new types of predators into islands or aquatic systems. Examples of catastrophic introductions include the stocking of Nile perch (*Lates niloticus*) into Lake Victoria and the accidental introduction of brown tree snakes (*Boiga irregularis*) onto the island of Guam. Lake Victoria, the world's largest tropical lake (one of the African Great Lakes shared by the countries of Uganda, Tanzania, and Kenya), is famous as a spectacular example of adaptive radiation (the evolution of large numbers of species from a single founder species) that created an assemblage of over 500 endemic cichlid fish. The cichlid fish community was devastated by the introduction of Nile perch, which resulted in the extinction of approximately 200 species (Witte et al. 2000).

A similar, but smaller-scale scenario played out on the island of Guam in the Mariana Islands south of Japan, which had 22 native bird species before brown tree snakes became established after World War II. Over a 40-year period, tree snakes eliminated 13 of the native bird species from Guam (Rodda and Savage 2007). The absence of these birds on Guam has impacted ecosystem dynamics on the island, with several tree species that relied on birds as seed dispersers having greatly reduced recruitment (Caves et al. 2013). While the loss of birds negatively impacted some forest trees, it seems to have led to increases in forest spiders that birds formerly preyed upon (Rogers et al. 2013). Invasive species that have been particularly important causes of extinctions include: Rats (*Rattus* spp.), cats (*Felis catus*), goats (*Capra hircus*), foxes (*Vulpes* spp.), pigs (*Sus domesticus*), Nile perch (*L. niloticus*), mosquito fish (*Gambusia affinis*), trout (multiple genera), and avian malaria (*Plasmodium relictum*).

2.5.3 OVERHARVESTING

Humans have a long history of overharvesting species to the point of extinction (Beacham 1997). Numerous flightless species of birds like the famous dodo (*Raphus cucullatus*), large island tortoises, and the sea mink (*Mustela macrodon*) fell to human exploitation. Once numbering approximately three billion birds, passenger pigeons (*Ectopistes migratorius*) were the most abundant bird in North America. Over-hunting coupled with habitat loss drove their extinction. The last of its species, Martha, died in 1914 at the Cincinnati Zoo (Yeoman 2014). American bison once numbered in the tens of millions of individuals (between 30 million and 75 million), but intense commercial hunting reduced the species to less than 300 animals and they were almost lost (U.S. Fish and Wildlife Service 1998). Even today, overharvesting is pushing species like rhinoceros, elephants, and gorillas towards extinction. With only 30 individuals remaining (World Wildlife Fund 2017; Center for Biological Diversity 2017), the world's smallest dolphin, the Vaquita (*Phocoena sinus*) is also the world's most endangered marine mammal. The Vaquita is on the brink of extinction as a result of being caught in illegal fish nets aimed at Totoaba (*Totoaba macdonaldi*), a fish prized for the presumed medicinal value of its swim bladder. Totoaba have declined to very low numbers and are now also an endangered species, further driving up its black market value and increasing poaching pressure.

2.5.4 CLIMATE CHANGE

There is little controversy in the scientific arena as to the causes of current and projected changes to Earth's climate (IPCC 2013). Human activity has resulted in large increases in atmospheric greenhouse gases like carbon dioxide and methane. Carbon dioxide is typically released in the burning of fossil fuels (IPCC 2013). Increases in atmospheric greenhouse gases are warming the Earth and acidifying the oceans (IPCC 2013, 2011). These, in turn, lead to sea level rise (IPCC 2013), spatial shifts in ecosystems (Pecl et al. 2017), numerous extinctions due to habitat loss (Fortini et al. 2013, 2015), and changes to coral reefs as a result of acidification (IPCC 2011). While many predictions of impacts to biodiversity are estimated to occur in the future, changes are underway now (Pecl et al. 2017). The first documented mammal extinction due to climate change occurred in 2014, when the Bramble Cay melomys (*Melomys rubicola*) was lost due to rising sea level that swamped its namesake island in the Great Barrier Reef (Gynther et al. 2016). This rodent-like species was the Great Barrier Reef's only endemic mammal and it had the most isolated and restricted distribution of any Australian mammal—only 2.2 hectares (5.4 acres) on a single small island (Gynther et al. 2016). Speciation of a mammal on such a small island is scientifically interesting and its loss hinders our ability to better understand evolutionary processes.

2.5.5 POLLUTION

Industrialization has led to the introduction of air and water pollution that has impacted both human health and biodiversity. Concerns in the 1950s and 1960s over the use of man-made pesticides like DDT led to calls for stricter regulation or elimination of some compounds (Carson 1962). The ban on most uses of DDT in the 1970s led to a rebound in populations of some birds like peregrine falcons, pelicans, and bald eagles that were threatened with extinction (U.S. Fish and Wildlife Service 1999). Pesticides continue to be a concern with respect to endangered species like the rusty-patched bumble bee (U.S. Fish and Wildlife Service 2017) and salmon (National Marine Fisheries Service 2009).

2.5.6 INTENTIONAL PERSECUTION

A number of species, especially top predators and species that damage agricultural crops have been intentionally targeted for extermination. The Carolina parakeet was considered an agricultural pest and essentially hunted to extinction, as was the Seychelles Alexandrine parrot that also ran afoul of agricultural interests and was destroyed (Becham 1997). Similarly, top predators like wolves, bears, lions, and tigers have been and continue to be hunted and poisoned to protect livestock and other interests (Beacham 1997). Top predators have been shown to have important impacts on ecosystem functioning and biodiversity (Terborgh 2015).

The removal of native predators from a co-evolved ecosystem can result in an overabundance of prey herbivores, with an accompanying negative impact on grazed plants and species utilizing those plants. For example, wolves (*Canis lupus*) were re-introduced to Yellowstone National Park in 1995, 70 years after they were purposefully extirpated. Since reintroduction, wolves, in conjunction with State hunting programs (MacNulty et al. 2016), have reduced the population of elk (*Cervus elaphus*), which in turn increased the re-growth of some, but not all, populations of browsed willows. Studies (Marshall et al. 2014) have shown that willows have not rebounded in areas where overbrowsing had resulted in the loss of both willows and beavers. The absence of beavers and willows changed local hydrology, which caused stream channels to incise and lower the water table of floodplains. For willows to rebound to former levels, there needs to be both a reduction of browsing and adequate water. In these areas, reduced browsing was not enough by itself; the restoration of water tables will be required (Wolf et al. 2007; Bilyeu et al. 2008;

Marshall et al. 2014). Returning a top predator in this situation did benefit the eco-system, but as with most ecological situations, it is rare that a single factor can fix all problems associated with degraded ecosystems. While re-establishing top preda-tors is appropriate in many instances, it should be remembered that adding a "new" predator that has not co-evolved to that ecosystem could result in catastrophic spe-cies and biodiversity loss (see section 2.5.2 on invasive species).

2.6   BIODIVERSITY LOSS: SHOULD WE CARE?

Is it important if elephants go extinct or if we lose redwood trees? Is it important if we no longer have dozens of different types of apples, or derive all of our corn from genetically modified varieties? Over 99% of all species that ever lived on Earth are now extinct (Barnosky et al. 2011), so do we really care if there is another mass extinction event? Consider the following:

1. The oxygen we breathe comes from both the ocean's phytoplankton (70%) and rainforests (29%) (Nelson 2017). If for no other reason than self-inter-est, it is important to pay attention to and support the functions of these important oxygen factories.
2. At least 40% of the world's economy is derived from biological resources (Organization for Economic Cooperation and Development 2002).
3. Native ecosystems provide important services—called "ecosystem ser-vices." The Millennium Ecosystem Assessment (2005) categorizes ecosys-tem services as provisioning (e.g., food, water, fiber, and fuel), regulating (e.g., climate regulation, pollination, pest regulation, pollution control, and erosion control), cultural (e.g., spiritual, aesthetic, recreational, and educa-tional), and supporting (e.g. primary production, oxygen production, and soil formation). We typically get these services for free, unless the systems become damaged and restorative actions are required.
4. One-quarter to one-half of medicines are derived from plants and animals and these represent between USD $160 billion to $320 billion annually in economic output (TEEB 2009). Losing species that we think may have medicinal benefits is unwise, and allowing undescribed or unevaluated spe-cies to go extinct is gambling with our health and that of future generations.
5. Many tourism and recreational opportunities are based on biodiversity, from fall colors to spectacular animal migrations to iconic species like redwoods and tigers. People are drawn to plants and animals. Economic activities associated with biodiversity are growing and represent an important source of income in many areas—approximately USD $880 billion to the U.S. economy alone (Outdoor Industry Association 2017). Outdoor recreation produces over 7.5 million jobs annually, more than the computer industry (6.7 million), construction (6.4 million), food and beverage (4.7 million), education (3.5 million), real estate (2.1 million), and lawyers (775,000).
6. Biodiversity is critical to agriculture (Council for Agricultural Science and Technology 1999) and is a key driver in the production of seeds for the USD $30 billion agricultural seed business (TEEB 2009).

7. Studies have shown that higher biodiversity increases ecosystem productivity (Tilman et al. 2012) and enhances ecosystem functioning (Leftcheck et al. 2015; Soliveres et al. 2016; Delgado-Baquerizo et al. 2016). Cloud forests comprised of native species retained more water than forests of introduced trees (Takahashi and Giambelluca 2011).

8. In many parts of the world, the harvesting of wild plants and animals is an important source of both subsistence and culture. The extinction or even reduced numbers of these species can impact local communities. For example, in the 1800s as part of the Government's efforts to subjugate Native American Plains Indians, it was thought that bison were specifically targeted for population reductions to damage tribal subsistence and culture (Smits 1994). Regardless of whether or not the slaughter of bison was intentional, the outcome did hurt tribes both culturally and economically. Similarly, salmon are intricately linked with a number of native cultures. The loss of salmon due to hydroelectric dams, deforestation, and overfishing has damaged tribes economically and culturally (Taylor 2009).

9. Wild relatives of domesticated organisms are important to breeding programs, especially in instances when there is a need to find genes that may provide resistance to diseases or pests (Council for Agricultural Science and Technology 1999). The world's plants and animals represent an immense and mostly untapped genetic resource. Losing this resource before we understand its value represents a huge future loss. This was recognized even back in the early 1900s when the U.S. Bureau of Plant Industry attempted to save Hawaii's spectacular red tree cotton (*Kokia drynarioides*) from extinction in the hopes that it could prove useful for breeding with domestic cotton (Young and Popenoe 1916; Rock 1919). This species is not yet extinct, but has fewer than five wild plants remaining (Figure 2.2).

10. Sandifer et al. (2015) state that "We are just beginning to appreciate the breadth of human health benefits of experiencing nature and biodiversity." They identified a number of studies that indicated the health benefits of interacting with nature. These included a reduction in certain allergies and respiratory diseases after exposure to microbial diversity; improved psychological health, positive effects on mental processes and cognitive ability; increased social interactions; reduced aggression; reduced pain; and better general health. Another study (Wolf et al. 2017) focusing on mental well-being found "benefits from natural environments that are rich in animal and plant species." Their research compared how people felt after exposure to high biodiversity images versus low biodiversity images. The results showed that after initial education about biodiversity, subjects that viewed high diversity images were generally more positive, more vital (energized), and less anxious than those seeing urban or low biodiversity images. Additionally, predators and scavengers are also thought to reduce some health risks to humans by removing dangerous organic wastes, controlling populations of disease vectors, or reducing populations of species that pose hazards to humans (O'Bryan et al. 2018).

11. Today's pending mass extinction is different from past extinction events that were caused by changing conditions or catastrophic events such as meteor strikes. The loss of species that we are seeing now is driven by habitat loss due to the appropriation of land and waters specifically for human use. Island biogeography studies have shown that the number of species in an area increases or decreases with the size of the area (MacArthur and Wilson 1967). Since we humans have appropriated half of the Earth just to support our own populations, the remaining half is all that is available to support the millions of wild species alive today or to serve as places where future natural evolution could occur. While evolution and speciation would still happen in urban, aquacultural, and agricultural settings, the evolutionary forces in these human-dominated systems would be vastly different than those found in natural coral reefs and rainforests.

12. For some, there is a moral obligation to protect nature and the species in it for future generations. This obligation is sometimes driven by a personal sense of what is right or by religious beliefs. Many religions consider the conservation of Earth's plants and animals to be important and have joined together to promote conservation through ARC—the Alliance of Religions and Conservation (http://www.arcworld.org/about_ARC.asp).

We cannot specifically predict which species will be important to people or to the world's functioning a hundred years from now. Aldo Leopold (Leopold 1953) said it best in "A Round River," one of his classic conservation essays, "To keep every

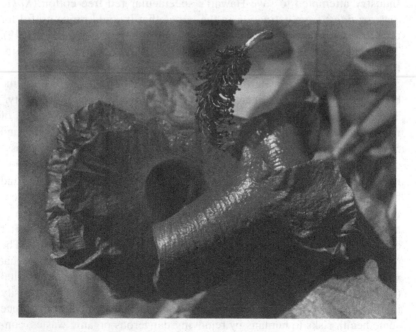

FIGURE 2.2 *Kokia drynarioides* (red cotton tree) Hawaii. (Photo courtesy of Dr. Loyal Mehrhoff, Center for Biological Diversity, Honolulu, Hawaii.)

cog and wheel is the first precaution of intelligent tinkering." Recently, over 3,000 scientists concurred with Leopold that it is important to prevent the unnecessary loss of species (Antonelli and Perrigo 2017). Humans have done a lot of tinkering, much of it with little regard for the plants and animals we share this planet with. It is time to start thinking for the future.

There are efforts currently underway to protect biodiversity. Based on our knowledge of biodiversity trends and gradients, scientists and conservation organizations have identified key areas of high biodiversity, or hotspots, to focus conservation efforts. Noted scientist and conservationist E.O. Wilson is advocating for the protection of half of the Earth's terrestrial and marine habitats in order to save the vast majority of our biodiversity (Wilson 2016). Based on island biogeography theory, such an effort could save 85% of the planet's plants and animals. Such efforts, if implemented, could greatly improve our ability to conserve biodiversity. But as scientists (Ripple et al. 2017) point out, humanity has been very slow to respond to environmental challenges such as biodiversity loss, climate change, and unsustainable resource use even when they negatively impact human society.

2.7 CONCLUSION

Life on Earth is amazing. It is a source of wonder and inspiration and a means to a healthy life. Regardless of whether you cherish or unknowingly benefit from biodiversity, it is vital. It keeps our economies running, feeds us, helps regulate the climate and other processes, provides recreational opportunities, and feeds the spirit of cultures throughout the world.

However, protecting biodiversity will not be easy.

As a society, we have undervalued biodiversity and placed short-term gains over long-term stewardship. Saving biodiversity will take becoming more informed and seeking additional information; making biodiversity-friendly choices; and creating change in one's own community. Some endeavors include volunteering with conservation organizations or supporting effective biodiversity conservation laws like the U.S. Endangered Species Act or the Canadian Species at Risk Act. Realizing our personal choices of food, clothing, housing, transportation, and family size can also make a difference in reducing impacts to biodiversity. We have an opportunity to not only sustain life on Earth, but to improve our future well-being, as well as that of all living organisms and the ecosystems that we are inextricably connected to.

REFERENCES

Antonelli, A., and A. Perrigo. December 15, 2017. We must protect biodiversity. *Washington Post*. https://www.washingtonpost.com/opinions/2017/12/15/53e6147c-e0f7-11e7-b2e9-8c636f076c76_story.html?utm_term=.bce37cd7df80.

Barnosky, A.D., N. Matzke, S. Tomiya, G.O.U. Wogan, B. Swartz, T.B. Quental, C. Marshall, et al. 2011. Has the Earth's sixth mass extinction already arrived? *Nature* 471: 51–57. http://www.nature.com/articles/nature09678.

Beacham, W. 1997. *The World Wildlife Fund Guide to Extinct Species of Modern Times*. Edited by W. Beacham. Osprey, FL: Beacham Publishing Co. https://archive.org/details/worldwildlifefun00worl_0.

Bilyeu, D.M., D.J. Cooper, N.T. Hobbs. 2008. Water tables constrain height recovery of willow on Yellowstone's northern range. *Ecological Applications* 18: 80–92, doi: 10.1890/07-0212.1. https://www.ncbi.nlm.nih.gov/pubmed/18372557.

Brown J.H. 2014. Why are there so many species in the tropics? *Journal of Biogeography* 41: 8–22. http://onlinelibrary.wiley.com/doi/10.1111/jbi.12228/full.

Carson, R. 1962. *Silent Spring*. Houghton Mifflin Co. https://archive.org/stream/fp_Silent_Spring-Rachel_Carson-1962/Silent_Spring-Rachel_Carson-1962_djvu.txt.

Caves, E.M., S.B. Jennings, J. Hille Ris Lambers, J.J. Tewksbury, and H.S. Rogers. 2013. Natural experiment demonstrates that bird loss leads to cessation of dispersal of native seeds from intact to degraded forests. *Plos One* 8(5): e65618. https://doi.org/10.1371/journal.pone.0065618.

Ceballos, G., P.R. Ehrlich, and R. Dirzo. 2017. Biological annihilation via the ongoing sixth mass extinction signaled by vertebrate population losses and declines. *Proceedings of the National Academy of Science* 114(30): E6089–E6096. www.pnas.org/cgi/doi/10.1073/pnas.1704949114.

Center for Biological Diversity. 2017. Vaquita. http://www.biologicaldiversity.org/species/mammals/vaquita/index.html.

Council for Agricultural Science and Technology. 1999. Benefits of biodiversity. Task force report no. 133. http://www.cast-science.org/publications/?benefits_of_biodiversity&show=product&productID=2839.

Delgado-Baquerizo, M. Fernando, T. Maestre, P.B. Reich, T.C. Jeffries, J.J. Gaitan, D. Encinar, M. Berdugo, C.D. Campbell, and B.K. Singh. 2016. Microbial diversity drives multifunctionality in terrestrial ecosystems. *Nature Communications* 7: 10541, doi: 10.1038/ncomms10541. https://www.nature.com/articles/ncomms10541?WT.ec_id=NCOMMS-20160203&spMailingID=50613647&spUserID=ODkwMTM2NjQyNgS2&spJobID=860336606&spReportId=ODYwMzM2NjA2S0.

Dodson, C.H. and A.H. Gentry. 1991. Biological extinction in western ecuador. *Annals of the Missouri Botanical Garden* 78(2): 273–295. https://www.jstor.org/stable/2399563.

Fortini, L., J. Price, J. Jacobi, A. Vorsino, J. Burgett, K. Brinck, F. Amidon, et al. 2013. A landscape-based assessment of climate change vulnerability for all native Hawaiian plants. Technical Report HCSU-044. Hawaii Cooperative Studies Unit, Hilo, HI. https://hilo.hawaii.edu/hcsu/documents/TR44_Fortini_plant_vulnerability_assessment.pdf.

Fortini, L.B., A.E. Vorsino, F.A. Amidon, E.H. Paxton, and J.D. Jacobi. 2015. Large-scale range collapse of Hawaiian forest birds under climate change and the need for 21st century conservation options. *Plos One* 10(10): e0140389. https://doi.org/10.1371/journal.pone.0140389.

Garcia, M. 2000. Melanoplus spretus. *Animal Diversity Web*. http://animaldiversity.org/accounts/Melanoplus_spretus/ Accessed October 2, 2017.

Global Footprint Network. 2018. https://www.footprintnetwork.org/our-work/ecological-footprint. Accessed January 21, 2018.

Gynther, I., N. Waller, and L.K.P. Leung. 2016. Confirmation of the extinction of the Bramble Cay melomys Melomys rubicola on Bramble Cay, Torres Strait: Results and conclusions from a comprehensive survey in August–September 2014. Unpublished report to the Department of Environment and Heritage Protection, Queensland Government, Brisbane. https://www.ehp.qld.gov.au/wildlife/threatened-species/documents/bramble-cay-melomys-survey-report.pdf.

Hochkirch, A. 2014. Melanoplus spretus. (errata version published in 2017). The IUCN Red List of Threatened Species 2014: e.T51269349A111451167. http://www.iucnredlist.org/details/51269349/0. Downloaded on October 3, 2017.

Hooke, R. LeB., J.F. Martin-Duque, and J. Pedraza. 2012. Land transformation by humans: A review. *GSA Today* 22(12), doi: 10.1130/GSAT151A.1. http://www.geosociety.org/gsa-today/archive/22/12/article/i1052-5173-22-12-4.htm.

IPCC. 2011. *Workshop Report of the Intergovernmental Panel on Climate Change Workshop on Impacts of Ocean Acidification on Marine Biology and Ecosystems*. Edited by C.B. Field, V. Barros, T.F. Stocker, D. Qin, K.J. Mach, G.-K. Plattner, M.D. Mastrandrea, M. Tignor, K. L. Ebi. Stanford CA: IPCC Working Group II Technical Support Unit, Carnegie Institution, 164 pp. https://www.ipcc.ch/pdf/supporting-material/IPCC_ IAOMBE_WorkshopReport_Japan.pdf.

IPCC. 2013. Summary for policymakers. In: *Climate Change 2013: The Physical Science Basis. Contribution of Working Group I to the Fifth Assessment Report of the Intergovernmental Panel on Climate Change*. Edited by T.F. Stocker, D. Qin, G.-K. Plattner, M. Tignor, S.K. Allen, J. Boschung, A. Nauels, Y. Xia, V. Bex, P.M. Midgley. Cambridge and New York, NY: Cambridge University Press. https://www.ipcc.ch/pdf/ assessment-report/ar5/wg1/WGIAR5_SPM_brochure_en.pdf.

Krausmann, F., K.H. Erb, S. Gingrich, H. Haberl, A. Bondeau, V. Gaube, C. Lauk, C. Plutzar, and T.D. Searchinger. 2013. Global human appropriation of net primary production doubled in the 20th century. *Proceedings of the National Academy of Science* 110(25): 10324–10329. doi: 10.1073/pnas.1211349110. https://www.ncbi.nlm.nih.gov/ pubmed/23733940.

Lawton, J.H. 1995. Population dynamic principles. In: *Extinction Rates*, edited by J.H Lawton and R.M May, 233 pp. New York, NY: Oxford University Press.

Leftcheck, J.S., J.E.K. Byrnes, F. Isbell, L. Gamfeldt, J.N. Griffin, N. Eisenhauer, M.J.S. Hensel, A. Hector, B.J. Cardinale, and J.E. Duffy. 2015. Biodiversity enhances ecosystem multifunctionality across trophic levels and habitats. *Nature Communications* 6. https://www.nature.com/articles/ncomms7936.

Leopold, L.B., ed. 1953. *Round River: From the Journals of Aldo Leopold*. New York, NY: Oxford University Press. https://global.oup.com/academic/product/round-river-9780195015638?cc=us&lang=en&.

Locey, K.J., and J.T. Lennon. 2015. Scaling laws predict global microbial diversity. *PeerJ PrePrints* 3:e1808. http://www.pnas.org/content/113/21/5970.full.

Lockwood, J.A. 2001. Voices from the past: What we can learn from the Rocky Mountain Locust. American Entomologist 47: 208–215. https://academic.oup.com/ae/article/47/ 4/208/2364751.

MacArthur, R.H. and E.O. Wilson. 1967. *The Theory of Island Biogeography*. Princeton, NJ: Princeton University Press. https://press.princeton.edu/titles/7051.html.

Marshall, K.N., D.J. Cooper, and N.T. Hobbs. 2014. Interactions among herbivory, climate, topography and plant age shape riparian willow dynamics in northern Yellowstone National Park, USA. *Journal of Ecology* 102: 667–677. doi: 10.1111/1365-2745.12225. http://onlinelibrary.wiley.com/doi/10.1111/1365-2745.12225/abstract.

May, R. 2010. Tropical arthropod species, more or less? *Science* 329: 41–42. http://science. sciencemag.org/content/329/5987/41.

MacNulty, D.R., C.T. Stahler, T. Wyman, J. Ruprecht, and D.W. Smith. 2016. The challenge of understanding Northern Yellowstone Elk dynamics after Wolf reintroduction. *Yellowstone Science* 24(1): 25–33. https://works.bepress.com/dan_macnulty/63/.

McCallum, M.L. 2015. Vertebrate biodiversity losses point to a sixth mass extinction. *Biodiversity and Conservation* 24: 2497–2519. https://link.springer.com/ article/10.1007/s10531-015-0940-6.

McGill, B.J., M. Dornelas, N.J. Gotelli, and A.E. Magurran. 2015. Fifteen forms of biodiversity trend in the anthropocene. *Trends in Ecology and Evolution* 30(2): 104–113. https:// doi.org/10.1016/j.tree.2014.11.006.

Millennium Ecosystem Assessment. 2005. *Ecosystems and Human Well-Being: Biodiversity Synthesis*. Washington, DC: World Resources Institute. https://www.millenniumassessment.org/documents/document.354.aspx.pdf.

Mora, C., D.P. Tittensor, S. Adl, A.G.B. Simpson, and B. Worm. 2011. How many species are there on earth and in the ocean? *PLoS Biology* 9(8): e1001127. https://doi.org/10.1371/journal.pbio.1001127.

National Marine Fisheries Service. 2009. Endangered Species Act Section 7 consultation biological opinion environmental protection agency registration of pesticides containing carbaryl, carbofuran, and methomyl. http://www.nmfs.noaa.gov/pr/pdfs/carbamate.pdf.

Nelson, D. 2017. Save the plankton, breathe freely. *National Geographic Society Education.* https://www.nationalgeographic.org/activity/save-the-plankton-breathe-freely/.

O'Bryan, C.J., A.R. Braczkowski, H.L. Beyer, N.H Carter, J.E.M. Watson, and E. McDonald-Madden. 2018. The contribution of predators and scavengers to human well-being. *Nature Ecology and Evolution* 2(2): 229–236. http://www.nature.com/articles/s41559-017-0421-2.epdf?author_access_token=8jhHXmykVkUztJisXmVu7dRgN0jAjWel9jnR3Z oTv0Og3FQwnhyVY0pNYXwMdT4GKts4p4U_TigjaVYeDCklajdt9we4VjZ-16gnqYi TFtMwQ5LZBmxBXYfN53JtheEmt2aJsbj4_pwse3DocQImtQ%3D%3D.

Organization for Economic Cooperation and Development. 2002. *The DAC Guidelines Integrating the Rio Conventions into Development Co-operation.* Paris, France. https://unfccc.int/files/meetings/workshops/other_meetings/application/pdf/dac.pdf.

Outdoor Industry Association. 2017. *The Outdoor Recreation Economy.* Boulder, CO. https://outdoorindustry.org/resource/2017-outdoor-recreation-economy-report/.

Pecl, G.T., M.B. Araújo, J.D. Bell, J. Blanchard, T.C. Bonebrake, I.-C. Chen, T.D. Clark, et al. 2017. Biodiversity redistribution under climate change: Impacts on ecosystems and human well-being. *Science* 355: 1389, doi: 10.1126/science.aai9214. http://science.sciencemag.org/content/355/6332/eaai9214.

Pimm, S., P. Raven, A. Peterson, C.H. Sekercioglu, and P.R. Ehrlich. 2006. Human impacts on the rates of recent, present, and future bird extinctions. *Proceedings of the National Academy of Sciences* 103(29): 10941–10946. http://www.pnas.org/content/103/29/10941.abstract.

Pimm, S.L., C.N. Jenkins, R. Abell, T.M. Brooks, J.L. Gittleman, L.N. Joppa, P.H. Raven, C.M. Roberts, and J.O. Sexton. 2014. The biodiversity of species and their rates of extinction, distribution, and protection. *Science* 344: 1246752. http://science.sciencemag.org/content/344/6187/1246752.

Ripple, W.J., C. Wolf, T.M. Newsome, M. Galetti, M. Alamgir, E. Crist, M.I. Mahmoud, and W.F. Laurance. 2017. World scientists' warning to humanity: A second notice. *Bioscience* 67(12): 1026–1028. https://doi.org/10.1093/biosci/bix125.

Rock, J. 1919. *The Hawaiian Genus Kokia: A Relative of the Cotton.* Honolulu, HI: Territory of Hawaii, Division of Forestry. https://catalog.hathitrust.org/Record/100423235.

Rodda, G.H. and J.A. Savage. 2007. Biology and impacts of Pacific Island invasive species. 2. Boiga irregularis, the Brown Tree Snake (Reptilia: Colubridae). *Pacific Science* 61(3): 307–324. https://www.fort.usgs.gov/sites/default/files/products/publications/21716/21716.pdf.

Rogers, H., J. Hille Ris Lambers, R. Miller, and J.J. Tewksbury. 2013. Correction: 'Natural experiment' demonstrates top-down control of spiders by birds on a landscape level. *PLoS One* 8(4). https://doi.org/10.1371/annotation/b294c406-c8ae-4c89-a083-5e6e26fb8f22.

Sandifer, P.A., A.E. Sutton-Grier, and B.P. Ward. 2015. Exploring connections among nature, biodiversity, ecosystem services, and human health and well-being: Opportunities to enhance health and biodiversity conservation. *Ecosystem Services* 12: 1–15. https://www.sciencedirect.com/science/article/pii/S2212041614001648.

Sax, D.F., and S.D. Gaines. 2003. Species diversity: From global decreases to local increases. *Trends in Ecology & Evolution.* 18: 561–566. https://www.sciencedirect.com/science/article/pii/S0169534703002246.

Sax, D.F., S.D. Gaines, and J.H. Brown. 2002. Species invasions exceed extinctions on islands worldwide: A comparative study of plants and birds. *American Naturalist* 160: 766–783. http://www.journals.uchicago.edu/doi/abs/10.1086/343877.

Smil, V. 2011. Harvesting the biosphere: The human impact. *Population and Development Review* 37(4): 613–636. http://vaclavsmil.com/wp-content/uploads/PDR37-4.Smil_.pgs613-636.pdf.

Smits, D.D. 1994. The frontier army and the destruction of the buffalo: 1865–1883. *Western Historical Quarterly* 25(3). http://www.jstor.org/stable/971110.

Soliveres, S., F. Van der Plas, P. Manning, D. Prati, M.M. Gossner, S.C. Renner, F. Alt, et al. 2016. Biodiversity at multiple trophic levels is needed for ecosystem multifunctionality. *Nature* 536 (7617): 456–459. https://www.nature.com/articles/nature19092.

Takahashi, M., T.W. Giambelluca, R.G. Mudd, J.K. DeLay, M.A. Nullet, and G.P. Asner. 2011. Rainfall partitioning and cloud water interception in native forest and invaded forest in Hawai'i Volcanoes National Park. *Hydrological Processes* 25: 448–464. doi:10.1002/hyp.7797. http://onlinelibrary.wiley.com/doi/10.1002/hyp.7797/abstract.

Taylor, J.E. 2009. *Making Salmon: An Environmental History of the Northwest Fisheries Crisis.* University of Washington Press, 488pp. http://www.washington.edu/uwpress/search/books/TAYMAK.html.

TEEB. 2009. The economics of ecosystems and biodiversity for national and international policy makers. http://doc.teebweb.org/wp-content/uploads/2014/04/TEEB-in-national-and-international-Policy-Making2011.pdf.

Terborgh, J.W. 2015. Toward a trophic theory of species diversity. *Proceedings of the National Academy of Sciences* 112: 11415–11422. http://www.pnas.org/content/112/37/11415.

Tilman, D., P.B. Reich, and F. Isbell. 2012. Biodiversity impacts ecosystem productivity as much as resources, disturbance, or herbivory. *Proceedings of the National Academy of Sciences* 109: 10394–10397. http://www.pnas.org/content/109/26/10394.full.

United Nations. 2017. *World Population Prospects: The 2017 Revision.* New York: United Nations Department of Economic and Social Affairs, Population Division. https://esa.un.org/unpd/wpp/publications/Files/WPP2017_KeyFindings.pdf.

U.S. Fish and Wildlife Service. 1998. American buffalo, *(Bison bison).* Species Accounts. https://www.fws.gov/species/species_accounts/bio_buff.html.

U.S. Fish and Wildlife Service. 1999. Endangered and threatened wildlife and plants; final rule to remove the American peregrine falcon from the federal list of endangered and threatened wildlife, and to remove the similarity of appearance provision for free-flying peregrines in the conterminous United States. *Federal Register* 64(164): 46542–46558. https://www.federalregister.gov/documents/1999/08/25/99-21959/endangered-and-threatened-wildlife-and-plants-final-rule-to-remove-the-american-peregrine-falcon.

U.S. Fish and Wildlife Service. 2017. Endangered and threatened wildlife and plants; endangered species status for rusty patched bumble bee. *Federal Register* 82(7): 3186–3208. https://www.federalregister.gov/documents/2017/02/10/2017-02865/endangered-and-threatened-wildlife-and-plants-endangered-species-status-for-rusty-patched-bumble-bee.

Vecchiato, M., E. Argiriadis, S. Zambon, C. Barbante, G. Toscano, A. Gambaro, and R. Piazza. 2015. Persistent organic pollutants (POPs) in Antarctica: Occurrence in continental and coastal surface snow. *Microchemical Journal* 119: 75–82. https://www.sciencedirect.com/science/article/pii/S0026265X14001969.

Vitousek, P.M., H.A. Mooney, J. Lubchenco, and J.M. Melillo. 1997. Human domination of earth's ecosystems. *Science* 277(5325): 494–499. http://science.sciencemag.org/content/277/5325/494.full.

Vitousek, P.M., P.R. Ehrlich, A.H. Ehrlich, and P.A. Matson. 1986. Human appropriation of the products of photosynthesis. *BioScience* 36(6): 368–373. https://academic.oup.com/bioscience/article-abstract/36/6/368/230276?redirectedFrom=fulltext.

Wackernagel, M., N.B. Schulz, D. Deumling, A.C. Linares, M. Jenkins, V. Kapos, C. Monfreda, et al. 2002. Tracking the ecological overshoot of the human economy. *Proceedings of the National Academy of Sciences* 99(4):9266–9271. http://www.pnas. org/content/99/14/9266.abstract#cited-by.

Wagner, W.L., D.R. Herbst, and D.H. Lorence. 2005. Flora of the Hawaiian Islands. http:// botany.si.edu/pacificislandbiodiversity/hawaiianflora/index.htm. Accessed October 2017.

Willis, K.J., M.B. Araújo, K.D. Bennett, B. Figueroa-Rangel, C.A. Froyd, and N. Myers. February 28, 2007. How can a knowledge of the past help to conserve the future? Biodiversity conservation and the relevance of long-term ecological studies. *Philosophical Transactions of the Royal Society B* 362: 175–187, doi: 10.1098/ rstb.2006.1977. https://www.ncbi.nlm.nih.gov/pmc/articles/PMC2311423/.

Wilson, E.O. 2016. *Half-Earth: Our Planet's Fight for Life.* New York, NY: Liveright Publishing Corporation, 256 pp. http://www.half-earthproject.org/book/.

Witte, F., B. Msuku, J. Wanink, O. Seehausen, E.F.B. Katunzi, P.C. Goudswaard, and T. Goldschmidt 2000. Recovery of cichlid species in Lake Victoria: An examination of factors leading to differential extinction. *Reviews in Fish Biology and Fisheries* 10: 233. https://doi.org/10.1023/A:1016677515930.

Wolf, E.C., D.J. Cooper, and N.T. Hobbs. 2007. Hydrologic regime and herbivory stabilize an alternative state in Yellowstone National Park. *Ecological Applications* 17: 1572–1587, doi: 10.1890/06-2042.1. https://www.ncbi.nlm.nih.gov/pubmed/17913124.

Wolf, L.J., S. Zu Ermgassen, A. Balmford, M. White, and N. Weinstein. 2017. Is variety the spice of life? An experimental investigation into the effects of species richness on self-reported mental well-being. *PLoS One* 12(1): e0170225, doi: 10.1371/journal.pone.0170225. http:// journals.plos.org/plosone/article?id=10.1371/journal.pone.0170225.

World Wildlife Fund. 2017. Vaquita. https://www.worldwildlife.org/species/vaquita.

Yeoman, B. 2014. Why the passenger pigeon went extinct. *Audubon.* http://www.audubon. org/magazine/may-june-2014/why-passenger-pigeon-went-extinct.

Young, R.A., and P. Popenoe. 1916. Saving the Kokio Tree: Wild relative of cultivated cottons becomes nearly extinct in Hawaii, but is rescued for plant breeders—may be of value in hybridization—other species similarly threatened. *Journal of Heredity* 7(1): 24–28. https://doi.org/10.1093/jhered/7.1.24.

3 Industrial Agriculture, Biodiversity, and Planetary Boundaries

Kumara Sidhartha

CONTENTS

3.1 INTRODUCTION

The Earth system is comprised of the interactions between physical, chemical, and biological processes, including the activities and systems of human societies and all other life forms of this planet. Among the many activities within this system, industrial-scale agriculture plays an important role in disrupting the Earth system. Scholars have designed a planetary boundaries framework (as discussed in Chapter 1) to quantify and monitor disturbances to the Earth system. This chapter explores the connection between industrial-scale agriculture and its impact on the planetary boundaries.

3.2   FOOD CHAIN AND ENERGY TRANSFER

Have you ever watched a nature video showing zebras feeding on grasses in the African savannah while a pride of lions steadily approaches downwind, scoping the most vulnerable zebra to capture? You may have seen a similar sequence with gazelles feeding on plants while a cheetah silently approaches. Eventually the predators run after their prey and, if they have made the right selection and are skillful enough, they will capture their prey and eat what they can before scavengers arrive to feast on the carcass. This feeding sequence, from plants to foraging animals to predators displays the flow of energy (calories) from one creature to the other.

Think about how many plants grow in the savannah compared with the number of animals feeding on them. Can you imagine a savannah with millions of lions or cheetahs? How about thousands of grazing animals among only twenty plants? It is hard to imagine that scenario because the laws of physics make it impossible to have a larger number of carnivores than herbivores, in the same way it's impossible to have a larger number of herbivores than plants. In reality, in any given food landscape, there are many more plants than there are herbivores, and many more herbivores than there are predators. This has a great deal of influence on the sustainability of food consumption and the demands placed on natural resources.

3.2.1   LAWS OF THERMODYNAMICS

The ecosystem would collapse without an abundance of plants for the foragers and an abundance of prey animals for the predators. This is reflected in some basic laws of physics. The first law of thermodynamics states that energy cannot be destroyed nor created; it can only be transformed from one state to another e.g., imagine the mechanical energy of cycling firing up the electrical energy for the headlight of the bicycle (Ritter 2006). The second law of thermodynamics states that when energy is transformed from one state to another, it always moves from a source of higher energy concentration to a lower concentration source (think solar energy moving to plants) and some of the energy in this process is wasted. This is known as entropy.

All living creatures require energy, and the greatest source of energy for our planet is the sun. Primary producers—plants, algae, and some bacteria—have the unique ability to convert solar energy into carbohydrates, which store and supply energy and heat. When we consume plants we replenish our energy, which we measure in terms of calories, directly from these primary producers. Similarly, grazing animals feed on plants to replenish their carbohydrates. In contrast, predators replenish their energy by eating herbivores (Ritter 2006). This pattern applies to aquatic life as well.

3.2.2   TROPHIC PYRAMID

This system of energy transfer from one level to the next is shown graphically in the trophic pyramid in Figure 3.1.

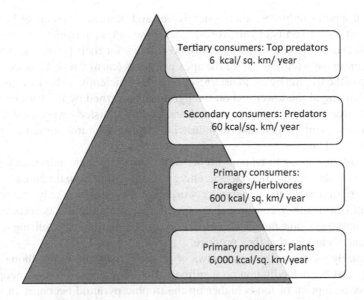

Tertiary consumers: Top predators
6 kcal/ sq. km/ year

Secondary consumers: Predators
60 kcal/sq. km/ year

Primary consumers:
Foragers/Herbivores
600 kcal/ sq. km/ year

Primary producers: Plants
6,000 kcal/sq. km/year

FIGURE 3.1 Trophic Pyramid: Energy transfer and efficiency at different trophic levels.

At the base of the pyramid—the largest segment—are the primary producers, which consume solar energy to produce carbohydrates. At the apex of the pyramid are the top predators, which consume other predators and herbivores.

There are two levels between the apex predators and the primary producers. In the lower middle, at the level just above the primary producers, are the herbivores, or primary consumers. In the upper middle level are those herbivores' predators, which, in turn, are prey for the predators at the apex.

Thus, all the solar energy that is converted by the primary producers becomes the source of life and sustenance for other living creatures, for the foragers that eat those plants, then for the animals that eat those herbivores, and finally for the animals that eat those predators. Remember, energy is never destroyed, it is only transformed, and this is one manifestation of the great cycle of life on this planet (Muir 2012).

The numbers in the Trophic Pyramid indicate the relative number of calories produced at each consumer level. The pyramid shows that primary producers can convert solar energy into 6,000 kcal per meter squared per year. Their consumers, the herbivores or primary consumers, produce one-tenth of the calories they consume, or 600 kcal; in other words, they require ten times the amount of energy that they produce. And it's ten times less efficient at the next level, where secondary consumers produce only one-tenth the amount of calories they consume. Finally, at the apex of the pyramid, tertiary predators produce only one-tenth the amount of energy that they consume. This is known as the "entropy" effect, the second law of thermodynamics.

What does this pattern say about the energy efficiency at each level of consumption? Only 10% of the calories produced at each trophic level is transferred to the next level. Thus, the plants' production of 6,000 kcal per meter squared per year is converted into only 600 kcal in the foragers (to put it another away, 1,000 units of plants can support only 100 units of herbivores and in turn, 100 units of herbivores can support only 10 units of carnivores). And those 600 kcal (which required 6,000 kcal from plants) are converted into only 60 calories for their predators. And those 60 kcal convert into only 6 kcal for the apex predators (carnivores). Thus, consuming at the top of the trophic pyramid uses resources less efficiently and is less sustainable than consuming at the lower end on the pyramid. Governed by the laws of physics, this holds true for all conditions of food and energy transfer—whether it is played out in factory farming operations of industrial-scale agriculture—or in backyards as free-range chickens.

This pattern applies to aquatic life as well. Aquatic plants, as primary producers, convert solar energy into caloric energy. Plant-eating aquatic animals are the primary consumers of the underwater world and they produce only one-tenth the amount of calories they consume. Likewise, larger sea animals, as secondary and tertiary consumers, consume smaller fish and aquatic mammals, requiring ten times the amount of calories that they produce.

Fortunately (or naturally, by the laws of physics), there are not millions of lions and tigers and bears feeding on prey animals. But there are millions of people who do. The consumption of foods higher up the trophic pyramid becomes an increasingly dire challenge as our population increases.

3.2.3 FOOD EFFICIENCY AND POPULATION GROWTH

Our population is growing at an explosive rate. There were one billion people alive in 1800 and that number tripled to three billion people in 1960. It is expected to triple again to an estimated nine billion by 2040. Each day we add over 130,000 people to our planet (Worldometers 2017).

Our growth and the consumption of animals are changing the balance of food production and consumption that has evolved over millions of years. In our brief period on this planet we have strengthened our ability to expand, extract, produce, and destroy to the point that we have modified the systems of life on the planet (Smil 2011). What was once a world teeming with wild and free animals several thousand years ago is now almost entirely filled with humans and the animals we raise for food (Smil 2011). Today, some seventy billion animals are killed annually for food around the world, including about one million killed every hour just in the United States alone (A Well-Fed World 2017).

When we eat a plant-based diet, there are more calories freed up to feed everyone—all living beings (Oppenlander 2012). The trophic pyramid shows the relative efficiency at each level of consumption: A plant-based diet, eating at the lower end of the trophic pyramid, is exponentially more efficient than a carnivorous diet (Campbell and Campbell 2006). A plant-based diet is the more efficient source of nourishment for humans, not only in terms of land use, but also in terms of animal welfare and healthcare costs (Campbell and Campbell 2006). Promisingly, there are areas such as in Mongolia and Iceland where people are diversifying their diets and consuming more plant-based nutrition (Hoag 2013; Bonhommeau 2013). However, the increase in plant-based consumption in those places is offset in other places, where people are consuming more animals because of their improved economic conditions such is the case in India and China (Hoag 2013).

3.3 INDUSTRIAL AGRICULTURE

3.3.1 OVERVIEW

In order to sustain a growing animal-consuming human population, growing numbers of livestock are used in the food industry, requiring land and plants to feed them. The Union of Concerned Scientists defines industrial agriculture as a system of "chemically intensive food production" using large-scale, intensive farming of a single crop, known as monoculture, and enormous animal production facilities (Union of Concerned Scientists 2017).

Planting rows of a single crop, acre upon square acre, simplifies farming. Monoculture allows farmers to apply a straightforward, assembly-line production method that accommodates routine tasks and machinery that can harvest faster than people, which also reduces human-related costs such as wages and healthcare. This practice is discussed in detail in Chapter 4 and is referenced in other chapters as well. In the United States, corn, soybeans, wheat, rice, and cotton are typically grown as monoculture crops. Corn and soybean are the two most abundant plant foods grown in monoculture to feed livestock (Union of Concerned Scientists 2017).

3.3.2 SOCIOECONOMIC IMPACT

Industrial agriculture is a multi-billion dollar industry in the United States. According to the U.S. Department of Agriculture's Economic Research Service, "agriculture, food, and related industries contributed $992 billion to U.S. gross domestic product (GDP) in 2015." That figure amounts to 5.5% of the GDP. Farming alone contributed $136.7 billion to the overall U.S. economy—about 1% of GDP (USDA Economic Research Service 2016).

The agro-food and related industries employ twenty-one million people (that are documented) for 11% of U.S. employment (USDA Economic Research Service 2016). Figures 3.2 and 3.3 identify the sectors associated with agricultural inputs, along with their contributions to the U.S. economy and employment, respectively.

3.3.3 CONCENTRATED ANIMAL FEEDING OPERATIONS

The livestock side of industrial agriculture involves Concentrated Animal Feeding Operations (CAFOs). The U.S. Environmental Protection Agency defines Animal Feeding Operations (AFOs) as agricultural operations where land animals are confined for at least forty-five days per year in lots or facilities that do not have sustained vegetation. The size of the operation usually determines whether the operation will be deemed a CAFO (EPA 2017a) but an operation of any size will be defined as a CAFO if it discharges manure or wastewater in a waterway, i.e., a man-made ditch, stream, river, etc. (USDA Natural Resources Conservation Service 2017). Whatever the size, these operations "generally congregate animals, feed, manure, dead animals, and production operations on a small land area" (EPA 2017b).

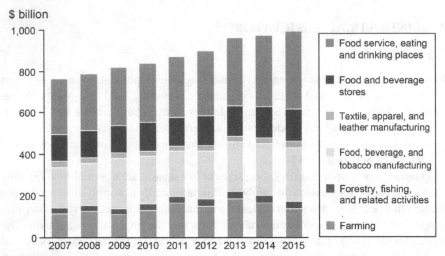

Value added to GDP by agriculture, food, and related industries, 2007-15

$ billion

Note: GDP refers to gross domestic product.
Source: USDA, Economic Research Service using data from U.S. Department of Commerce, Bureau of Economic Analysis, *Value Added by Industry* series.

FIGURE 3.2   Value of industrial agriculture added to GDP.

The animals' movements are restricted and they are fed high-calorie, grain-based food that is often supplemented with hormones in order to enlarge them before slaughter for maximum profits (Union of Concerned Scientists 2017). Overcrowding, high stress, and unsanitary conditions lead to reliance on large amounts of antibiotics not only to treat unhealthy animals but also to prevent disease and promote more growth in relatively healthy animals (Gurian-Sherman 2008).

In 2000, 16,000 tons of pharmaceuticals were produced in the United States, and 70% of that was used in the food animal industry to control bacteria and increase growth rates (Martin et al. 2010). In 2014, 14,000 tons of antimicrobials alone were approved for use in the industry, 98% of which was approved for use on domestic animals (U.S. Dept. of Health and Human Services 2014). More than half the antibiotic groups used in agriculture are critical for human use (Silbergeld 2008). For further discussion of antibiotic resistance see Chapter 8.

Industry leaders have lobbied—often successfully—for state laws to prevent whistleblowers from taking photographs or shooting videos without the farmer's consent (Potter 2014). This so-called "ag-gag" legislation treats whistleblowers as criminals, describing them as "terrorists". In Australia, similar legislation was proposed but did not pass (Schilling 2016). While federal judges have struck-down ag-gag laws in two states citing them as unconstitutional, six states have upheld them (Humane Society of the United States 2018).

Today, the majority of the U.S. meat, dairy, and poultry production is concentrated in these large facilities. Dairies with over 2,000 cows, hog houses with over 10,000

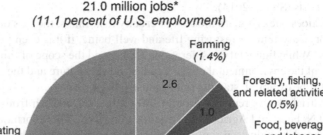

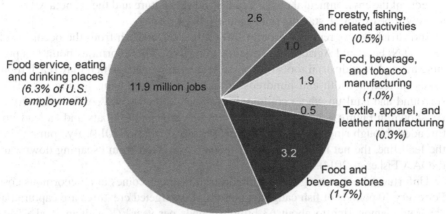

Employment in agriculture, food, and related industries, 2015

21.0 million jobs*
(11.1 percent of U.S. employment)

Farming
(1.4%)

2.6

1.0

Forestry, fishing,
and related activities
(0.5%)

Food service, eating
and drinking places
*(6.3% of U.S.
employment)*

11.9 million jobs

1.9

Food, beverage,
and tobacco
manufacturing
(1.0%)

0.5

Textile, apparel, and
leather manufacturing
(0.3%)

3.2

Food and
beverage stores
(1.7%)

*Full- and part-time jobs. Categories do not sum to totals due to rounding.
Source: USDA, Economic Research Service using data from U.S. Department of
Commerce, Bureau of Economic Analysis.

FIGURE 3.3 Employment in industrial agriculture.

pigs, and broiler houses with over 10,000 chickens are common (EPA National Risk Management Research Laboratory 2004).

The marine equivalent is aquaculture, in which aquatic animals are farmed and stocked. According to the United Nations, the aquaculture industry is growing faster than all other animal food-producing sectors, prompting concerns about environmental degradation (U.N. Environment Programme 2017).

3.3.4 ECONOMIES OF SCALE AND EXTERNALIZED COSTS

Industrial agriculture is intended to build economies of scale in the production of agricultural commodities. Economies of scale—higher production, lower costs per output, and higher profits—seem like an ideal solution for a growing world population. But the perceived value of industrialized agriculture is in its convenience and efficiency for the farmer and low consumer prices. However, it is not efficient. It only appears efficient because many of the costs are externalized (Gurian-Sherman 2008).

Externalized costs are the negative impacts that are excluded from consideration by an economic entity. For example, if a business operation pollutes the environment but neglects to clean it up, the burden imposed on the community and the environment. Thus, externalized costs are those incurred by third parties rather than the entities that caused them. While externalized costs are difficult to quantify, it has been estimated that industrial agriculture incurs over $400 billion in externalized costs that included healthcare, subsidies, damage to the environment, cruelty, and fishing-related costs (Simon 2014).

How does one calculate the cost of cruelty to animals, the loss of an ancient rain-forest or ecosystem, or restoring life and well-being, if it is even possible to correct the loss? While financial considerations are beyond the scope of this chapter, several aspects of the environmental costs of industrial agriculture and the planetary bound-aries will be explored, starting with industrialized fishing.

Industrial fishing removes around 100 million tons of fish from the oceans each year (U.N. Food and Agriculture Organization 2012). This enormous bounty is pos-sible as modern industrial tools like purse seine fishing nets, which may reach thou-sands of feet in width and hundreds of feet in depth, allowing fishing vessels to surround and haul up whole communities of sea animals (NOAA Fisheries 2014). As shown in Figure 3.4, the seine has a top line attached to floats and "a lead line threaded through rings along the bottom" (NOAA Fisheries 2014). By "pursing" in the lead line, the net is closed off and fish are prevented from escaping downward (NOAA Fisheries 2014).

Unfortunately, capturing fish with industrial methods comes at an enormous cost. For every 10 pounds of fish caught, 4 pounds of untargeted creatures are captured as "by-catch, amounting to about 63 billion pounds per year" (Keledjian et al. 2014). According to a 2010 estimate, as much as 2.7 trillion animals are hauled out of the ocean each year, and commercially caught fish are likely to die from asphyxiation or live gutting (Mood 2010). Millions of pounds of fish are discarded every day (Keledjian et al. 2014). Hundreds of thousands of mammals—whales, dolphins, and seals—are killed by drowning or are crushed by the weight of the catch (Keledjian et al. 2014).

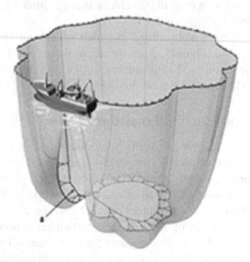

FIGURE 3.4 Purse seine fishing net. (Credit: National Marine Fisheries Service/ National Oceanic and Atmospheric Administration. [http://www.nmfs.noaa.gov/pr/interactions/gear/purseseine.htm].)

Three-quarters of the world's fisheries have been threatened by exploitation or depletion (U.N. FAO 2017). Scientists have found that with the loss of biodiversity, "rates of resource collapse increased and recovery potential, stability, and water quality decreased exponentially" (Worm et al. 2006). If we continue to exploit marine animals at an accelerated pace, there will be a total collapse of these eco-systems, not to mention that the ocean's food will cease to exist (Worm et al. 2006). What will life be like with such empty oceans, not only for humanity but for other species that depend on the ocean's abundance, such as polar bears? Examining industrial agriculture from the perspective of externalized costs allows us to keep in mind questions such as: Who pays for the loss of dead whales? Who pays for the loss of entire species or ecosystems? How efficient are current practices of indus-trial agriculture? What is the impact of our choices as consumers, as shareholders, as stewards of our domain?

3.4 PLANETARY BOUNDARIES

3.4.1 BIODIVERSITY AND BIOSPHERE INTEGRITY

Biodiversity loss is among the most significant externalized costs of industrial agriculture. Species diversity ensures that ecosystems function with resilience (Hooper 2005). When one species disappears, in most cases its predators can simply search for other sources of food, and its prey have their populations con-trolled by other predator species. In time, the ecosystem adapts. But if multiple species become extinct or if a keystone species or ecologically important carni-vores have declined, their predators face extinction and their prey may grow out of control, leaving the ecosystem out of balance (Hooper 2005). Thus, biodiver-sity loss increases the vulnerability of natural systems, threatening biosphere integrity (Steffen et al. 2015; Hooper 2005). While the link between industrial agriculture and biodiversity loss is vast, examples in this section will focus on monoculture, declining bee colonies, soil microorganisms, and disturbing wild animals.

Monoculture, by design, excludes or deliberately kills living organisms as a method to minimize pests and maximize yield. In this way, monoculture is the antithesis of biodiversity. To a bee in search of nectar, a field of corn is akin to a desert. The bee must find nectar-producing flowers for its survival, and if the farmer has successfully eradicated all plants other than corn, there will be no food available for the bee. Even if the bee does find a monoculture crop that provides nectar, it still will find it difficult if not impossible to find the vari-ety of foods necessary to meet its nutritional needs (Di Pasquele 2013). Another challenge for the bee is that if the nectar-producing crops are treated with pesti-cides, the larvae's mortality rate increases within six days of low-dose exposure (Zhu 2014). A third threat the bee faces is the genetic material in Genetically Modified Organism (GMO) crops, which is believed to make the bee vulnerable to parasites (Simon 2014).

Millions of bee colonies have collapsed in recent years, a phenomenon known as Colony Collapse Disorder. At the end of World War II, before pesticides were mainstreamed, there were an estimated 5.9 million bee colonies (Simon 2014). In 2008, that number declined to 2.4 million (Simon 2014). While the reasons for the loss may be debated, there is no doubt that these creatures are in trouble and the die-off has grown at an accelerated rate in recent years (Simon 2014). When the bees are in trouble, other living creatures are in trouble, since bees are pollinators. In fact, one-third of the food we consume is pollinated by bees (Simon 2014).

Unlike diverse, self-sustaining, and stable ecosystems, growing one plant repeatedly on the same land depletes the soil of nutrients, making the plants weak and vulnerable to pests. As a consequence, monoculture *requires* the use of pesticides to manage weeds and pests, along with fertilizers to replenish the soil (Union of Concerned Scientists 2017).

When left alone to thrive without human intervention, soil is teeming with life. A spoonful of healthy garden soil contains a microcosm where billions of microorganisms live (Herring 2010). In fact, the world beneath our feet may account for as much as 95% of the Earth's species biodiversity, "...as many as 75,000 species of bacteria in [a] teaspoon, along with 25,000 species of fungi, 1,000 species of protozoa, and 100 species of tiny worms called nematodes" (Ohlson 2014). Further details are offered in Chapter 4.

Each microorganism in the soil contributes to the ecosystem in its own way. For example, soil bacteria convert airborne nitrogen into nutrients for the plants, a process known as nitrogen fixation (Herring 2010). It is in bacterial nodules in the roots of leguminous plants, such as beans and locust trees, where nitrogen fixation takes place (Oregon State University Forage Information System 2017).

As for fungi in the soil, scientists increasingly realize their value in the ecosystem. Fungal mycorrhizae develop on plants to form a symbiotic relationship between the plants and fungi. The mycorrhizal structures then help the plants and fungi take in nutrients and resist pathogens (Koide and Haider 2017). The structures help the soil absorb and store water and prevent erosion. Plowing tears apart this living structure and leaves the soil exposed to the sun (Ohlson 2014). Leaving the soil bare and exposed to the sun harms the soil ecosystem and further contributes to biodiversity loss.

With a growing human population, more land is being cleared, not just for human food but also to grow livestock and the crops to feed them. In the United States, the top three crops are corn, soybeans, and hay, with most grown for livestock (Simon 2014). More than 400 million acres in the United States are used for cropland and more than 600 million are used for grazing (Nickerson et al. 2011). With livestock comes the desire to protect the animals from predators. For example, in 2012 an entire pack of wolves in Washington State was killed off after cattle ranchers had lost some head of cattle (Maughan 2012).

In other cases, wild animals are herded up and moved away from their natural habitat. The U.S. Bureau of Land Management has the authority to "remove excess wild horses and burros from the range to sustain the health and productivity of the public lands" (U.S. Bureau of Land Management 2017). Today, there are more wild horses in government holding facilities than roaming free (costing U.S. taxpayers $49 million per year). Since the animals are struggling to survive in an increasingly limited habitat, the Bureau is working on ways to reduce their population because it is "far exceeding what is healthy for the land and animals" (U.S. Bureau of Land Management 2017).

What is the impact of habitat loss on biodiversity? In a message for the United Nations Environmental Programme, the Secretariat of the Convention on Biological Diversity, Ahmed Djoghlaf, stated:

> [T]he ability of the planet to provide the goods and services that we, and future generations, need for our well-being is seriously and perhaps irreversibly jeopardized. We are indeed experiencing the greatest wave of extinctions since the disappearance of the dinosaurs. Extinction rates are rising by a factor of up to 1,000 above natural rates. Every hour, three species disappear. Every day, up to 150 species are lost. Every year, between 18,000 and 55,000 species become extinct. The cause: human activities
>
> **Djoghlaf 2007**

Our demand for animal food is fueling the destruction of habitats that so many species depend on for survival. Argentina has lost two-thirds of its forests since the mid-20th century, harming over 40% of its plant and animal species (Oppenlander 2013). Africa is losing some ten million acres of forest per year, including an estimated 140,000 lions and leopards plus countless foragers and microscopic creatures that comprise forest ecosystems (Oppenlander 2013). Zimbabwe alone has lost over 85% of its forests, and continues to lose 1% per year, primarily for animal agriculture (Oppenlander 2013).

3.4.2 LAND-SYSTEM CHANGE AND HABITAT LOSS

When human beings impose dramatic change on a landscape, turning rainforests, prairies, or swampland into fields for grazing or growing crops (or building cities), we destroy established, vibrant, resilient ecosystems. Unfortunately, the prevailing assumption, which strengthened with the growth of Western capitalism in the 20th century, is that growth is good because it is good for the economy.

Consider the value of a wooded habitat. Aside from sustaining biodiversity, forests produce rain. Trees hold water and release it into the air through a process called transpiration (U.S. Geological Survey 2016b). Researchers observed that the Amazon rainforest makes its own rain; fungi and plants contribute to the formation of condensation nuclei that ultimately lead to mist and clouds (Pöhlker 2012). Another study showed that the Amazon rainforest actually puts *more* water into the atmosphere than the Amazon River pours into the ocean (Loomis 2017). Further information is discussed in the vignette in Chapter 11.

In the last few hundred years, humans have cleared some 4.5 billion acres of land in order to grow animals for food (U.N. Food and Agriculture Organization 2006). Today, nearly one-third of the Earth's land is used for animal agriculture, and feed crop production alone accounts for one-third of the arable land (U.N. Food and Agriculture Organization 2006).

Over 185 million acres of the Amazon rainforest, once considered impenetrable, have been cleared since 1978 (Butler 2017). Almost 90% of deforestation in the Amazon rainforest is attributed to animal agriculture (Oppenlander 2013). The destruction continues today at an astounding rate of nearly 20 million acres per year, over 37 acres per minute (Butler 2017). People have tried to stop the destruction, but at the risk of losing their lives. Over a thousand environmental activists have been killed trying to save the Amazon (Batty 2009).

Indonesia is losing more of its rainforests despite a moratorium. The country has lost 26 million acres of its rainforests because of global demand for palm oil (USDA Foreign Agricultural Service 2013). Palm oil will be discussed in further detail in Chapter 9.

It is not only forests that hold moisture. The Dust Bowl in the 1930s taught America that deep plowing destroys the deep-rooted grasses that stop erosion and hold water in the land even during droughts. Tragically, the Great Plains' vulnerable topsoil turned to dust and filled the air, killing animals and people and displacing farmers and families. During one dust storm in 1935, the region lost an estimated three million tons of topsoil (History.com 2009).

We can expect more destruction of natural ecosystems as long as our demand for meat continues to grow (Oppenlander 2013). Globally, the average person consumes 75 pounds of meat per year, with the highest rates in Australia and the United States, where the average person eats about 200 pounds of meat per year (Gould and Friedman 2015).

3.4.3 BIOCHEMICAL FLOWS

The U.S. meat industry produces approximately 130 times more waste than the amount produced by humans (U.S. General Accounting Office 1999). Each CAFO may produce as much waste as a small city; an operation with 2,500 cows, for example, produces as much waste as a city with 411,000 people (EPA National Risk Management Research Laboratory 2004). Since the volume of manure exceeds what the land can absorb, the water table and surrounding environment are polluted. (EPA National Risk Management Research Laboratory 2004; Muir 2012).

In the case of industrial cropland, the soil is burdened with fertilizers and pesticides and is susceptible to erosion. Under natural conditions, soil erodes and is replenished at a rate of less than one inch per century. However, because of industrial agricultural practices, globally we lose about 1% of the earth's topsoil per year (Verso 2015). The natural replenishing rate is far behind the rate of human-induced loss of topsoil, which is ten times the amount replenished in the United States, and thirty to forty times the amount that is replenished in India and China (Verso 2015).

The loss of topsoil has been described as "the biggest environmental problem the world faces" second only to population growth (Verso 2015). Again, details follow in Chapter 4.

In the United States, tons of topsoil, filled with excess nutrients—particularly nitrogen and phosphorous—enter the Mississippi River through erosion and form what is known as a "dead zone" in the Gulf of Mexico. The tilled soil travels downriver to the gulf, where the nutrients feed algae and form algal blooms (Virginia Institute of Marine Science 2017). The explosion of algae die and fall to the bottom where bacteria consume them, depleting the surrounding oxygen and suffocating marine life in the area. In 2017, the dead zone grew to over 8,700 square miles (Callum 2017).

Unfortunately, nearly 400 dead zones have been identified in the world, along the coasts of South America, South East Asia, Europe, and eastern North America (Scientific American 2018). Runoff from industrial agriculture contributes to dead zones in areas such as the Chesapeake Bay and elsewhere along the east coast of the United States near Virginia (Gurian-Sherman 2008) and the Gulf of Mexico.

Globally, industrial agriculture is responsible for more than 400 nitrogen-flooded dead zones in the oceans, and they are likely to expand because of global warming (Zielinski 2014). Reducing our nutrient pollution will reduce the dead zones (Zielinski 2014).

3.4.4 FRESHWATER USE

Only 2.5% of the planet's water is fresh water, and of that, only 0.3% is surface water, such as in rivers and lakes (U.S. Geological Survey 2016a). The rest is in glaciers, underground, and moving elsewhere in the water cycle. Water-insecure areas are growing with over a third of the world's population now living in areas with water scarcity (Jalava 2014).

Animal agriculture accounts for as much as one-third of all freshwater consumption (Mekonnen and Hoekstra 2012). On average, one dairy cow will consume over 543,000 gallons of water per year. It takes 1,847 gallons of water to produce one pound of beef, 665 gallons to produce one pound of butter, and 391 gallons to produce one pound of eggs (Mekonnen and Hoekstra 2012). In the U.S., agriculture accounts for over 80% of water use (USDA Economic Research Service 2017). Researchers have found that a 50% decrease in animal product consumption will reduce total water usage in agriculture by 37% (Jalava 2014).

Industrial agriculture requires energy for irrigation and harvesting, and for the manufacture of chemical fertilizers and pesticides which is also energy-intensive—especially in the form of natural gas (Post Carbon Institute 2011). Natural gas is extracted through a process called hydraulic fracturing, or fracking, for short. Fracking takes enormous amounts of freshwater, mixes it with chemicals, and injects the mixture into the Earth to grow targeted fractures and extract gas; the later stages include collecting the wastewater and reusing or disposing of it (EPA 2016). However, the U.S. EPA reports that fracking can pollute drinking water (EPA 2016). It is estimated that fracking uses some 70–140 billion gallons per year (EPA Office of Research & Development 2011).

3.4.5   CLIMATE CHANGE

The atmosphere surrounding our planet is critical to life as we know it. Greenhouse gases (GHGs) trap heat in the atmosphere, leading to global warming and climate change. According to the U.S. EPA, the main greenhouse gases are carbon dioxide (CO_2), methane (CH_4), nitrous oxide (N_2), and fluorinated gases. The gases' effect on the climate depends on their abundance in the atmosphere, how long they stay there, and how potent they are i.e., how effectively they warm the planet (EPA 2017c).

Figure 3.5 shows that in the United States, carbon dioxide accounts for 82% of greenhouse gas emissions caused by humans (EPA 2017c). This is due primarily to burning fossil fuels for transportation, energy, and industry (EPA 2017c).

We are not just adding CO_2 to the atmosphere; our activities are also undercutting the ability of natural sinks such as the oceans and forests to absorb CO_2. A 2016 study found that although the Amazon rainforest continues to be a long-term sink, its ability to accumulate carbon is declining because of deforestation (Brienen 2015). Furthermore, rising CO_2 levels weaken plants. Research has shown a link between increased CO_2 levels and declines in the nutrient values in plants (Evich 2017).

Photosynthesis allows plants to transfer atmospheric carbon to the soil. This is vital as carbon makes the soil more fertile and gives it a structure that helps the soil absorb and retain water, critical during droughts and floods alike (Ohlson 2014). However, plowing releases the stored carbon, and released carbon combines with oxygen to form carbon dioxide (Ohlson 2014).

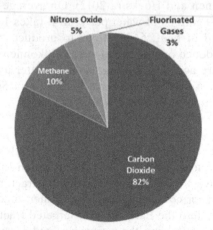

U.S. Environmental Protection Agency (2017). *Inventory of U.S. Greenhouse Gas Emissions and Sinks: 1990-2015.*

FIGURE 3.5 Greenhouse gas emissions, inventory of U.S. greenhouse gas emissions and sinks: 1990–2015 by the U.S. Environmental Protection Agency (2017).

In places where cultivation has gone on for thousands of years, as much as 80% or more of the soil's carbon has been depleted (Ohlson 2014). In just two hundred years, the state of Ohio lost half of its soil carbon (Ohlson 2014). Today, the misuse of land accounts for 30% of the carbon entering the atmosphere (Ohlson 2014).

The next most abundant GHG is methane, which accounts for 10% of greenhouse gas emissions. It stays in the atmosphere for less than two decades, but it traps heat 25–100 times faster than CO_2 (Vaidyanathan 2015). At the end of its supercharged lifetime, methane decays into CO_2 (Vaidyanathan 2015).

According to the U.S. EPA, human activities are responsible for more than half of global methane emissions each year (EPA 2013). Livestock is the primary source of anthropogenic methane, followed by natural gas production and distribution, landfills, and coal mining (EPA 2013).

Globally, animal agriculture accounts for 18% of greenhouse gas emissions. In comparison, the entire transportation sector accounts for 13% of greenhouse gases (U.N. Food and Agriculture Organization 2006; Walsh 2013). Figure 3.6 illustrates the various sources of greenhouse gases originating from livestock farms.

Nitrous oxide accounts for only about 5% of greenhouse gas emissions, but it is 296 times more effective than carbon dioxide at warming the atmosphere and stays in the atmosphere for more than 100 years (EPA 2017c; U.N. Food and Agriculture Organization 2006). The majority of GHG emissions from the livestock sector originate from enteric fermentation of food in the intestines (39%), manure (26%), and from the production of feed (21%) (Chatham House 2014).

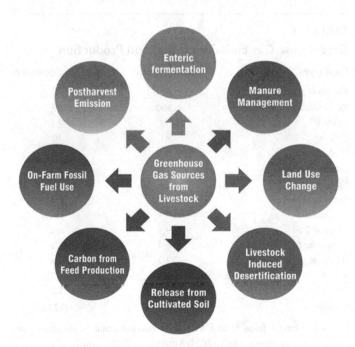

FIGURE 3.6 Different sources of GHGs from livestock farms. (Credit: Jose, S. *Frontiers in Environmental Science* 4, 27, 2016.)

The livestock sector of agriculture is responsible for 65% of the atmospheric nitrous oxide emissions and, compared to 1995, is estimated to double by year 2055 if the global trend of meat and dairy consumption continues as projected (Chatham House 2014). The main source of nitrous oxide is manure and fertilizers used in producing feed for livestock.

The global treaties on climate change such as the Copenhagen Protocol, Cancun Agreement, and the subsequent Paris Agreement led to a consensus target for limiting the rise of average global temperatures to no more than two degrees Celsius, compared to the pre-industrial era. Among the various scenarios called Representative Concentration Pathways (RCP), only the lowest risk pathway (known as RCP 2.6) projected by the Inter-governmental Panel on Climate Change has the best-case scenario outcomes of meeting this target. Researchers analyzed the food sectors' contribution to climate change using various diet scenarios that included varying amounts of animal products and concluded that only vegetable protein sources achieved the RCP 2.6 target if they were not transported or grown in heated greenhouses (Girod 2014).

Other researchers in the U.K. calculated that an average 2,000 kcal high meat diet had 2.5 times as many GHG emissions than an average 2,000 kcal vegan diet (Scarborough 2014). The amount of GHG emissions from various food sources is listed in Table 3.1.

TABLE 3.1

Greenhouse Gas Emissions from Food Production

Food Types	g CO_2eq/kcal	g CO_2eq/g-protein
Ruminant meat	330	62
Recirculating aquaculture	160	39
Dairy	74	9.1
Pork	61	10
Poultry	52	10
Butter	33	n/a
Eggs	24	6.8
Rice	14	6.5
Vegetables	14	n/a
Tropical fruit	9.1	n/a
Temperate fruit	6.4	n/a
Oil crops	7.2	n/a
Wheat	5.2	1.2
Maize	3	1.2
Legumes	1.9	0.25

Source: Adapted from Global diets link environmental sustainability and human health, Tilman 2014, *Nature.* 515(7528): 518–22.

Overall, vegetable sources of protein generally contribute fewer GHG emissions than animal products (Tilman 2014).

Fluorinated gases make up only about 3% of greenhouse gases. Unlike the others, fluorinated gases are man-made and emitted through industrial processes, including transportation, refrigeration, etc. Generally, they are considered the most potent and long lasting of the greenhouse gases, since some may remain in the atmosphere for thousands of years (EPA 2017c).

Ultimately, the impact and growth in the livestock sector must be considered in policy decisions and professional practice guidelines to reduce GHG emissions.

3.4.6 Ocean Acidification

Ocean acidification is a continually and rapidly unfolding process in the ocean's chemistry with an uncertain future. The primary driving force behind this anomalous process is an excess of anthropogenic CO_2 in the atmosphere. Hence, the term "the other CO_2 problem" used by some scientists to refer to ocean acidification (Doney 2009). In both climate change and ocean acidification—the common biochemical change is an increase in CO_2 fueled in part by animal agriculture. In this setting, oceans act as a carbon sink and absorb close to 30% of the atmospheric CO_2. This increase in ocean CO_2 leads to changes in sea chemistry in the form of excess hydrogen ions. The result is a decrease in ocean pH relative to the baseline pH number, a process called acidification (Doney 2009).

If the rise in atmospheric CO_2 continues in its current trajectory without successful mitigation efforts, by the end of the 21st century, the ocean pH is projected to drop 0.3–0.4 units in the pH scale, pushing the acidity (and hydrogen ions) up by 100%–150% of current levels (Woods Hole Oceanographic Institute 2010).

Increases in acidity and hydrogen ions lead to a decrease of calcium carbonate in the oceans, which in turn impacts marine life that depend on calcium carbonate for their survival, as in the case of crustaceans that need stable shells to thrive (Figure 3.7).

Scientists are beginning to investigate this effect mostly in controlled settings. One such study involved assessing the effects of ocean acidification on the integrity of coral reefs (Anthony 2008). Coral reef ecosystems such as the Great Barrier Reef off the coast of Australia are known for their vast benefits to human and marine life: For protecting the coastlines from the effects of storms; for providing nitrogen for the marine food chain; providing habitat to shelter numerous marine species; and even assisting with nutrient cycling in the oceans (Scripps Institution of Oceanography 2018). Three groups of reef building species were studied to see: (1) bleaching of the reefs; (2) the organic productivity by the reefs; and (3) calcification of the reef builders. The study found that all three outcomes used as proxy markers of coral reef health were negatively impacted by ocean acidification (Anthony 2008).

To close this research gap, another study off the coast of British Columbia found that while a few species such as phytoplankton and microalgae may benefit from the high levels of hydrogen ions, other species will be negatively impacted (Haigh 2015).

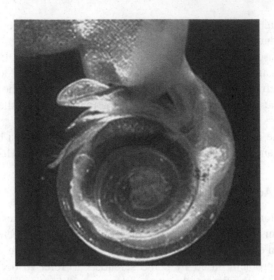

FIGURE 3.7   Acidification interferes with calcification of the shells and skeletons essential for the survival many of marine organisms. Pictured here is a shell that is transparent due to lack of calcium carbonate because of ocean acidification. (Photo credit: NOAA 2017.)

In sum, the ability to regenerate the health of our oceans remains largely unknown. However, the likelihood of continued negative impacts is guaranteed if this current trajectory continues (Doney 2009).

3.4.7   STRATOSPHERIC OZONE DEPLETION

Ozone is a molecule containing three oxygen atoms. It is found naturally in the stratosphere layer (10–50 km above the Earth's surface). It goes through natural cycles of creation and breakdown (EPA 2017b, 2017c). The ozone layer in the stratosphere helps to absorb and prevent excessive ultra-violet B (UV-B) rays from the sun reaching the Earth's surface. Excess UV-B rays are harmful to humans because of their potential to cause melanoma and non-melanoma cancers and cataracts. They can also affect plants and marine ecosystems. Anthropogenic ozone-depleting substances (ODS) have had a destructive impact on the ozone layer.

Beginning in the 1970s, scientists discovered that the depletion rate of ozone was happening at a rate well beyond that of natural processes recorded in the past. Further findings revealed that chlorine and bromine atoms encountering ozone destroyed the latter. One chlorine atom can destroy 100,000 molecules of ozone. Bromine is 40 times more potent than chlorine in this effect. Common sources of bromine that affect the ozone are halons and methyl bromide. The use of methyl bromide as a fumigant in industrial agriculture has largely decreased thanks to the Montreal Protocol (UNEP 2017). Nitrous oxide is projected to be the dominant ozone-depleting substance of the future (Ravishankara 2009).

As mentioned earlier in this chapter, the livestock industry contributes the most (65%) to anthropogenic nitrous oxide released into the atmosphere. This chemical is 296 times more potent than carbon emissions in increasing the global average temperature.

3.4.8 ATMOSPHERIC AEROSOL LOADING

Aerosols are tiny particles such as dust, chemicals, and fungi that enter the atmosphere and affect cloud formation. Industrial agriculture releases ammonia, which is an aerosol. Though atmospheric ammonia is part of natural nitrogen cycle, the use of chemical fertilizers and livestock waste, both rich in nitrogen, have increased the airborne ammonia levels to excess. Higher than normal levels of gaseous ammonia in the air can be harmful to humans and plants and can also pollute the waterways, leading to nitrogen flux into rivers and oceans and causing algal blooms and 'dead zones' as aforementioned. Researchers reported an increasing pattern of airborne ammonia concentration over the agricultural centers in the United States, Europe, India, and China from 2002 to 2016 (Warner 2017). "Little ammonia comes from tailpipes or smokestacks. It's mainly agricultural, from fertilizer and animal husbandry," reports Dr. Russell Dickerson (Warner 2017). Dr. Juying Warner of the same research team believes the excess ammonia "hotspots" seen over China are due to the growing demand for meat in Chinese diets, "as people shift from a vegetarian to a meat-based diet, ammonia emissions will continue to go up" (Warner 2017).

3.4.9 NOVEL ENTITIES

Among the nine planetary boundaries proposed by the original work of Rockstrom et al. (2009), the "novel entities" is a placeholder for problems that we are ignorant about. Sometimes such deficits lend to identifying the issues only after global-scale damage has occurred. One classic example is the industrial use of halocarbons that led to ozone depletion. By the time this connection was recognized between the anthropogenic use of this chemical and impact in the ozone layer, the damage was done (Rockstrom 2009). Novel entities include newly engineered materials previously unknown to the Earth system—including chemicals and novel organisms. The three conditions for novel entities to pose a planetary boundary threat are: (1) the novel entity has a disruptive effect on a vital Earth system process (2) the disruptive effect is not discovered until it is, or inevitably will become, a problem at a planetary scale and (3) the effect of the novel entity cannot be readily reversed (Steffan 2015).

Chemical pollution is one of the novel entities considered here. The large scale impact of chemical pollution is difficult to quantify due to the vast number used across industries. There are more than 100,000 synthetic chemicals currently used in the global economy with new chemicals introduced every year (Persson 2013). *Risk* involves the probability of harm being posed while the term *hazard* refers to the potential for harm. David Gee further clarifies the differences between risk, uncertainty, and ignorance and the potential actions respectively using the table below (Gee 2006) (Table 3.2).

The distinction between prevention and precaution is worth mentioning. In prevention, the risk is known (e.g., tobacco use and lung cancer). Precaution, in contrast, involves avoidance of tobacco before the large-scale damage to public health occurs. One example of where the principle of precaution was used involves ships, marine life, and a chemical called tributylin [TBT] (Gee 2006). This chemical was mixed in paints used on the hull of ships. Growth of marine organisms in the hull of the ships is a common occurrence. To avoid this bioflouling, the bottom of the ships were painted with the anti-floulant chemical, TBT. In the early 1980s, the discovery that oyster beds were collapsing in Arachon, France, led to the suspicion that TBT leaching from the paint was the cause. This was based on the observation that the increased use of TBT paints in boats correlated with the collapse of local oyster beds. During that period, technology had not advanced enough to carry out risk assessment and causal analysis of TBT and the death of oysters, yet TBT was banned based on observation and precaution. The oyster beds recovered. In this instance, a large-scale, irreversible damage from chemical pollution was avoided due to precautionary action.

Gee proposed four strategies (three apply to novel entities such as chemical pollution) that may be applied to governing threats for which humans are ignorant of the full-scale impact on planetary boundaries:

1. Reducing specific exposures to potentially harmful agents on the basis of credible early warnings of initial harmful impacts, thus limiting the size of any other surprise impacts from the same agent (such as the asbestos cancers that followed asbestosis).

TABLE 3.2
Difference between Prevention and Precaution.

Situation	State and Dates of Knowledge	Examples of Action
Risk	Known impacts; known probabilities, e.g., cigarette smoking	Prevention: action taken to reduce known hazards, e.g., eliminate exposure to nicotine
Uncertainty	Known impacts; unknown probabilities, e.g., antibiotics in animal feed and emergence of drug-resistant bacteria	Precautionary prevention: action taken to reduce exposure to potential hazards
Ignorance	Unknown impacts and therefore unknown probabilities, e.g., the surprise of chlorofluorocarbons (CFCs), pre-1974.	Precaution: action taken to anticipate, identify, and reduce the impact of surprises

Source: Adapted from Gee, D. *Environmental Health Perspectives*, 2006, doi:10.1289/ehp.8134.

---

2. Limiting technological monopolies in order to promote a diversity of adaptable alternatives to meet the same needs served by the monopoly (such as asbestos, chlorofluorocarbons [CFCs], etc.).
3. Using forecasting scenarios and predictive computer-based modeling to anticipate surprises.

3.5 CONCLUSION

The growth and development of human-made systems and processes has rapidly expanded over the past 200 years at the expense of the life-supporting natural systems of the Earth. The nine planetary boundaries provide a framework to analyze the damage incurred to the Earth system and can offer a guide for change on multiple levels (policy, community, individuals). Industrialized agriculture including livestock and feed production are negatively impacting the biosphere. What is produced to feed growing populations and how it is distributed will determine if the current trajectory of this planet will change. Shifting dietary consumption patterns towards a plant-based diet grown to regenerate the natural processes of the Earth can have an important and positive impact on the planetary boundaries and biodiversity loss.

REFERENCES

Anthony K.R.N., D.I. Kline, G. Diaz-Pulido, S. Dove, O. Hoegh-Guldberg. 2008. Ocean acidification causes bleaching and productivity loss in coral reef builders. *Proceedings of the National Academy of Sciences of the United States of America.* 105(45):17442–17446

A Well-Fed World. 2017. Factory farms. http://awfw.org/factory-farms/. Accessed September 22, 2017.

Batty, D. April 8, 2009. Brazilian faces retrial over murder of environmental activist nun in Amazon. *TheGuardian.com*. Accessed September 25, 2017. https://www.theguardian.com/world/2009/apr/08/brazilian-murder-dorothy-stang.

Bonhommeau, S., Dubroca, L., le Pape, O., Barde, J., Kaplan, D.M., Chassot, E., and Nieblas, A-E. (2013). Eating up the world's food web and the human trophic level. PNAS, December 17, 2013. Vol. 110(51): 20617–20620. www.pnas.org/cgi/doi/10.1073/pnas.1305827110

Brienen, R.J.W., O.L. Phillips, T.R. Feldpausch, E. Gloor, T.R. Baker, J. Lloyd, G. Lopez-Gonzalez, et al. 2015. Long-term decline of the Amazon carbon sink. *Nature* 519(7543): 344–348.

Butler, R. January 26, 2017. Amazon destruction. *Rainforests.Mongabay.com.* https://rainforests.mongabay.com/amazon/amazon_destruction.html. Accessed September 25, 2017.

Callum, R. August 4, 2017. Opinion: Industrial meat production is killing our seas. It's time to change our diets. *The Guardian, U.S. Edition.* https://www.theguardian.com/commentisfree/2017/aug/04/meat-industry-gulf-mexico-dead-zones-pollution?CMP=Share_iOSApp_Other. Accessed August 4, 2017.

Campbell, T.C., and T.M. Campbell. 2006. *The China Study: Startling Implications for Diet, Weight Loss and Long-Term Health*. Dallas, TX: Benbella Books.

Ceballos, G., P.R. Ehrlich, A.D. Barnosky, A. García, R.M. Pringle, and T.M. Palmer. June 19, 2015. Accelerated modern human–induced species losses: Entering the sixth mass extinction. *Science Advances*, 1400253 ed.

Chatham House: The Royal Institute of International Affairs. December 2014. *Livestock: Climate Change's Forgotten Sector.* Available at https://www.chathamhouse.org/sites/default/files/field/field_document/20141203LivestockClimateChangeForgottenSector BaileyFroggattWellesleyFinal.pdf Accessed January 10, 2018.

Di Pasquale, G. et al. 2013. Influence of Pollen Nutrition on Honey Bee Health: Do Pollen Quality and Diversity Matter? *PLoS ONE* 8(8): e72016. doi: 10.1371/journal.pone.0072016

Djoghlaf, A. May 22, 2007. Message from Mr. Ahmed Djoghlaf on the occasion of the international day for biological diversity. *CBD.int.* https://www.cbd.int/doc/speech/2007/sp-2007-05-22-es-en.pdf. Accessed September 25, 2017.

Doney S.C., V.J. Fabry, R.A. Feely, J.A. Kleypas. 2009. Ocean Acidication: The Other CO2 Problem. *Annual Review of Marine Sciences.* 1:169–192. https://doi.org/10.1146/annurev.marine.010908.163834

EPA. 2013. Inventory of U.S. greenhouse gas emissions and sinks: 1990–2011. Washington.

EPA. December 13, 2016. EPA releases final report on impacts from hydraulic fracturing activities on drinking water. *EPA.gov.* https://www.epa.gov/newsreleases/epa-releases-final-report-impacts-hydraulic-fracturing-activities-drinking-water. Accessed September 19, 2017.

EPA. June 20, 2017a. Agriculture: Animal production. https://www.epa.gov/agriculture/agriculture-animal-production. Accessed July 16, 2017.

EPA. January 17, 2017b. National pollutant discharge elimination system (NPDES). https://www.epa.gov/npdes/animal-feeding-operations-afos. Accessed May 29, 2017.

EPA. 2017c. Overview of greenhouse gases. https://www.epa.gov/ghgemissions/overview-greenhouse-gases. Accessed September 20, 2017.

EPA National Risk Management Research Laboratory. May 2004. EPA National Service Center for Environmental Publications (NSCEP). *nepis.epa.gov.* https://nepis.epa.gov/Exe/ZyNET.exe/901V0100.TXT?ZyActionD=ZyDocument&Client=EPA&Index=2000+Thru+2005&Docs=&Query=&Time=&EndTime=&SearchMethod=1&TocRestrict=n&Toc=&TocEntry=&QField=&QFieldYear=&QFieldMonth=&QFieldDay=&IntQFieldOp=0&ExtQFieldOp=0&XmlQuery=&File=D%3A%5Czyfiles%5CIndex%20Data%5C00thru05%5CTxt%5C00000011%5C901V0100.txt&User=ANONYMOUS&Password=anonymous&SortMethod=h%7C-&MaximumDocuments=1&FuzzyDegree=0&ImageQuality=r75g8/r75g8/x150y150g16/i425&Display=p%7Cf&DefSeekPage=x&SearchBack=ZyActionL&Back=ZyActionS&BackDesc=Results%20page&MaximumPages=1&ZyEntry=1&SeekPage=x&ZyPURL. Accessed May 29, 2017.

EPA Office of Research & Development. February 7, 2011. Draft plan to study the potential impacts of hydraulic fracturing on drinking water resources. *EPA.gov.* https://www.epa.gov/sites/production/files/documents/HFStudyPlanDraft_SAB_020711.pdf. Accessed September 22, 2017.

Evich, H.B. September 13, 2017. The great nutrient collapse. *Politico.com.* http://www.politico.com/agenda/story/2017/09/13/food-nutrients-carbon-dioxide-000511. Accessed September 14, 2017.

Gee, D. 2006. Late Lessons from early warnings: Toward realism and precaution with endocrine-disrupting substances. *Environmental Health Perspectives.* 114(Suppl 1): 152–160, doi: 10.1289/ehp.8134.

Girod B., D.P. van Vuuren, E.G. Hertwich. 2014. Climate policy through changing consumption choices: Options and obstacles for reducing greenhouse gas emissions. *Global Environmental Change.* 25:5–15.

Gould, S., and L.F. Friedman. September 26, 2015. The countries where people eat the most meat. *BusinessInsider.com.* http://www.businessinsider.com/where-do-people-eat-the-most-meat-2015-9. Accessed September 27, 2017.

Gurian-Sherman, D. April 2008. CAFOs uncovered: The untold costs of confined animal feeding operations. *ucsusa.org*. Union of Concerned Scientists. http://www.ucsusa.org/sites/default/files/legacy/assets/documents/food_and_agriculture/cafos-uncovered.pdf. Accessed July 21, 2017.

Haigh R., D. Ianson, C.A. Holt, H.E. Neate, A.M. Edwards. 2015. Effects of Ocean Acidification on Temperate Coastal Marine Ecosystems and Fisheries in the Northeast Pacific. *PLoS ONE* 10(2): e0117533. https://doi.org/10.1371/journal.pone.0117533.

Herring, P. February 2, 2010. The secret life of soil. *extension.oregonstate.edu*. http://extension.oregonstate.edu/gardening/secret-life-soil-0. Accessed July 9, 2017.

History.com. 2009. Dust bowl. *History.com*. http://www.history.com/topics/dust-bowl. Accessed September 27, 2017.

Hoag, H. December 2, 2013. Humans are becoming more carnivorous. *Nature News*, doi: 10.1038/nature.2013.14282.

Hooper, D.U., F.S. Chapin, J.J. Ewel, A. Hector, P. Inchausti, S. Lavorel, J. H. Lawton, et al. 2005. Effects of biodiversity on ecosystem functioning: A consensus of current knowledge. *Ecological Monographs* 75: 3–35.

Humane Society of the United States. (2018). *Ag-Gag Laws Keep Animal Cruelty Behind Closed Doors*. http://www.humanesociety.org/issues/campaigns/factory_farming/factsheets/ag_gag.html Retrieved Friday June 22, 2018.

Jalava M., Kummu, M., Porkka, M., Siebert, S., and Varis O. (2014). Diet change – a solution to reduce water use? *Environmental Research Letters* 9: 074016 https://doi.org/10.1088/1748-9326/9/7/074016

Jose, S., V. Sejian, M. Bagath, A.P. Ratnakaran, A.M. Lees, Y.A.S. Al-Hosni, M. Sullivan, R. Bhatta, and J.B. Gaughan. 2016. Modeling of greenhouse gas emission from livestock. *Frontiers in Environmental Science* 4: 27, doi: 10.3389/fenvs.2016.00027.

Keledjian, A., G. Brogan, B. Lowell, J. Warrenchuk, B. Enticknap, G. Shester, M. Hirshfield, and D. Cano-Stocco. March 2014. Wasted catch. *Oceana.org*. http://oceana.org/sites/default/files/reports/Bycatch_Report_FINAL.pdf. Accessed September 22, 2017.

Koide, R., and K. Haider. 2017. Mycorrhizal fungi and field crops. *extension.psu.edu*. http://extension.psu.edu/plants/crops/cropping-systems/documents/mycorrhizal-fungi-and-field-crops.pdf. Accessed August 11, 2017.

Loomis, I. August 17, 2017. Trees in the Amazon make their own rain. *ScienceMag*. http://www.sciencemag.org/news/2017/08/trees-amazon-make-their-own-rain.   Accessed September 19, 2017.

Martin, D.F., D.R. Ward, and B.B. Martin. 2010. Agricultural pharmaceuticals in the environment: A need for inventiveness. *Technology and Innovation* 12: 129–141. http://chemistry.usf.edu/faculty/data/Martin-Publication2.pdf.

Maughan, R. September 22, 2012. Wedge wolf pack will be killed because of its increasing beef consumption (Update 9/25 – 28). *The Wildlife News*.

Mekonnen, M.M., and A.Y. Hoekstra. 2012. A global assessment of the water footprint of farm animal products. Ecosystems 15: 401–415.

Mood, A., and Brooke, P. July 2010. *Estimating the Number of Fish Caught in Global Fishing Each Year*. http://www.fishcount.org.uk/published/std/fishcountstudy.pdf. Accessed September 22, 2017.

Muir, P. November 21, 2012. Human impacts on ecosystems: Trophic issues. *OregonState.edu*. people.oregonstate.edu/~muirp/trophic.htm. Accessed August 6, 2017.

Nickerson, C., R. Ebel, A. Borchers, and F. Carriazo. December 2011. Major uses of land in the United States, 2007. *Economic Research Service*. https://www.ers.usda.gov/webdocs/publications/44625/10649_eib89_reportsummary.pdf?v=41055.

NOAA Fisheries. January 30, 2014. Purse seine: Fishing gear and risks to protected species. http://www.nmfs.noaa.gov/pr/interactions/gear/purseseine.htm. Accessed September 16, 2017.

Ohlson, K. 2014. *The Soil Will Save Us*. New York, NY: Rodale.

Oppenlander, R. 2013. *Food Choice and Sustainability*. Minneapolis, MN: Langdon Street Press.

Oppenlander, R. April 22, 2012. The world hunger-food choice connection: A summary. http://comfortablyunaware.com/blog/the-world-hunger-food-choice-connection-a-summary/. Accessed September 27, 2017.

Oregon State University Forage Information System. 2017. Define biological nitrogen fixation (BNF) and explain its importance. *Oregon State University National Forage & Grassland Curriculum*. http://forages.oregonstate.edu/nfgc/eo/onlineforagecurriculum/instructor-materials/availabletopics/nitrogenfixation/definition. Accessed August 10, 2017.

Persson, L.M., et al. 2013. Confronting Unknown Planetary Boundary Threats from Chemical Pollution. *Environmental Science and Technology* 47 (22):12619–12622.

Pöhlker, C., K.T. Wiedemann, B. Sinha, M. Shiraiwa, S.S. Gunthe, M. Smith, H. Su, et al. 2012. Biogenic potassium salt particles as seeds for secondary organic aerosol in the Amazon. *Science* 337(6098): 1075. https://www.mpg.de/6329380/plants_fungi_salt-aerosol. Accessed September 19, 2017.

Post Carbon Institute. June 1, 2011. Natural Gas Report Supplements: Public Health, Agriculture, Transportation. Available at http://www.postcarbon.org/publications/natural-gas-report-supplements/ Accessed February 6, 2018.

Potter, W. May 1, 2014. Australia risks copying US 'ag-gag' laws to turn animals activists into terrorists. *The Sidney Morning Herald*. http://www.smh.com.au/environment/animals/australia-risks-copying-us-aggag-laws-to-turn-animal-activists-into-terrorists-20140501-37k8i.html. Accessed July 13, 2017.

Ranganathan, J., and F. Irwin. October 21, 2010. Biodiversity summit must tackle destructive impacts of food production. *WRI.org*. http://www.wri.org/blog/2010/10/biodiversity-summit-must-tackle-destructive-impacts-food-production. Accessed September 25, 2017.

Ravishankara A.R., J.S. Daniel, R.W. Portmann. 2009. Nitrous oxide (N2O): the dominant ozone-depleting substance emitted in the 21st century. *Science* 326(5949): 123–125. doi: 10.1126/science.1176985

Ritter, M.E. 2006. The physical environment: An introduction to physical geography. *EarthOnlineMedia*. http://www.earthonlinemedia.com/ebooks/tpe_3e/biogeography/trophic_levels_and_food_chains.html. Accessed July 18, 2017.

Rockstrom J., et al. 2009. Planetary Boundaries: Exploring the Safe Operating Space for Humanity. *Ecology and Society* 14(2): 32. http://www.ecologyandsociety.org/vol14/iss2/art32/

Scarborough P. et al. 2014. Dietary greenhouse gas emissions of meat-eaters, fish-eaters, vegetarians and vegans in the UK. *Climatic Change* 125(2): 179–192.

Schilling, N. May 18, 2016. Australia says NO to ag-gag. *In Defense of Animals*. http://www.smh.com.au/environment/animals/australia-risks-copying-us-aggag-laws-to-turn-animal-activists-into-terrorists-20140501-37k8i.html Accessed July 13, 2017.

Scientific American. 2018. *What Causes Ocean "Dead Zones"?* https://www.scientificamerican.com/article/ocean-dead-zones/ Accessed February 1, 2018.

Scripps Institution of Oceanography. 2018. Value of Corals. Available at https://scripps.ucsd.edu/projects/coralreefsystems/about-coral-reefs/value-of-corals/ Accessed on January 20, 2018.

Silbergeld E.K., Graham, J., Price, L.B. 2008. Industrial food animal production, antimicrobial resistance, and human health. *Annual Review of Public Health*. 29: 151–169.

Simon, D.R. April 12, 2014. Are big macs killing bees? https://meatonomics.com/tag/externalized-costs/. Accessed September 18, 2017.

Smil, V. 2011. Harvesting the biosphere: The human impact. *Population and Development Review*, December 13: 613–636. http://vaclavsmil.com/wp-content/uploads/PDR37-4.Smil_.pgs613-636.pdf.

Steffen, W., K. Richardson, J. Rockström, S.E. Cornell, I. Fetzer, E.M. Bennett, R. Biggs, et al. 2015. Sustainability Planetary boundaries: Guiding human development on a changing planet. *Science*. February 13: 736–746.

Tilman D., M. Clark. 2014. Global diets link environmental sustainability and human health. *Nature*. 515(7528): 518–22. doi: 10.1038/nature13959.

U.N. Environment Programme. 2017. Overfishing: A threat to marine biodiversity. *UN.org*. http://www.un.org/events/tenstories/06/story.asp?storyid=800#. Accessed September 24, 2017.

U.N. Environment Programme. 2017. The Montreal Protocol: triumph by treaty. Available at https://www.unenvironment.org/news-and-stories/story/montreal-protocol-triumph-treaty Accessed on January 21, 2018.

U.N. FAO. 2017. General situation of world fish stocks. *FAO.org*. http://www.fao.org/news-room/common/ecg/1000505/en/stocks.pdf. Accessed September 24, 2017.

U.N. Food and Agriculture Organization. 2006. *Livestock's Long Shadow: Environmental Issues and Options*, 390 p. Rome: UNFAO.

U.N. Food and Agriculture Organization. 2012. *The State of World Fisheries and Aquaculture*. Rome: UNFAO.

U.S. Bureau of Land Management. June 24, 2017. *Wild Horse and Burro: Program Data*. https://www.blm.gov/programs/wild-horse-and-burro/about-the-program/program-data. Accessed September 18, 2017.

U.S. Department of Health and Human Services. September 2014. *Summary Report on Antimicrobials Sold or Distributed for Use in Food-Producing Animals*. https://www.fda.gov/downloads/ForIndustry/UserFees/AnimalDrugUserFeeActADUFA/UCM231851.pdf. Accessed September 14, 2017.

U.S. General Accounting Office. July 26, 1999. Animal agriculture: Waste management practices. *GAO.gov*. http://www.gao.gov/archive/1999/rc99205.pdf. Accessed September 27, 2017.

U.S. Geological Survey. December 2, 2016a. How much water is there on, in, and above the earth? https://water.usgs.gov/edu/earthhowmuch.html. Accessed September 19, 2017.

U.S. Geological Survey. December 2, 2016b. Evapotranspiration – The water cycle. *Water. USGS.gov*. https://water.usgs.gov/edu/watercycleevapotranspiration.html. Accessed September 27, 2017.

Union of Concerned Scientists. (2017). Food and agriculture. http://www.ucsusa.org/our-work/food-agriculture/our-failing-food-system/industrial-agriculture#.WXEcSMaZORt. Accessed April 12, 2017.

Union of Concerned Scientists. (2017). Prescription for trouble: Using antibiotics to fatten livestock. *ucsusa.org*. http://www.ucsusa.org/food_and_agriculture/our-failing-food-system/industrial-agriculture/prescription-for-trouble.html#.WXJdl8aZORs. Accessed July 21, 2017.

Union of Concerned Scientists. 2017. Hidden costs of industrial agriculture. http://www.ucsusa.org/food_and_agriculture/our-failing-food-system/industrial-agriculture/hidden-costs-of-industrial.html#.WXEkbsaZORs. Accessed April 12, 2017.

USDA Economic Research Service. April 28, 2017. How important is irrigation to U.S. agriculture? https://www.ers.usda.gov/topics/farm-practices-management/irrigation-water-use/background.aspx. Accessed September 22, 2017.

USDA Economic Research Service. October 14, 2016. What is agriculture's share of the overall U.S. economy? https://www.ers.usda.gov/data-products/chart-gallery/gallery/chart-detail/?chartId=58270. Accessed July 14, 2017.

USDA Foreign Agricultural Service. June 26, 2013. Indonesia: Palm oil expansion unaffected by Forest Moratorium. Accessed September 19, 2017. https://ipad.fas.usda.gov/highlights/2013/06/indonesia/

USDA Natural Resources Conservation Service. 2017. Animal feeding operations: Animal feeding operations (AFO) and concentrated animal feeding operations (CAFO). *ncrs.usda.gov*. https://www.nrcs.usda.gov/wps/portal/nrcs/main/national/plantsanimals/livestock/afo/.

Vaidyanathan, G. December 22, 2015. How bad of a greenhouse gas is methane? *ScientificAmerican.com.* https://www.scientificamerican.com/article/how-bad-of-a-greenhouse-gas-is-methane/. Accessed September 27, 2017.

Verso, E. December 9, 2015. Topsoil erosion. *large.stanford.edu.* http://large.stanford.edu/courses/2015/ph240/verso2/. Accessed August 13, 2017.

Virginia Institute of Marine Science. 2017. Dead zone formation. *VIMS.edu.* http://www.vims.edu/research/topics/dead_zones/formation/index.php. Accessed July 9, 2017.

Walsh, B. December 16, 2013. The triple whopper environmental impact of global meat production. *Science.Time.com.* http://science.time.com/2013/12/16/the-triple-whopper-environmental-impact-of-global-meat-production/. Accessed September 25, 2017.

Warner, J.X. et al. 2017. Increased atmospheric ammonia over the world's major agricultural areas detected from space. *Geophysical Research Letters* 44(6): 2875–2884. doi:10.1002/2016GL072305

Woods Hole Oceanographic Institution. 2010. FAQs about Ocean Acidification. Available at http://www.whoi.edu/page.do?pid=83380&tid=7342&cid=131410 Accessed on January 20, 2018.

Worldometers. 2017. World population. *Worldometers.info.* http://www.worldometers.info/world-population/. Accessed May 28, 2017.

Worm, B., E.B. Barbier, N. Beaumont, E. Duffy, C. Folke, B.S. Halpern, J.B.C. Jackson, et al. 2006. Impacts of biodiversity loss on ocean ecosystem services. *Science* 314(5800): 787–790.

Zhu, W., D.R. Schmehl, C.A. Mullin, and J.L. Frazier. 2014. Four Common Pesticides, Their Mixtures and a Formulation Solvent in the Hive Environment Have High Oral Toxicity to Honey Bee Larvae. *PLoS ONE* 9(1): e77547. doi: 10.1371/journal.pone.0077547

Zielinski, S. November 10, 2014. Ocean dead zones are getting worse globally due to climate change. *Smithsonian.com.* http://www.smithsonianmag.com/science-nature/ocean-dead-zones-are-getting-worse-globally-due-climate-change-180953282/. Accessed September 22, 2017.

4 Our Soils in Peril

Anandi Gandhi

CONTENTS

> "The story of our relationship to the earth is written more truthfully on the land than on the page. It lasts there. The land remembers what we said and what we did."
>
> **Robin Wall Kimmerer, 2013**

4.1 INTRODUCTION

Past civilizations from the valley of the Nile, Central and Southern America, China, North America, Soviet Russia, and Europe all share a similar story. In his book "Dirt: The Erosion of Civilizations", David R. Montgomery writes about how each civilization in its own way has known the importance of fertile soil as the key to agricultural productivity and yet has repeatedly made the mistake of mistreating and relentlessly mining precious top soil.

Early groups of hunter-gatherer humans figured out how to take care of the plants that fed them and kept them alive. Soon they discovered how to grow vegetables, tubers, and grains through the sowing of seeds in the soil. Thus began the process of farming or altering existing landscapes for human food. It wasn't long before they learned how to store surplus food and had enough to eat all year-round, providing a sense of security that led to larger families. Within just a few hundred years the small groups exploded into large and prosperous regions. A large population led to centralized systems of governance and economics. Despite becoming accustomed to their lifestyle, war and death brought an abrupt end to past civilizations.

What really happened to these societies? The question more accurately is, what has happened again and again to so many different civilizations that have existed through-out history? To understand this mystery, one needs to look a little closer at these highly evolved and well-organized societies to read the story that is hidden between the lines. This forgotten story is about the most neglected, exploited, and abused foundation of all civilizations: soil. Our repeated failure over the last 10,000 years to take care of the "living skin" of the Earth—the very basis for existence of all life on Earth—may lead us in the same direction of our predecessors (Montgomery 2007).

4.2   SOIL: THE FOUNDATION OF LIFE AND AGRICULTURE

To understand how the lack of soil conservation can destroy civilizations it is important to grasp what soil truly is and why it is so important. Only over the last few decades have scientists discovered and confirmed that soil is actually alive, extremely complex, and comprised of astounding biodiversity. Montgomery and Bilke (2016) defines fertile soils as, "the frontier between geology and biology; a mix of weathered rock fragments and organic matter". Often misunderstood as dead or inert, soil is actually bursting with soil dwellers and microbial life. We are only just beginning to understand the importance of what soil biologist Elaine Ingham calls the "soil food web" (USDA 1999). According to Ingham, the five main types of microorganisms found in the soil are bacteria, fungi, nematodes, protozoa, and microarthopods, which are abundant in both numbers and species (USDA 1999).

As mentioned in Chapter 3, a teaspoon of soil, depending on its fertility, may have between 1 billion and 7 billion organisms within which there may exist 75,000 species of bacteria, 25,000 species of fungi, 1,000 species of protozoa, and 100 species of nematodes (Ohlson 2014). Added to these microorganisms are other soil dwellers such as earthworms, beetles, voles, etc. and together they form the soil food web. There may be differences in the composition of these microbial species depending on different environments and soil types, but they perform similar functions everywhere. They play the role of decomposing organic matter, purifying water, and renewing soil fertility through nutrient cycling. Nutrient cycling refers to the ability of these microorganisms to convert decaying and dead organic matter (leaf litter, plant detritus, dead animals, etc.) into nutrients that the plants require for their growth (Ohlson 2014). In addition to decomposition, many microorganisms are capable of extracting minerals from rocks and subsoils thereby making those available to plants as well. This process of mineral mining and nutrient extraction by microorganisms had been occurring in the soil long before plants evolved on Earth. With the appearance of plants, however, the process of cooperation and symbiosis between plant and soil organisms began.

Plants help maintain the biology in the soil through exudates which are sugars, carbohydrates, and proteins that the plant releases through its roots to feed beneficial organisms (USDA 1999). These organisms, in turn, provide the plant with the nutrients through a complex web of interactions. Plants exudate one-third or 40% of their food to attract the microorganisms that will provide the plant with the specific nutrients it needs (Ohlson 2014). The zone near plant root tips is an area of intense soil organism activity called the rhizosphere. Unlike what is widely professed, plants need more than just nitrogen, phosphorus, and potassium. In healthy living soils, they receive all the fertilization they need through indirect processes in the rhizosphere. Soils that do not have organic matter cannot provide the food that soil dwellers need to survive, thus leading to degraded soils where plants are unable to thrive (Ohlson 2014). Nutrients from organic matter and plant exudates are first ingested by bacteria, which are then preyed upon by protozoa, nematodes, or microarthopods. These larger organisms, through their excretion, produce a chemical version of the nutrients that are finally available to the plant in a form it can absorb. Nutrients are distributed by mychorrhizal fungi that form symbiotic relationships with plant roots; the fungi are responsible for reducing plant competition through equitable distribution of those nutrients throughout the plant community (FAO and ITPS 2015).

Specific microorganisms are adapted to specific plant communities and environments. This specialization means that if you place a healthy plant in degraded soil, it will show signs of struggle because it is missing its special soil dynamics. Soil dwellers and microorganisms not only help plants access nutrients from the air (such as nitrogen), rocks, and organic matter—they also build soil structure by anchoring themselves to particles of sand, clay, and silt, gluing them together and building aggregates (Ohlson 2014). These aggregates allow for spaces in the soil for gases and water to move through without taking the soil apart and destroying the homes of these creatures. Earthworms and other larger organisms are well known for their process of aeration by moving up and down through the soil while eating and releasing nutrient-rich excretions. The benefits of having this healthy soil structure is that the ground becomes a large sponge capable of holding just the right amount of moisture and air that plants require. Their roots systems have the space and ease to grow in volume and length, which is the best sign of a healthy and productive plant.

Another important element of soil is carbon. Organic matter in soil contains 55%–60% of carbon by mass (FAO and ITPS 2015). Plants use carbon dioxide from the air for the process of photosynthesis. However, not all of it is used by the plant; some carbon gets stored in the soil as humus (Ohlson 2014). Plants growing on living, healthy soil can steadily remove carbon dioxide from the atmosphere, which is then sequestered in the soil (Ohlson 2014). Soils are capable of storing large quantities of carbon and are only second to oceans in being a carbon sink. Healthy soil can nourish plants leading to the maximization of carbon fixation with the added effect of reducing carbon dioxide in the atmosphere. These benefits depend on the organisms of the soil food web (Shiva 2017). Carbon stored in soil organic matter has helped determine essential soil properties and functions such as pH balance, nutrient storage and availability, and regulating soil moisture. When there is adequate soil carbon content, it has a positive impact on soil structure, particle agglomeration, and stability, as these properties influence water infiltration rates and create resistance to water and wind erosion (FAO and ITPS 2015). Healthy soils are key to sustaining soil fertility for thousands of years, making plants naturally resilient to environmental fluctuations, pests, and disease. Healthy soils can also prevent the release of carbon from soil into the atmosphere.

4.2.1 Learning from History

It was 5000 BC when agriculture first started in the fertile floodplains of the mighty Nile River valley. The floodplains were blessed with fresh silt deposits, which meant that soil nutrients were being renewed every year. For many years balance and prosperity prevailed through simple technologies, such as minimally modified seasonal irrigation overflow channels that were locally controlled (Montgomery 2007). By 3000 BC, surplus food production and storage led to the centralization of economics and governance, creating the desire to export. This led to a few key changes in the traditional agricultural practices. Irrigation changed from being seasonal to becoming more aggressive and year-round with cash crops grown for export. Over time this excessive irrigation led to the increase of salts in the soil, diminishing plant yields and degrading the fertility of the land (Montgomery 2007).

The Yao dynasty in China started around 2357 BC. As favorable agricultural conditions led to population growth, the demand for agricultural land increased. This led to deforestation on the surrounding hills for farming. Very quickly, intensive farming and grazing on the hills led to severe soil erosion on sloped hillsides. Less than 100 years after its establishment, the Yao dynasty collapsed (Montgomery 2007).

The story of ancient Rome, though much more complex, has a very similar story. The main impact in this case was through the introduction of the metal plow. Early Roman farms were multilayered, diverse, and farmers tended them by hand. When the metal plow was introduced, it allowed for deep subsoil digging and plowing of the hillsides. As productivity skyrocketed, severe soil erosion began within a few seasons of farming on fragile sloping lands. Philosophers Plato and Aristotle both posited the degradation of the land was due to the land-use practices of the Bronze Age (Montgomery 2007). Despite these warnings, the health of the soil was ignored. Farmers were encouraged to continue plowing and in less than a thousand years, the Roman heartland had lost all its precious topsoil (Montgomery 2007).

Loss of soil organic matter is what defines the story of the Mayan civilization. In 2000 BC the Mayans traditionally used the slash and burn method that involved deforesting a small area, farming the land for a couple of years, and then leaving the land fallow for 10 to 20 years, allowing the soil and ecosystem to regenerate during their absence (Montgomery 2007). This was a stable system that worked when there was access to large sections of land and a rather small population. But as the population started increasing from 200,000 in 600 BC to 1 million in 300 AD, the Mayans stopped moving from one piece of land to another and instead settled down, farming in the same spots (Montgomery 2007). This new intensive and extractive farming practice did not return any organic matter back to the soil and led to stripping the soil down to the bedrock. The Mayan civilization collapsed in 900 AD (Montgomery 2007).

The Egyptian, Yao, Roman, and Mayan civilizations degraded their topsoil and did not attempt to conserve the soil until it was impossible to reverse the damage in their lifetimes. Low-impact farming techniques supported smaller populations and healthy soils. High-impact methods introduced major changes that caused deforestation including new technologies like the plow, over-irrigation, and monocropping (cultivating just a single crop on a piece of farmland), which in turn caused increases in food productivity for short periods leading to population growth. However, the living topsoil steadily disappearing. Even if some efforts were made to save the soil in the end, it was too late for fertility to return quick enough to ensure their civilization's survival. Without anthropogenc involvement, soil rebuilding occurred at a rate that was too slow to sustain humans for thousands of years. Moving forward, erosion had degraded half of Australia's soils by the mid-1980s (Montgomery 2007). West Africa also experienced its own dust bowl in the 1970s (Montgomery 2007). This is the history of the human impact on soil in almost every part of the world.

4.3   MODERN AGRICULTURE AND SOIL

"Death of soil is like a disease that remains undetected until the last stages when it has already become a crisis"

David Montgomery, 2007

Presently, 38% of land on Earth is agricultural (FAO and ITPS 2015). The global population is expected to grow to 9.6 billion by 2050 (FAO and ITPS 2015). In the 21st century, our relationship with soil is greatly determined by our population densities and available cultivable land. Cultivated area per capita is expected to decrease by 50% by 2050 in less developed countries (FAO and ITPS 2015). It has been reported that food production will have to increase by 70%–100% to meet the population demands (FAO and ITPS 2015). However, approximately 20% of the Earth's vegetated surface shows persistent declining trends in productivity (UNCCD 2017). One-third of Earth's soils are severely degraded and fertile soil is being lost at an extremely high rate (UNCCD 2017). Only 28% of land still remains forested (FAO and ITPS 2015). These facts and figures convey that our population is growing—cultivable land is shrinking—and food productivity is reaching its limit. We are currently experiencing a silent global ecological crisis: the death of soil.

The major anthropogenic reasons for the loss of soil biodiversity according to *The Status of the World Soil Resources* report are: Intensive human exploitation, reduced soil organic matter and carbon, soil erosion, soil pollution, soil salinization, soil compaction, land-use change, and climate change (FAO and ITPS 2015). Purported solutions include intensification and expansion. Intensification would mean increasing the use of chemical fertilization, irrigation, tillage, and increased livestock density. Increasing these practices however will further diminish soil productivity due to the extractive nature of these practices. Expansion of agricultural land from an environmental and ethical perspective is no longer possible because it results in unfair land-grabs, rapid and irreversible deforestation of the last remaining forests, and worsening climate change (FAO and ITPS 2015). Many of the technologies that modern and industrial agriculture employs are directly or indirectly responsible for poor soil health and biodiversity loss.

Soil erosion is a global ecological crisis faced by almost every country in the world. The rate of soil erosion is naturally quite slow. The current rate of soil erosion on intensely farmed agricultural and pasture land is between 100 and 1,000 times faster than in natural landscapes such as forests and grasslands. Globally, 20–200 gigatons of soil erode every year through water and wind due to agricultural practices that expose soil (FAO and ITPS 2015). For agricultural productivity to sustain itself, soil erosion must be eliminated altogether. In other words, for farming to be sustainable the rate of soil erosion needs to be the same as the rate of soil creation. Soil erosion directly impacts soil organic matter content. If it runs off or blows away, it reduces water infiltration capacity of the remaining soil due to diminished microbial activity, and leaves behind an inhospitable environment for plants to survive in.

Soil salinization indicates elevated salt content in soil. Salinization increases osmotic pressure, diminishing the soil moisture and deteriorating the soil structure, allowing very little permeability of air and water. When soil structure collapses and moisture content is reduced, plants are inhibited due to lack of water and root growth, apart from being unable to process the high salt content. Soil salinization affects more than 100 countries and 1 billion hectares of soil all over the world (FAO and ITPS 2015). Salinization occurs due to poor management of salts and sodium in soils through the use of irrigated water with high salt and sodium content—and through bringing up deep groundwater to the soil surface. The impact of these practices is exacerbated by the replacement of deep-rooted plants with others that have shallow root systems (UNCCD 2017).

Soil acidification refers to the pollution of the soil due to the excessive use of ammonium-based fertilizers and removal of biomass through constant harvesting (FAO and ITPS 2015). It results in reduced microbial activity in soil. Thirty percent of all topsoil and 75% of all subsoil is affected by soil acidification.

Soil contamination is yet another result of excessive use of fossil fuels, pesticides, and other pollutants. Even though the extent of soil contamination is difficult to assess or quantify, the extensive use of pesticides and nutrients in soil are a problem in many parts of the world (UNCCD 2017). Genetically modified (GM) seeds are also a source of soil pollution through seeds that are left behind in the soil after a harvest. They also have unknown effects on soil microorganisms, such as bacteria that are capable of capturing and using genetic material from other plant matter. This may lead to genetic contamination (Damato 2009).

Loss of soil organic matter and carbon from soil occurs due to deforestation, land-use changes, and tilling of the soil. Carbon loss from soil is highest where land-use changes from native perennial or forest cover to agricultural land (FAO and ITPS 2015). Conversion of land from native forest to cropland can result in a 42% loss of carbon while the conversion from pasture to cropland can result in a 59% loss of carbon from the soil (FAO and ITPS 2015). On lands where agriculture has been performed for millennia, the loss of soil carbon can be as high as 80% (Ohlson 2014). Globally the world's soils have lost up to 80 billion tons of carbon (Ohlson 2014). Lost soil carbon transforms into carbon dioxide and is released into the atmosphere and exacerbates the effects of climate change.

Soil erosion, salinization, acidification, and the loss of soil organic matter and carbon are linked to modern agricultural practices. Some of the most harmful and widespread agricultural technologies that impact soil biodiversity and fertility are mechanized tiling, use of chemicals fertilizers and pesticides, and large-scale monocropping.

Tilling or plowing has been practiced through the different ages of agriculture, from Neolithic to post-Industrial Revolution. Hence, it is not a new technology but ends up destroying soil structure and hastening soil erosion. While breaking up the soil creates more aeration, tilling or plowing causes more soil compaction by the weight of the plow, making it much harder for plant roots to penetrate. In soils that are plowed over and over again, this compaction makes it almost impenetrable for plant roots (Montgomery 2007). Roots may travel deep into the subsoil to access nutrients through the help of soil dwellers who can make minerals available from the bedrock and subsoil. Compaction due to the plow cuts this access for plants and the shallow root system leads to weak plants with lowered productivity. Breaking up the soil structure contributes to decreased organic matter due to exposed soil that releases carbon into the atmosphere and reduced microbial activity. Less organic matter means less food for soil biodiversity and fewer nutrients for plants. Tilling can lower yields by up to 60% (FAO and ITPS 2015). Dr. Rattan Lal says, "Nothing in nature repeatedly turns over the soil to the specified plow depth of fifteen to twenty centimeters. Therefore, neither plants nor soil organisms have evolved or adapted to this drastic perturbation" (Ohlson 2014).

The impacts of tilling can be large-scale and devastating as witnessed in the U.S. during the dustbowls of 1933–1935. The mechanized steel plow was introduced by John Deere in 1838 (Montgomery 2007). The difference between the non-mechanized and mechanized plow was that it allowed one farmer to till very large pieces of land, turning them into industrial-sized farms. The 20th-century farmer could work 15 times more land that a 19th-century farmer. With mechanized plows, agricultural land multiplied rapidly and many fields were plowed and left open without any crops or weeds to hold the soil down. Severe droughts hit the Southern Plains of the U.S. where the highest concentration of farms existed. Without water and vegetation, strong winds created the famous dust bowls, taking away almost all the topsoil from several farms in a single day. More than 3 million people left the plains in the 1930s (Montgomery 2007). Despite the negative impacts of plowing, most farmers all over the world routinely plow their land, leaving the soil completely bare and exposed to the elements, killing the soil life that survives in the darkness of soil rich in organic matter.

How are high yields obtained from soil that has become degraded? This brings us to the other widespread technologies: synthetic fertilizers and pesticides. If the soil is unable to naturally provide the nutrients a plant needs, then the plant will be weak, susceptible to pests, and will probably produce very little food. Instead of taking care of the soil, industrial agriculture focuses on feeding the plant. This creates short-term yields while ignoring the needs of the soil. The use of synthetic fertilizers is so intensive that 30% of topsoil and 75% of subsoil globally has become too acidic to allow for sustainable plant growth (FAO and ITPS 2015). The agrichemical industry has isolated three macronutrients that plants need: nitrogen (N), phosphorus (P), and potassium (K) (referred to as NPK). However, the use and application of them is problematic. First, plants need a diversity of nutrients and minerals in addition to NPK. Isolating these nutrients chemically and then applying them over and over in large quantities deteriorates the soil quality and diminishes the availability of other key minerals that plants need (Montgomery and Biklé 2016). Another critical issue is that providing plants these nutrients in large quantities destroys the nutrient cycling that typically takes place underground between the plant roots, soil organisms, fungi, and other creatures (Montgomery and Biklé 2016). Chemicals destroy soil biodiversity and do not create biodiversity. Thus, soil is no longer living and cannot offer nourishment to the plant apart from what was artificially added by the farmer.

Agrichemicals not only disrupt symbiotic relationships and nutrient transfers, but they also disable the plants internal defense system making it vulnerable to pests and pathogens, thereby increasing the need of chemical pesticides (FAO and ITPS 2015). The heavy use of pesticides can cause populations of beneficial soil microorganisms to decline (Aktar 2009).

While the literature on the impact of pesticides on soil microorganisms is growing, there is enough evidence to show that changes in soil biodiversity impacts the entire food chain. Once soil has lost all its nutrients and the plants are dependent on chemical fertilizers, more and more application is required to obtain the same yield. Chemicals often require more irrigation, causing soil salinization in addition to acidification. Chemical fertilizers and pesticides reduce soil organic matter and soil life, which causes compaction and soil erosion that, in turn, reduces water infiltration and moisture availability for plants.

Both mechanized tilling and applications of large amounts of chemicals are used on large-scale farms that grow only a single crop variety year after year on the same land. This practice of monocropping is used to align mechanization and market-focused efficiencies. However, monocropping has a negative impact on soil and plant health and facilitates erosion. Monocropping involves growing seasonal cash crops such as grains soy, fodder, and biofuels that replace the existing perennial native vegetation. The damage that monocropping has on soil, on both the macro and micro level, is immense. In most parts of the world, agricultural land replaces whatever natural ecosystem existed on that land previously, including forests. Forests, whether temperate or tropical, consist of perennial vegetation, which means that soil is never exposed at any time and nutrient cycling occurs continuously in the soil. In this situation there is almost no loss of soil and plenty of organic matter constantly replenishing the soil through falling leaves, dying plants, animals, and organisms of all kinds. When temperate forests are converted into agricultural lands, the soil loses more than half of its organic matter (FAO and ITPS 2015). The rate of soil organic matter loss is highest in monocropped industrial farms that regularly practice tilling and chemical application (FAO and ITPS 2015). "Changes in soil diversity modify vegetation dynamics directly through associations of symbionts and pathogens with plant roots and indirectly, by modifying nutrient availability to plants" (FAO and ITPS 2015). The symbiotic connections between plant roots and fungal networks either becomes severely diminished or non-existent in monocropped farms due to the lack of both plant and soil biodiversity. In a perennially vegetated world every plant has evolved to have its own set of adapted underground relationships. But in a field with row after row of the same type of seasonal plant which in a few months is completely removed, the soil is bereft of life and nutrients. Planting the same type of vegetable or crop also enhances pest problems causing further use of agrichemicals on crops and vegetables.

Agribusinesses have also produced GM seeds. In India over the last 20 years, nearly 300,000 farmers have ended their lives by ingesting pesticides or by hanging themselves (Umar 2015). These suicides have been linked to the failure of the crop they have purchased (Bt Cotton, a GM cotton seed) on credit or through the accumulation of life time savings. Unable to withstand the drought as well as native seed crops could, the monocropped Bt Cotton crops failed in these areas. Biodiverse vegetation can adapt to stresses better than GM crops.

The fundamental issue with the agricultural practices of tilling, chemical use, monocropping, and genetic modification is that they are counterproductive to soil health. These practices may boost plant productivity in the short-term, but leave behind degraded land and tragic consequences for some farmers. Other large-scale impacts include: other desertification, which is the loss of cultivable land; diminishing groundwater tables due to intensive irrigation; land sinking in areas where the aquifers have been depleted, and dust bowls.

4.4 THE FUTURE OF SOIL

When we look back at the history of our predecessors, one glaring truth is that agriculture can be purely extractive by destroying the soil. The subsequent loss of soil organic matter deprives food for soil life, which leads to the collapse of soil structure. The plants surviving in this hard, dry land without their underground allies struggle to establish deep and strong root systems. They are plagued by pests and disease, as well as unprecedented climate conditions of droughts and floods. Without organisms to hold the soil together, cultivable lands are being rapidly lost due to intensive human exploitation. No technology in modern industrial agriculture is capable of reversing soil erosion or maintaining a balance between soil erosion and soil creation. Soil is being mined as an infinite resource when it should be recognized as finite and vulnerable.

Although some farmers know that their soils have been degraded, there may be no incentive to conserve and amend their soil.

4.5 CONCLUSION

Soils are a major reservoir of global biodiversity that are essential to preserve and restore. The importance of soil biodiversity is becoming increasingly clear and the repercussions of human activities on soil health are vast. Research has demonstrated that exposing and disturbing the soil takes away organic matter and destroys a diversity of life in the soil. As long as soil erosion continues to exceed soil formation, we continue with practices that are unfavorable and potentially devastating to all of humanity. We live in a time where climate change, extreme weather events, and the overexploitation of natural resources including living soil impedes the health and well-being of both humans and the living systems of the planet.

REFERENCES

Aktar, W., D. Sengupta, and A. Chowdhary. 2009. Impact of pesticides use in agriculture: their benefits and hazards. *Interdisciplinary Toxicology* 2(1): 1–12.
Damato, G. June 17, 2009. The devastating effect of GMOs on the future of soil. *NW Resistance Against Genetic Engineering*. http://nwrage.org/content/devastating-effects-gmos-future-soil-0. Accessed September 15, 2017.

Food and Agriculture Organization of the United Nations and Intergovernmental Technical Panel on Soils. 2015. *Status of the World's Soil Resources (SWSR) – Main Report.* Rome: FAO http://www.fao.org/documents/card/en/c/c6814873-efc3-41db-b7d3-2081a10ede50/ Accessed July 3, 2017.

Kimmerer, R.W. 2013. *Braiding Sweetgrass: Indigenous Wisdom, Scientific Knowledge and the Teachings of Plants.* Minneapolis, MN: Milkweed Editions.

Montgomery, D.R., and A. Biklé. 2016. *The Hidden Half of Nature: The Hidden Roots and Life and Health.* New York: W. M. Norton & Company, Inc..

Montgomery, D.R. 2007. *Dirt: The Erosion of Civilizations.* Berkeley, CA: University of California Press.

Ohlson, K. 2014. *The Soil Will Save Us: How Scientists, Farmers, and Foodies Are Healing the Soil to Save the Planet.* New York, NY: Rodale Inc.

Shiva, V. 2017. *Seeds of Hope, Seeds of Resilience.* New Delhi: Navdanya/RESTE.

Umar, B. May 18, 2015. India's shocking farmer suicide epidemic. *Aljazeera.* http://www.aljazeera.com/indepth/features/2015/05/india-shocking-farmer-suicide-epidemic-150513121717412.html. Accessed August 29, 2017.

United Nations Convention to Combat Desertification. 2017. *The Global Land Outlook,* first edition. Bonn, Germany: UNCCD.

5 The Far-Reaching Impact of Disposable Plastic

Rebecca Prince-Ruiz

CONTENTS

5.1 INTRODUCTION

It is difficult to imagine a world without plastic. Plastics are now used in everything from the packaging of food and medical supplies to communication devices and even clothing. Rapid growth in the use of plastics over the last century has seen the production of plastics surpass all other man-made materials except steel and cement (Geyer et al. 2017). The durability of plastics when combined with its limited recapture and reuse of materials has resulted in a growing problem. As plastic waste enters the environment, using a material that is essentially designed to last forever to produce disposable items has consequences far beyond anything imaginable.

5.2 HISTORY AND BACKGROUND

Since the invention of the first synthetic plastics in the early 20th century, plastics have rapidly become part of daily life. Almost every person in the world will encounter plastic (especially disposable, single-use plastic packaging) on a daily basis. Yet plastics were originally designed to replace a growing demand for limited resources including ivory and tortoiseshell, and used to manufacture durable items such as billiard balls and hair combs (Freinkel 2011). Large-scale production and widespread use of plastics in consumer markets began after World War II (Freinkel 2011).

Plastics are cheap to produce, lightweight yet strong, and can be flexible and durable. They are made from synthetic polymers that are mostly derived from fossil hydrocarbons and petroleum by-products. When combined with plasticizers, stabilizers, and other chemicals, plastics can take on an infinite number of forms, with tens of thousands of different plastics now being made. Early plastics manufactured in the United States created celluloid (created from a natural polymer, cellulose in cotton) and Bakelite that was manufactured entirely in the laboratory from phenol (a waste product of coal) and formaldehyde (Freinkel 2011).

During the first half of the 20th century there was a shift in the use of plastics to create entirely new material types and products such as polystyrene, nylon, PVC, and Teflon. During World War II, plastic production nearly quadrupled as not only were most existing resources put into the war effort but the military monopolized most of the new plastics invented ranging from plastic pocket combs that were issued to each member of the armed forces to gun turrets and helmet liners (Freinkel 2011). In the 1950s new markets for plastic production were required and thus plastics began to be increasingly used in civilian markets.

Plastics enabled the invention of "disposable" items such as packaging, containers, bags, plastic wrap, and food-serving wares. For societies raised on a scarcity of resources and a culture of reuse, the new "disposable culture" required education in order to encourage the public to throwaway items after a single use. In August 1955, *Life* magazine published an article "Throwaway Living" that celebrated this new lifestyle and depicted a modern American family throwing disposable tableware and other consumer goods into the air, enjoying their newfound freedom from domestic chores such as washing dishes (Cosgrove 2014).

In the first global analysis of all plastics ever manufactured, Geyer et al. (2017) reported that plastic production has outpaced most other man-made materials. An estimated 7,800 million metric tons of virgin plastics were manufactured from 1950 to 2015 while half of this (3,900 million metric tons) was produced in the last 13 years (Geyer et al. 2017). Plastic production now represents approximately 6% of global oil consumption (World Economic Forum et al. 2016). Increasing rates of consumption and population growth means rates of plastic production will likely increase in the future.

5.3   THE ENVIRONMENTAL IMPACTS OF PLASTIC WASTE

The appropriate disposal of plastic waste presents challenges to municipalities around the world, particularly in countries with limited resources or substandard waste management infrastructure. Geyer et al. (2017) estimated that of the total metric tons of plastic waste that has been generated globally, a massive 79% of this has been accumulating in landfills and, worse, elsewhere in the natural environment. Of the remainder, 12% was incinerated while a mere 9% has been recycled. Of that 9% which has been recycled, only 10% has been recycled more than once (Geyer et al. 2017). This small fraction of recycled plastics are technically *downcycled*, meaning that materials are recycled into products of lesser quality which are less likely to be further recycled.

Comparing the low plastic recycling rates to the much higher global recycling rates of iron and steel (70%–90%) or paper (58%) that have the potential to be recycled continuously, a stark picture of the problems associated with disposable plastic begins to emerge (World Economic Forum et al. 2016). Recycled plastics are usually low value materials due to mixing of polymers types and the plethora of chemicals and additives such as stabilizers and colorants in the original materials. Producers and manufacturers of plastic goods largely prefer virgin plastics due to low cost and purity of material type. While plastics are manufactured with the potential to last a lifetime—the majority of products are designed for single use. Data available on recycling rates shows Europe has the highest recycling rate of 30%, followed by China at 25% while the United States has plateaued at 9% (Geyer et al. 2017). Recycling plastic will be challenging in the future; in 2017 China announced a series of bans and restrictions on importing foreign waste, including plastics (de Freytas-Tamura 2018).

Consumers are often surprised at the low global rates of plastic recycling. In 1988, the Society of the Plastics Industry introduced a plastic resin identification code consisting of the numbers 1–7 to indicate the plastic type enclosed within the universal triangular recycling symbol (three chasing arrows). Although this symbol on plastic packaging does not indicate whether it will be recycled—consumers have considered it a symbol of recycling (Freinkel 2011).

Our current system of production and manufacturing is based on one-way or linear systems. The World Economic Forum et al. (2016) estimates that after a brief first use cycle, 95% of the plastic packaging material value is lost to the economy. Unlike organic materials that cycle through natural ecosystems, the most commonly used plastics are fossil fuel-based and are not biodegradable. Plastic waste that is not captured by collection systems accumulates in the natural environment such as the marine environment and other waterways.

Each year an estimated eight million metric tons of plastic enters the world's oceans, the majority originating from land-based sources (Jambeck et al. 2015). On shorelines and in oceans—from the equator to the poles—and from the sea surface to the sea floor—marine habitats have been polluted by man-made debris of which plastic is the most abundant (Thompson et al. 2009). Plastics are transported to the ocean via wind, rain and tides, through storm water systems, streams, rivers, and wastewater treatment systems. Weathering causes plastic debris to break down into smaller and smaller pieces resulting in marine microplastics (<5mm diameter) that are distributed throughout the world's oceans (Clark et al. 2016). Covering about two-thirds of the Earth's surface, oceans generate oxygen, absorb carbon dioxide, provide food, and regulate the climate too. Plastic pollution is yet another pressure taking a significant toll on oceans already threatened by climate change, ocean acidification, fishing pressures, and other anthropogenic causes (United Nations Environment n.d).

Cleanup efforts provide information on the types of litter most commonly found on beaches and waterways. Of the top ten items collected over 30 years of annual international coastal cleanups coordinated by Ocean Conservancy, eight are disposable food-serving plastics including beverage bottles and bottle caps, food wrappers, grocery bags, lids, straws, stirrers, and polystyrene foam containers (Ocean Conservancy 2017). Almost 700 species are known to interact with marine debris (Gall and Thompson 2015). Marine debris has been listed among the major threats to biodiversity in the marine environment (Gall and Thompson 2015).

Marine organisms are impacted by plastic pollution via entanglement and ingestion (Wilcox et al 2015). Images of seabirds, turtles, and marine mammals entangled in plastic debris such as fishing line, ropes, plastic bags, and balloons have become frequent in the media. Experts have identified items commonly littered that pose a high risk to marine wildlife via ingestion that includes: Plastic food packaging, straws, stirrers, and plastic utensils (Wilcox et al. 2015). The impact of plastics in the marine environment extends to organisms at the base of the marine food web with mussels, worms, and zooplankton ingesting microplastics (Cole et al. 2013).

Consumption of plastic debris also exposes marine organisms to contamination from toxicants, which are either added to the plastics during production (e.g., flame retardants) or adsorbed to the surface of plastic when in the water (e.g., persistent organic pollutants such as DDT and trace metals) (Rochman et al. 2013).

Overlooked and infrequently publicized, the ingestion of plastic by land-based animals including goats, cows, and even camels is disconcerting. Seattle-based photographer Chris Jordan created an art piece "Gastrolith"—a striking mass of over 500 plastic bags and other pieces of litter taken from the stomach of a dead camel found in the desert near Dubai (Jordan 2016).

Both the scale and impact of the plastics pollution problem are difficult to comprehend. It is difficult to visualize the enormity of eight million metric tons of plastic entering the world's oceans each year and the impact it has on marine wildlife. In a study on the impacts of plastic ingestion by Flesh-footed Shearwaters (a sea bird), Lavers et al. (2014) investigated the stomach contents of seabird fledglings living on the World Heritage-listed Lord Howe Island in the Tasman Sea, between Australia and New Zealand. At approximately 80 days old these fledglings have been fed by their parent birds from food foraged at sea with 90% having plastic in their stomach. One bird had 276 pieces of plastic in its stomach, accounting for 14.4% of its body mass (Lavers et al. 2014).

If "business as usual" continues, it is predicted that by the year 2050 not only will plastic waste outweigh fish in the oceans (World Economic Forum et al. 2016) but 99% of all seabirds species will have ingested plastic (Wilcox et al. 2015).

5.4   THE ROLE OF DISPOSABLE PLASTIC IN FOOD SYSTEMS

The largest application of plastics, about 26% of the total volume used, is for packaging (World Economic Forum et al. 2016). Since the 1950s the rise of disposable plastic packaging has had far-reaching impacts on the development of modern food systems, providing a lightweight, cheap, and convenient material to preserve and transport food items. The principal purpose of packaging is to protect food from external influences or damage—to contain it—and to provide the consumer with information about contents, origins, and nutritional information. Plastic packaging further enabled the transportation of large-scale quantities of food over long distances, a system initially progressed by advances in food preservation techniques and transportation methods. A visit to a modern supermarket reveals fruit and vegetables packaged in plastic in the fresh produce aisles as well as in the deep-freeze section, including "out of season" produce which has been transported long distances or from other countries. Extreme examples of packaging such as individual pieces of fruit which have been peeled and packaged as single items in clear plastic containers show the extent to which retailers are utilizing this material.

Plastic packaging doesn't simply contain food and beverages, but has also enabled the emergence of new markets. For example, the invention of the polyethylene terephthalate (PET) bottle in 1973 has made water available for "new forms of branded exchange and new practices of drinking" (Hawkins et al. 2015). Convenience foods such as ready-made meals can be stored, chilled, frozen, and reheated all in the same plastic packaging with virtually no preparation. Popular single-serve coffee brewing pods made from plastic and aluminum allow consumers to brew espresso style coffee in their own homes each day. Plastics have also enabled the creation of small packaging sizes providing consumers with a diversity of products as well as affordability—particularly in the case of developing countries. Plastic can also be found in the lining of metal cans or combined with a layer of aluminum in potato chip packets—or coating paper tubs of ice cream.

Consumer interest in processed foods and pre-prepared meals in the home is matched by the increasing demand for "to-go" food and beverages. The growth in this market has been fueled by "time-poor" lifestyles, global food transitions, and new technologies for ordering, payment, and delivery. No longer just the domain of weekend take-out meals, consumers are now wanting "to-go" food regularly—from takeout coffees to fresh juices and smoothies—sushi for lunch—or snacks. All of these items require some form of container in order to be transported and often come with additional packaging such as straws, utensils, carrier bags and sachets. Apart from compostable containers, cardboard pizza boxes and paper takeout containers, most "to-go" food containers are now plastic. As the name would suggest "to-go" food is often consumed in public places and work environments rather than in the home. Providing appropriate waste disposal facilities in public places for this food packaging waste challenges local authorities. Challenges to recycling include contamination by food in containers and the low value of the product altogether. The lightweight nature of plastic packaging often results in unintentional littering as containers are blown out of bins, adding to the burden of debris intentionally discarded. As described in Section 5.2, these items are problematic for marine wildlife.

Potential human health impacts from plastics is an area of emerging concern and research attention, both in terms of our exposure to microplastic pollution and via contamination from food packaged in plastic. Microplastics have been reported in food destined for human consumption such as seafood and processed food as well as air samples (Wright and Kelly 2017). A range of chemicals used in the manufacture of plastic packaging, including additives such as phthalates and BPA, are known to be concerning (Thompson et al. 2009). Chapter 8 offers further details about the implications of BPA in public health.

5.5 HEADING UPSTREAM TOWARDS SOLUTIONS

Given the benefits of plastic and the downstream impacts of waste and pollution, it is important to find solutions that respond to the scale and complexity of the problem. The problem of plastic waste on beaches and in the oceans can't be solved by clean-ups; plastic pollution is a symptom of problems upstream and reflects the flaws in the current systems of design and use of this material.

5.5.1 EDUCATION AND POLICY ACTIONS

There is a growing realization of the impact of plastics and other wastes that accu-mulate in oceans and waterways. This has been achieved via a range of awareness-raising initiatives, grassroots organizations, education and outreach campaigns, scientific research, media coverage, engagement by high profile individuals, and social media. Documentary films exploring the problems of plastic waste and pol-lution have reached a wide audience including *A Plastic Ocean*, *Albatross*, *Bag It*, *Blue The Film*, *Straws*, and *Tapped*.

Around the world, not-for-profit organizations, community groups, and gov-ernment programs increase awareness of the plastic pollution problem and pro-mote solutions. Organizations working to eliminate plastic waste is provided in Table 5.1.

The categories in Table 5.1 are intended as an informal guide. As most organiza-tions working on plastic waste issues conduct some form of education and awareness raising, most organizations traverse more than one category. Data collected during research and cleanups is used to raise awareness and advocate for policy change, such as the successful campaign to ban plastic microbeads organized by The 5 Gyres Institute and the *Story of Stuff* team, which led to the U.S. Microbead-Free Waters Act of 2015.

5.5.2 CONSUMER ACTION

Public concern about the growing levels of waste and pollution can be seen in the rising visibility of "plastic-free" and "zero-waste" activities. Activists are taking steps to reduce their waste and share their stories online and beyond. Although these labels of "plastic-free" and "zero-waste" are self-prescribed and definitions may vary, some people are aspiring to live "plastic-free" by eliminating single-use disposable plastics. A "zero-waste" lifestyle aims to eliminate creating any trash destined for the landfill or incinerator. Two leaders of these movements live in the San Francisco Bay area in California and have inspired people to re-evaluate the way they approach consumption habits and trash by sharing practical ways to make a difference.

In 2007 after seeing a photo of a decomposed carcass of a Laysan Albatross filled with plastic trash, Beth Terry vowed to purchase as little new plastic as possible, find

TABLE 5.1

Non-governmental Organizations Working to Eliminate Plastic Pollution

Focus	Organizations
Advocacy and policy	City to Sea (UK), Ocean Conservancy (USA, global), Ocean Recovery Alliance (Hong Kong, global), Parley for the Oceans (USA), Plastic Soup Foundation (Netherlands, global), Story of Stuff (USA, global), Upstream (USA)
Behavior change	Plastic-Free Tuesdays, Plastic Free July (Australia, global)
Circular Economy	Ellen McArthur Foundation (UK, global)
Cleanups and data collection	International Coastal Cleanup Day (USA, global), Litterati (USA, global), The Ocean Cleanup (Netherlands), Sea Shepherd Marine Debris Campaign (Australia), Surfrider Foundation (Global), Sustainable Coastlines Hawaii (USA), Take 3 (Australia), Tangaroa Blue (Australia), Two Hands Project (Australia, global)
Collaboration	Boomerang Alliance (Australia), Break Free From Plastic (global), Plastic Pollution Coalition (USA, global)
Education and awareness raising	Kōkua Hawaiʻi Foundation (USA), Plastic Free Seas (Hong Kong)
Research and communication	5 Gyres Institute (USA), Algalita Marine Research and Education (USA)
Specific plastic packaging e.g., bags, balloons, bottles, cups and straws	Balloons Blow (USA, global), Boomerang Bags (Australia, global), Bye Bye Plastic Bags (Indonesia), Refill Bristol (UK), Responsible Cafes (Australia), Rethink the Bag (South Africa), The Last Plastic Straw (USA)

alternatives, and share her discoveries on a blog. Her subsequent book *Plastic Free: How I Kicked the Plastic Habit and How You Can Too* (2012) examined plastics pollution problems and offers guidance to live plastic-free. For zero-waste lifestyle expert Bea Johnson, the choice was a conscious move by her family towards simplicity. An active blogger, public speaker, and author of *Zero Waste Home* (Johnson 2013), Johnson has inspired and educated people around the world on what has become a global movement.

An example of a program sharing solutions with a wider audience is the "Plastic Free July" campaign that originated in Australia (Plastic Free July 2017). This behavior change campaign raises awareness of the disposable plastics problem and challenges people to choose to refuse single-use plastic during the month of July and beyond. Started in 2011 and originally sponsored by the Western Metropolitan Regional Council with 40 people in Perth, Western Australia, this movement has grown to over two million individuals, schools, and organizations from 159 countries worldwide by the year 2017 (Plastic Free July 2017). It is now a non-profit organization.

The campaign provides individuals with information, ideas, and even recipes to avoid disposable plastics. Plastics Free July has a toolbox of resources for organizations, schools, and businesses to reduce their use of disposable plastics as well to share the campaign with the wider community. Its continued growth demonstrates that consumers are increasingly aware of the plastics problem and are willing to engage in solutions and choose alternatives. A 2017 survey of participants in the state of Western Australia revealed that significant levels of waste were avoided through the challenge, with an estimated 17,000 metric ton reduction in waste generated each year in that state alone (Western Metropolitan Regional Council 2017).

Additionally, food purchasing was the most commonly cited challenge for people trying to avoid single-use disposable plastic packaging. Many solutions to avoid disposable plastic closely align with the sustainable solutions to promote biodiversity. From growing their own food to supporting local (and therefore seasonal) food systems, Plastic Free July participants reported avoiding shopping at larger retail outlets that rely on heavily packaged foods in favor of supporting local food systems by shopping at farmer's markets, small grocery and produce stores, fishmongers, and butchers where they are able to take their own reusable produce bags and refillable containers (Plastic Free July 2017). For many Plastics Free July participants, eliminating disposable plastic packaging involved avoiding heavily processed foods which meant shifting to a healthier diet by cooking with fresh local produce and unpackaged ingredients from whole food stores (Rebecca Prince-Ruiz, pers. comm.). Thus, participants discovered unexpected co-benefit that included positive health and lifestyle outcomes (Rebecca Prince-Ruiz, pers. comm.). Participants interacted with growers, producers, independent retailers, and community members more. These additional unexpected benefits of a "low plastic lifestyle" assist in supporting local economies, building social capitol, and creating further actions to reduce plastics waste.

Although food shopping in this style can take more time, taking this extra effort and buying only what is needed and in the amount required sometimes results in cost savings and less impulse buying while eating more whole foods. Many Plastic Free July participants report efforts to cook from scratch once again by collaborating with a growing online community of plastic-free and zero-waste enthusiasts and also attend community events and workshops. At venues from farmer's markets, community centers, council offices, and universities, enthusiastic participants have demonstrated how to make kitchen staples such as crackers, yogurt, granola, pasta, and cheese without plastic packaging. These workshops are often organized by community groups, as participants in the Plastic Free July challenge are keen to share their skills and connect with other like-minded people in the community.

5.5.3   PUBLIC POLICY

Responding to problems of plastic pollution in the environment as well as growing public concern, some governments and municipalities are taking measures to reduce the impact of plastic waste with the focus on disposable food packaging. Legislative and regulatory measures to minimize plastic pollution include plastic bag bans; fees for plastic bags; bans on plastic disposable food-service wares; and container deposit legislation, whereby refunds are given for returned beverage containers to increase recycling and reduce littering. The City of San Francisco in California established legislation in 2003 adopting a zero waste to landfill goal by 2020 that is comprised of innovative policies to reduce plastic waste including: Mandatory recycling and composting, plastic bag bans, food-service ware ordinances and a ban on polystyrene and non-recyclable food-service wares, a cigarette litter fee, and restrictions on the sale of bottled water (SF Environment).

When considering alternatives to single-use disposable plastic, it is important to consider the end-of-life impacts of alternative products in waste management facilities as well as their unintended consequences. A 2016 report on the most harmful disposable plastic products used in California determined the most effective means of solving the plastic pollution problem is to substantially reduce the use of single-use disposable plastic items by replacing them with reusable or refillable alternatives and avoiding disposable materials altogether (Eriksen et al. 2016).

Because there is no universal definition or certification for "biodegradable" single-use plastic-type alternatives, there is confusion surrounding which materials are *truly* biodegradable and under what conditions they will break down, etc. (Eriksen et al. 2016). For instance, biodegradable plastics (made from biomass or fossil fuels) have also been suggested as one of the solutions to plastic pollution. However, the degree to which biodegradable plastics actually break down in the natural environment is the subject of much debate and is dependent on a number of factors, including the temperature and conditions altogether.

In 2015, the United Nations Environment Programme (UNEP) concluded that "complete biodegradation of plastics occurs in conditions that are rarely, if ever, met in marine environments, with some polymers requiring commercial composting facilities and prolonged temperatures of above 50°C to disintegrate" (UNEP 2015). Additionally, some plastics labeled as biodegradable such oxo-biodegradable plastics are fossil-fuel derived plastics containing additives to allow them to fragment more quickly in the presence of oxygen into smaller pieces, creating microplastics that can persist in the environment. The UNEP report concluded, "the adoption of plastic products labelled as 'biodegradable' will not bring about a significant decrease either in the quantity of plastic entering the ocean or the risk of physical and chemical impacts on the marine environment."

5.5.4 CREATING UPSTREAM CHANGES

Public actions in response to plastic pollution include participating in beach clean-ups and personal behavior change. However, as seen in Figure 5.1, we need to move beyond the ocean and beaches to the source.

The actions which occur upstream, including product design and manufacturing, impactful government policies and regulations, and creating waste management infrastructure are all critical. The "Heading Upstream" graphic provides a useful framework to create a shared picture of the complexity of the issue—and the range of stakeholders required for far-reaching solutions. This concept can be used to underpin efforts to transform the current linear flow of plastic packaging materials and ultimately develop a circular economy to recapture and reuse materials that prevent plastics pollution altogether.

While recognizing the complexities of the plastic pollution problem, what can no longer be denied is the impact on biodiversity. Plastic waste that is already in the

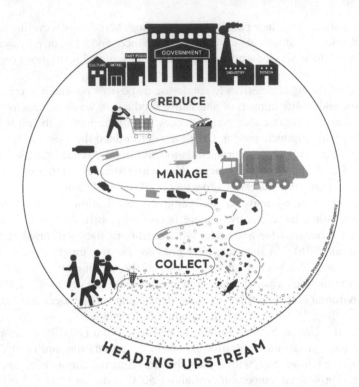

FIGURE 5.1 Heading upstream towards plastic waste solutions. (From R. Prince-Ruiz, Graphic: Cogency 2016)

environment will continue to cause harm to biodiversity and ecosystems for years to come. This is a driving force behind consumer-led plastic avoidance strategies such as the Plastic Free July campaign. We all need to do our part; that much is clear. There is no one perfect solution. Instead, a wide spectrum of interconnected and bold actions from the public, industry, scientists, and government policy-makers are necessary to create and sustain the change we need to see. How we act now to prevent and eliminate plastics pollution will determine the environment that future generations will inherit.

5.6   CONCLUSION

Since the invention of plastics one hundred years ago, this material has become a part of modern life. Rapid increases in production and the growing use in packaging, combined with low levels of material reuse and the lack of containment in our collection systems has resulted in massive amounts of plastic waste in the environment with devastating impacts. Single-use disposable plastic packaging is pervasive in modern food systems yet the material has the potential to last a lifetime. Heading upstream to reduce the plastic waste problem at the source requires collaboration and a range of solutions to avoid a future where there would be more plastic than fish in the world's oceans. Through personal responsibility and restructuring manufacturing, shifting away from disposable plastics can ultimately help to support healthy food systems and ecosystems while protecting and promoting biodiversity.

REFERENCES

Clark, J.R., M. Cole, P.K. Lindeque, E. Fileman, J. Blackford, C. Lewis, and T.M. Lenton, et al. 2016. Marine microplastic debris: A targeted planform understanding and quantifying interactions with marine life. *Frontiers in Ecology and the Environment* 14 (6): 317–324. doi:10.1002/Fee.1297.

Cole, M., P. Lindeque, E. Fileman, C. Halsband, R. Goodhead, J. Moger, and T.S. Galloway. 2013. Microplastic ingestion by zooplankton. *Environmental Science and Technology* 47 (12): 6646–6655. doi:10.1021/es400663f.

Cosgrove, B. 2014. Throwaway living: When tossing out everything was all the rage. *Time Life*. http://time.com/3879873/throwaway-living-when-tossing-it-all-was-all-the-rage/.

De Freytas-Tamura, K. 2018. Plastics pile up as China refuses to take the west's recycling. *New YorkTimes Website*. https://www.nytimes.com/2018/01/11/world/china-recyclables-ban.html.

Eriksen, E., M. Prindiville, and B. Thorpe. 2016. The plastics BAN (Better Alternatives Now) list. https://static1.squarespace.com/static/5522e85be4b0b65a7c78ac96/t/581cd663d2b857d18a7db3fd/1478284911437/PlasticsBANList2016-11-4.pdf.

Freinkel, S. 2011. *Plastic: A Toxic Love Story*. Boston: Houghton Mifflin Harcourt.

Gall, S.C. and Thompson, R.C. 2015. The impact of debris on marine life. *Mar Pollut Bull*. Mar 15; 92(1–2): 170–179.

Geyer, R., J.R. Jambeck, and K. Lavendar Law. 2017. Production, use, and fate of all plastics ever made. *Science Advances* 3 (7).

Hawkins, G., E. Potter, and K. Race. 2015, *Plastic Water: The Social and Material Life of Bottled Water*. Cambridge, MA: MIT Press.

Jambeck, J.R., R. Geyer, and C. Wilcox et al. 2015. Plastic waste inputs from land into the ocean. *Science* 347 (6223): 768–771.

Johnson, B. 2013. *Zero Waste Home: The Ultimate Guide to Simplifying Your Life*. New York: Scribner.

Jordan, C. 2016. Camel gastrolith. http://www.chrisjordan.com/gallery/camel/#gastrolith.

Lavers J.L., A.L. Bond, and I. Hutton. 2014. Plastic ingestion by flesh-footed shearwaters (*Puffinus carneipes*): Implications for fledgling body condition and the accumulation of plastic-derived chemicals. *Environmental Pollution* 187: 124–129.

Ocean Conservancy. (2017). Together for our Ocean: International Coastal Cleanup Report 2017. Washington, DC. https://oceanconservancy.org/wp-content/uploads/2017/06/International-Coastal-Cleanup_2017-Report.pdf

Plastic Free July. n.d. About plastic free July. http://www.plasticfreejuly.org/about.html. Accessed August 1, 2017.

Rochman, C.M., E. Hoh, T. Kurobe, , and S.J. The. 2013. Ingested plastic transfers hazardous chemicals to fish and induces hepatic stress. *Scientific Reports* 3: 3263. https://www.nature.com/articles/srep03263.

SF Environment. Legislation related to zero waste. https://sfenvironment.org/zero-waste-in-SF-is-recycling-composting-and-reuse. Accessed September 14, 2017.

Terry, B. 2012. *Plastic-Free: How I Kicked the Plastic Habit and How You Can Too*. New York: Skyhorse Publishing.

Thompson, R.C., C.M. Moore, F.S. vom Saal, and S.H. Swan. 2009. Plastics, the environment and human health: Current consensus and future trends. *Philosophical Transactions of the Royal Society B* 364: 2153–2166.

United Nations Environment. Why do oceans and seas matter? https://www.unenvironment.
    org/explore-topics/oceans-seas/why-do-oceans-and-seas-matter. Accessed February 6,
    2018.
United Nations Environment Programme (UNEP). 2015. *Biodegradable Plastics and Marine
    Litter: Misconceptions, Concerns and Impacts on Marine Environments*. Nairobi:
    United Nations Environment Programme (UNEP).
Western Metropolitan Regional Council. 2017. Plastic free July communications toolbox
    development. Report to the Waste Authority of Western Australia.
Wilcox, C., E. Van Sebille, and B.D., Hardesty. 2015. Threat of plastic pollution to seabirds is
    global, pervasive, and increasing. *PNAS* 112 (38):11899–11904.
World Economic Forum, Ellen MacArthur Foundation and McKinsey & Company. 2016. The
    new plastics economy — Rethinking the future of plastics. http://www.ellenmacarthur-
    foundation.org/publications.
Wright, S.L., and F.J. Kelly. 2017. Plastic and human health: A micro issue? *Environmental
    Science & Technology*, 51 (12): 6634–6647.

6 Just Food—Sustenance, Fairness, and Biodiversity

Valerie J. Stull and Michael M. Bell

CONTENTS

6.1 INTRODUCTION AND THE RIGHT TO FOOD

All creatures need to eat. The question is: How can we provide food for all life without compromising the livelihoods of either human or non-human beings? Justice requires that we provide for all, but we are not doing a very good job of it.

A persistent misconception regarding human hunger is that it stems from inadequacies in food production (Patel 2012). In reality, humans are producing more food than ever before (World Bank 2007), and there are ample calories to feed everyone on the planet today. The flaw lies not in a want for food, but in what Amartya Sen describes as the *entitlement to eat* (Sen 2013). Human food—and unavoidably agriculture—is entangled with social and political arrangements of social *power*. Injustices in food distribution, production, trade, exploitation of environmental resources, and pervasive poverty interfere with the entitlement to food. Also, a vast amount of human food is wasted, never reaching a human mouth—as much as 40% in the United States (Hall et al. 2009). Addressing these human injustices would go a long way, and perhaps even far enough, toward addressing the right to food for non-humans as well.

Part of the problem is that the principles of justice do not fit easily together into clear answers for the food system. On the one hand, food is widely considered a fundamental human right and is defined as such in Article 23 of the 1948 United Nations (UN) Declaration of Human Rights—but is not met in practice. The Special Rapporteur on the Right to Food to the UN describes this right as "regular, permanent and unrestricted access" to sufficient food "corresponding to the cultural traditions of the people to which the consumer belongs, and which ensure a physical and mental, individual and collective, fulfilling and dignified life free of fear" (OHCHR 2017). This right protects the most vulnerable and gives autonomy in food consumption, production, and access. Unfortunately, the human right to food is not met for more than 795 million people who regularly experience hunger today (FAO et al. 2015). Simply put, making this right a reality is clearly not universally available.

On the other hand, the case for biodiversity could be seen as entailing a right to food for non-human creatures, and hinging on providing the means, such as habitat protection, for their attaining that right. The obvious dilemma is that human sustenance may often impinge on those means, for example through deforestation and agricultural pesticides. A less obvious dilemma is that we typically regard humans as also having a right to individual autonomy and decision-making. In the words of Article 3 of the UN Declaration of Human Rights, "Everyone has the right to life, liberty and security of person." Although animal rights activists extend this right to all animals and some traditions such as the notion of *jiva* in Jainism extend it even further, we regard biodiversity as pertaining at the level of species, not for individual members of a species. Hawks may hunt rabbits, but the habitat that both require to continue their species must be maintained under most views of biodiversity. Yet in human rights, one individual cannot be sacrificed for another, even if such sacrifice maintains a larger community or even the human species as a whole. Human rights are not a matter of greatest good for the greatest number. Rights are about maintaining the greatest good for all, and are a necessary corrective to utilitarian thinking (Ashwood 2018). We cannot blithely turn farmland or fisheries back to the wild, even if the human species would be maintained—and perhaps more easily maintained—without considering the effect on individual humans. The UN Declaration of Human Rights does not allow for "life boat ethics," nor should it.

This chapter proposes a view of food justice that includes a concern for both human and non-human sustenance, while recognizing the right to food at the individual level for humans and at the species level for non-humans. The authors offer this view in the spirit of a post-humanist philosophy which does not put the human species ahead of other species, yet also envisions individual human consciousness as a special experience worthy of special consideration. Others might want to carry the argument further, especially with regard to the individual consciousness of other large vertebrates. The authors invite further conversation on that question, but feel that this chapter's framing requires less contentious debate given relatively widespread agreement with the UN Declaration of Human Rights and the principle of the ecological rights of biodiversity.

As well, the authors offer this notion of food justice as a way to assist in the resolution of another contentious debate: between the importance of *food security* and *food sovereignty* and between the importance of food provisioning and food control. A post-humanist vision of food justice requires food security and food sovereignty for both humans and non-humans. But, as the chapter will describe, the power dynamics of the current *corporate food regime* in human affairs undermines the food security and sovereignty of humans and non-humans alike.

6.2   BACKGROUND & WHERE WE ARE TODAY

Agriculture is the cornerstone of human society and advancement. Emerging around 10,000–12,000 years ago (at the start of the Neolithic period, in the Fertile

Crescent), the practice of cultivating and producing food has enabled humankind to alter ecosystems and increase population size. It allowed people to develop permanent settlements and acquire reliable food supplies and even surplus, fundamentally shaping socio-ecological change. Despite its seemingly slow evolution, dramatic methodological changes to agriculture in the second half of the 20th century have completely transformed it. Modern agriculture relies heavily on industrial methods that utilize monoculture, energy-intensive inputs, technology, and only a few specific crop varieties to maximize yield—methods that are now so widespread that they are often called "conventional agriculture."

One primary motivation behind efforts to maximize yield is a desire to promote *food security* for all humans. *Food security* implies that a person must have "physical and economic access to sufficient, safe, and nutritious food to meet dietary needs and food preferences for an active and healthy life" (FAO 1996). Resultantly, mechanization, strategic adoption and development of certain crop varieties, use of chemical fertilizers, and global trade have sprouted since the Green Revolution (GR)—a period of much agricultural research and technology transfer spearheaded by Norman Borlaug between 1940 and 1970. The GR leveraged concentrated investment to develop high-yield hybrid seeds with increased planting densities, shorter time to maturity, and the application of both chemical fertilizers and irrigation to radically increase crop productivity (Pingali 2012). As a result, cereal crop production tripled over 50 years, while the areas of land cultivated increased by only 30% (Wik et al. 2008). Techniques, seeds, patents, and infrastructure from the GR can now be found throughout the world.

Benefits from these technological advancements have included dramatic increases in global yields of a handful of crops—especially rice, wheat, and maize (FAO et al. 2004). It is often said that the GR saved millions of lives by preventing starvation through these dramatic increases in agricultural yield. The share of malnourished people fell significantly between 1960 and 1990 (Stevenson et al. 2011). During that time, crop improvement networks were created and spread around the globe, which allowed breeding materials and knowledge to be widely adopted in developing countries (Morris et al. 1994; Maredia and Byerlee 1999). As such, during the 1970s, the calories per person available globally increased by nearly 30%; across Asia, cereal production rates doubled from 1970 to 1975 while the land area under cultivation increased by only 4% (Hazell 2003).

While booms in food production since the GR have been considerable, these gains have not been equally distributed or consistent across regions (Pingali 2012; Foley et al. 2011). First, the GR privileged men over women due to reliance on machinery, high-energy, and extensive inputs, as well as patented seeds requiring more capital than women generally had available (Doss 1999; IAASTD 2009). Second, it often left poorer farmers behind due to inequitable rights to land, poor access to credit, and discriminatory policies (Hazell 2003). As well, many rural workers lost their jobs and livelihoods due to agricultural mechanizations (Scott 1985). Third, regional variability in the appropriateness and adoption of high-yield crop varieties meant that Africa stood as an exception to the success of the GR among developing areas. Much of the continent did not have adequate agricultural resources to support GR technologies. Overall contributions of the GR to improve yields and poverty reduction were also lower in marginally productive environments, because it depended on intensification in amenable areas (Pingali 2012). For example, rain-fed agriculture systems in Southeast Asia were unresponsive to GR strategies; this contributed to broadening regional disparities and poverty (Fan and Hazell 2001).

The environmental legacy of the GR is tenuous, as there are have been consequences from the energy- and land-intensive agricultural management practices, the policy atmosphere that fostered imprudent use of inputs, as well as cropping system expansion in areas unsuitable for intensification (Pingali 2012). For example, price protections and input subsidies for fertilizers, pesticides, and irrigation outpaced incentives for farm-level adoption of more efficient management mechanisms (Pingali 2012). GR practices have influenced water quality, soil degradation, chemical runoff, and have impacted areas not even cultivated (Matson et al. 1997; Tilman et al. 2002). Greenhouse gas emissions from agricultural production and land-use change have also been problematic (Wise et al. 2009).

Likewise, the GR nurtured an ideal climate for industrialized and profit-driven agriculture to thrive. Some of this industrial expansion has come by way of the erosion of local control as well and biodiversity loss. Field crop diversity in developing contexts has shifted with the commercialization and intensification of agriculture. Through public sector research and donor agency support, the GR promoted the global trade of hybrid seed varieties to farmers in developing economies, particularly for crops that respond positively to increases in inputs, such as staple grains. The dominant germplasm in many cereal growing areas shifted from locally adapted populations selected by farmers from the seeds they save ("landraces"), to seed types generated by commercial and research breeding programs that farmers must buy. The GR stimulated universal monoculture systems crowded out traditional crops. For example, traditional millets and pulses in South Asia were shifted out in favor of intensive rice and wheat (Pingali 2012). Farmer decision-making was undervalued in policy and practice compared to GR technologies and trade, and some farmers lost the ability to save seeds for the future use due to seed patents. As well, industrialized forms of livestock rearing spread, often compromising animal welfare and livestock genetic diversity.

On a global scale, efforts to protect food security have largely concentrated on simply producing more food through agricultural intensification—evidenced by the GR itself. It can be argued that the GR ignored underlying contexts of poverty, inequality, and imperialism that dictate access to food. While the productivity increases of the GR are undeniable, there have be three massive shifts in the agricultural landscape with outsized influence on food justice: (1) a shift in production methods toward monoculture and agricultural intensification, (2) a loss in agrobiodiversity, and (3) a stripping away of local autonomy due to agricultural commodification. The GR shaped the current food system in undesirable ways.

6.3   THE FOOD REGIME AND AN EMERGING FOOD CRISIS

The modern food system favors conventional, commercial scale agriculture by way of policy, research, and economic structures. But the word *system* implies an orderly set of guidelines with explicit rules or frameworks. Many scholars argue that through globalization and the rise of capital-intensive agriculture, a *corporate food regime* has emerged. This regime rewards industrial models of agriculture at the expense of ecosystems and the stewards of those ecosystems, including peasant farmers (McMichael 2014). The regime pushes agricultural methods that value yield and profit above all else. It privileges the wealthy who can afford expensive food products and ignores the poor. The corporate food regime does not care about protecting biodiversity or even producing nutritious food. It cares about production and profit.

A modern food crisis exists alongside of and in part because of the food regime. Pressures on agriculture will intensify in the next 40 years (Godfray et al. 2010), as the population will likely reach 9.7 billion by 2050 (UNDESA 2015). Without changing current distribution, waste, and agricultural management, crop production will likely need to be 60% higher by weight than it was in 2005 to satisfy food requirements (Alexandratos and Bruinsma 2012). Yet, nearly 795 million people worldwide remain chronically undernourished today (FAO et al. 2015) and face substantial increases in morbidity and mortality (Blossner 2015). Currently, developing nations, who are experiencing the highest rates of food insecurity, are at risk of major challenges due to climate change moving forward. Climate change is expected to have variable, but overall negative impacts on agricultural productivity around the globe (Lobell and Field 2007); these impacts will likely include enhanced pest and pathogen pressure, temperature variability and warming, extreme weather events, and increasing CO_2 in the atmosphere (IPCC 2014).

Concurrently, agriculture contributes significantly to climate change, presenting challenges both to human and non-human livelihoods. It is responsible for more non-CO_2 greenhouse gas emissions (GHGE) than any other sector, contributing about 54% in 2005 (including methane) (EPA 2012). In 2012, agriculture generated almost 10% of all GHGs emitted in the United States, stemming primarily from livestock such as cattle, soil management, and rice production (EPA 2012). Simply producing more food using current methods is imprudent. Additionally, food waste results in substantial GHGE, further contributing to the global food crisis (Porter et al. 2016).

Many solutions to address the global food crisis stem from the corporate food regime and principles of the GR; they are "productionist" in nature. International agencies, non-profit organizations, governments, and corporations appear focused on producing *more food* in order to *feed the world*. Proponents aim to address lofty food security goals, but these initiatives seem to benefit major players including large agrichemical and seed producers over the beneficiaries. Productionist strategies simply cannot address underlying causes of malnutrition—nor do they typically account for the potential social and ecological penalties that come from concentrating solely on crop yield. There are four primary pitfalls of this productionist approach.

First, an under-recognized product of the rise of industrial agriculture and the current food regime has been the concurrent loss of autonomy among many communities over their own food production, including losses of traditional food crops and methods of production. Scholars have argued that seed control has evaded farmers over recent decades, as it has become the prerogative of commercial producers, distributers, breeders, genetic engineers, and politicians regulating the seed market. The adoption of commercial crop varieties also undermines women's role in crop and seed management and influences agrobiodiversity (Pionetti 2005).

Second, agricultural intensification and land clearing have detrimental environmental tradeoffs that have not yet been fully explored, including losses in biodiversity (Godfray et al. 2010). Through high-input monoculture, soil fertility is declining as described in Chapter 4. Moreover, trade policies that favor export-driven production are closely tied to environmental degradation. Over time, a focus on producing a handful of profitable crops has led to biodiversity loss. Since the 1970s, loss of genetic diversity of thousands of plants and crops has been well documented. This is the result of epistemological and "political economic conditions" of the GR (Jacques and Jacques 2012). Since the 1900s, the FAO reports that 75% of all agricultural plant genetic material has been lost (FAO 1999) which is discussed in further detail in Chapter 11.

Third, by prioritizing both crop production and profit, the current food regime propagates the notion that a capitalistic system of agricultural intensification, with only a minority of the world participating, is the panacea for ensuring global food security. In reality, the current regime may actually impede food security, ecosystem restoration, democracy, and well-being (Lappe 1991; Duncan 1996). The food regime alleges that the market—above all else—is the most efficient supplier of food security (Friedmann 2005). Major players in the regime generate massive profits; agrichemical and seed companies gain economically where others cannot. The focus on export-driven agriculture is especially problematic as it discounts land stewardship, land tenure, agroecosystem biodiversity, and even diet diversity to produce surplus of a very limited number of cash-value crops. Export-driven agriculture has led to the displacement of producers via land grabbing and predation of the market (McMichael 2014), and it often relies on the exploitation of farm workers and animals to meet profit margins. As a result, we see the fracturing of rural societies—the very same communities that are primary managers of farmland and biodiversity. The combination of agricultural intensification and integration into the global market are socio-ecological drivers of poverty traps and biodiversity loss (Chappell et al. 2013).

Fourth, some have argued the food regime has contributed to a landscape of consumer blindness. As food chains lengthen, consumers become distanced from food production itself and are subsequently blinded to the associated "ecosystem plundering" and "biophysical override" of agriculture (Weis 2007). Likewise, with fewer people working in agriculture, the plight of farmers and farm workers is unknown to many consumers. Current conditions faced by peasant farmers are a good gauge of the combination of consumer ignorance regarding the ecological and social harms of industrial agriculture and the neoliberal policies that make industrial agriculture thrive (McMichael 2008).

There are both winners and losers in a capitalist food regime—and the poor and vulnerable often stand to lose. For example, Haiti, once a net exporter of food, is now a net importer due to measures imposed from outside (Schuller 2008). Frequent dumping of cheap, subsidized food from developed economies into developing countries disrupts local markets and can leave people financially vulnerable (McMichael 2014). Land grabbing for agricultural development through both direct and indirect means intensifies the over/under-consumption relationship organizing the food regime (Patel 2012) whereby millions of people go hungry despite a surplus in net calories produced. Non-human species suffer too, as they face habitat loss or degradation.

6.4 RISE OF THE COUNTERMOVEMENT (FOOD SOVEREIGNTY)

The impacts of the food regime are far reaching, and people have reacted by developing a wide range of movements pushing against it—movements emphasizing that food justice is more than food security, and more than food security for humans alone. These movements advocate for what has come to be called *food sovereignty*—focusing on ensuring personal and community autonomy over one's own food and agriculture policies. Central to food sovereignty is that it is not enough that people be fed. The human right to food depends as well on providing individual human control and autonomy over their food circumstances and the same goes for non-human animals.

Small-scale agriculture persists today despite the rise of large-scale commercial agriculture. Most of the world's food is grown, collected, and harvested by over 2.5 billion small-scale farmers, pastoralists, forest dwellers, and fisher folk—the majority of whom are women (Patria 2013). More than 1 billion people are engaged in agriculture across levels (ILO 2017) and many of these people retain traditional farming methods. The voices of these farmers have largely been muted under the guise of modernization and technological advancement for agriculture. Today, farmers are fighting for their rights to autonomy and control over their food production and food policies.

Founded at a meeting of small-scale farmers from across the globe in 1993, La Via Campesina ("the peasants' way") spearheaded one of the world's largest social movements and coined the term *food sovereignty* (*News & Views* 2005). A history of Via Campesina was provided by Food First: News & Views in an anonymous article entitled "Global Small-Scale Farmers" Movement Developing New Trade Regimes (*News & Views* 2005). The concept was later introduced at the 1996 World Food Summit and has been adopted by organizations across the globe. In the original vision of Via Campesina, food sovereignty centers on authentic agrarian reform fostering ecological agriculture and biodiversity, and equitable policies for small farmers everywhere. Importantly, it aims to address economic and political systems that reward transnational companies at the expense of peasants. Note that the food sovereignty literature frequently references peasants, which broadly includes farmers, landless, and indigenous people who work the land themselves. In 2002, La Via Campesina defined *food sovereignty* to mean:

the "right of peoples, communities, and countries to define their own agricultural, labor, fishing, food and land policies, which are ecologically, socially, economically and culturally appropriate to their unique circumstances. It includes the true right to food and to produce food, which means that all people have the right to safe, nutritious and culturally appropriate food and to food-producing resources and the ability to sustain themselves and their societies" (La Via Campesina 2002).

This is a compelling vision that has become very influential. However, the right to food of even the middle-class household in a city depends on more than having supermarket shelves with placeless, faceless, and traceless food wrapped in plastic, known only by its corporate logo. To cede control over one's food security is actually to compromise one's food security. Some scholars see food security as being antithetical to food sovereignty because the current means to address each seem at odds (McMichael and Schneider 2011; Windfuhr and Jonsen 2005). Food security tailors approaches to address the ability of people or households to purchase food on the market. Food sovereignty aims to ensure that households can access resources needed to control their food security, either through independent production on the part of the peasant or through what is sometimes called "political consumerism" that shapes the stream of products that fill the shelves (Micheletti 2003). If your food comes from a package that you do not control, it cannot be seen as secure. Many efforts to foster food security have ignored elements of food sovereignty; the authors suggest this is precisely the reason such initiatives have failed. Food sovereignty is antithetical to corporate industrial agriculture. It struggles for a resilient, democratic, sustainable means of food production by farmers who have rights (La Via Campesina 2000).

Keep in mind the central ethos of food justice is that food is a human right, not a commodity; food justice values human security over national security and pushes back against the corporate food regime (McMichael 2014). It advocates for land management in the hands of those who produce the food, and food policy driven by those who eat the food. By syncing decision-making with food production and policy, farmers and consumers are empowered to protect biodiversity for their own health and well-being. True food sovereignty degrades power hierarchies that allow governments, agricultural technology companies, and other stakeholders to take advantage of local communities' labor, environmental resources, and other assets for profit. It promotes locally driven agricultural management and land stewardship. As such, food sovereignty reconnects farmers to their land and surrounding ecosystems; it rearranges social power such that peasant farmers maintain their entitlement to eat—and it welcomes consumers to be involved in the myriad processes that yield their food.

To date, the food sovereignty movement has taken action in a number of ways and embodies an active struggle (Ajl 2014). First, it is advocating for policy change and raising awareness regarding the rights of peasant famers; this serves as a challenge to the dominant model of export-driven, large-scale, capitalistic agriculture (Wittman 2009). Second, it is using farming and agricultural training to address social inequalities. The movement has coordinated ecological farming initiatives around the globe (Rosset and Martínez-Torres 2012). For example, it is developing agroecological schools and networks to assist farmers in conversion to or consolidation of ecological farming—and advocating publicly for reorientation of research and extension systems to support agroecological innovation and scaling up via farmer organizations (McMichael 2014). Third, it is pushing to eliminate poverty among peasant farmers, and fourth, it seeks to reverse the urban bias against rural peoples. The movement is raising awareness of and problematizing how the food regime pushes for movement of food on a massive scale, forming increased movement of people and displacement of farmers due to inequitable trade. Lastly, it is pushing back against the view that what you can eat is only what is on the supermarket shelves.

6.5   FOOD SOVEREIGNTY, AGROECOLOGY, AND BIODIVERSITY PRESERVATION

By definition, there is no exclusive set of agricultural methods that meet all constructions of food justice because they are defined by communities and individuals themselves. However, agroecology offers a relevant approach to agriculture that is transdisciplinary, action-oriented, and participatory (Méndez et al. 2015). Agroecological methods blend modern agricultural science with indigenous knowledge and improved food security while protecting ecological resources and preserving agrobiodiversity in the developing world (Altieri et al. 2012). Likewise, because agroecology emphasizes participatory approaches, it is sensitive to the voices, opinions, and belief systems of all participants in variable contexts, and thus inherently embraces their sovereignty. In contrast to the corporate food regime, agroecological paradigms of development seek to revitalize and empower small farmers through processes that value diversity, recycling, community participation, and synergy that is viable for meeting current and future food demand (Altieri et al. 2012). They also offer a buffer against climate change because they strengthen farmer resilience through diversification of the agriculture system via polycultures, agroforestry, and mixed crop-livestock systems; these tactics are implemented in tandem with organic soil management, enhanced water harvesting and conservation, and an overall boost in agrobiodiversity (Altieri et al. 2015).

Crops are direct products of human intervention and selection based on wild plant diversity (Vigouroux et al. 2011). Not surprisingly, traditional farms typically have more diversity in staple crop varieties than non-staples, indicating traditional agriculture cultivates variation and difference at the farm and community levels (Jarvis et al. 2008; Jacques and Jacques 2012). Conventional agriculture, however, typically proceeds by overwhelming the variability of context, including biodiversity, with inputs of chemicals, machinery, and mass-produced seeds that seek ensure a predictable and high yield (Bell et al. 2008). An agroecological approach, on the other hand, seeks to recover a contextual view of agriculture that embraces variation in time and space, attuning agriculture to season and place (Bell and Bellon 2018). This is discussed further in Chapter 10. It is a "many kinds of eggs in many kinds of baskets" approach that farmers consider a productive advantage over attempting to grow the same crop year after year—or attempting to grow the same crop everywhere. With that variation comes opportunity for both the sovereignty of human and non-human concerns alike. In this sense, a food justice approach is necessarily an agroecological approach, and vice versa.

6.6   A REASON FOR HOPE

There is reason to hope for food justice moving forward. Communities are developing adaptive strategies that benefit humans and non-humans alike, whether or not they call it food justice, food security, food sovereignty etc. (McMichael 2014). The following examples outline efforts to empower communities by providing autonomy and control over food production and agriculture policy. Tactics differ, but the ultimate goal is the same: To fight for food justice such that food truly is a human and non-human right attainable to all. Simultaneously, these efforts promote biodiversity in food production, agroecosystems, and the environment at large.

Food sovereignty became a fundamental human right in Nepal in 2007, signifying an extraordinary achievement for peasant movements across the globe. This shift came after peasants unified and participated in the peoples' revolt of 2006, bringing their voice to the political scene. A peasant-supported Constituent Assembly was elected in 2008 (Pokharel 2013) increasing the inclusion of previously marginalized voices. Similarly, Ecuador, Venezuela, Mali, Bolivia, and Senegal have made food sovereignty part of their national policies, representing a crucial first step in changing food and agriculture policies to better represent poor and agrarian communities.

Across India, Dr. Vandana Shiva's organization, Navdanya, is creating a network of seed keepers and organic producers living in 22 states. Navdanya has established 122 seed banks and trained more than 900,000 farmers in seed and food sovereignty and sustainable agriculture in the last 20 years. The organization helped create the largest fair-trade, organic, and direct marketing network in India and is involved in biodiversity conservation, organic farming, and the rejuvenation of indigenous knowledge and culture (Navdanya 2017). An issue of particular importance to Dr. Shiva and Navdanya is genetic engineering and biopiracy that both threaten the right to food.

Elsewhere in southern India, women are taking control over seeds through management of a "seeds common" in the Deccan Plateau. Through this continuous local crop seed exchange, varieties circulate their genetic resources across and within fields, villages, and territories. According to Pionetti (2005), the "dynamic management of genetic resources enhances the stability of traditional agrosystems, increases the adaptation potential of local crops to evolving environmental conditions and limits the risk of genetic erosion" (Pionetti 2005).

These movements are growing in North America as well. In South Central Los Angeles, Ron Finley, sometimes called the "Gangsta Gardner," has initiated a wave of urban gardening in unused spaces such as parkways, vacant lots, and roadway medians. Finley's initial gardening efforts faced legal challenges, but along with support from Councilman Herb Wesson, a new ordinance was instated allowing gardens to be planted in public areas without a permit. Finley aims to empower youth and communities with gardening skills and to fight against oppressive forces that limit the ability of urban residents to cultivate their own food. Ultimately, he envisions urban gardens as gathering places and community hubs, where people can share, learn about nutrition, work the soil, and unwind. Finley is working so that everyone has the option of choosing health promoting foods over "junk foods" ("The Ron Finley Project" 2018).

Facing similar circumstances, the Detroit Black Community Food Security Network (DBCFSN) is responding to a history of inequalities that have generated food deserts in the city with the aims of addressing food insecurity through strategic organization of people using urban agriculture to gain more control over the food system and build self-reliance. DBCFSN played a crucial role in engineering a thorough food policy promoting nutrient-dense and culturally appropriate food to citizens at all times. This policy was unanimously adopted by the Detroit City Council, and ultimately the organization developed a seven-acre model urban farm project (D-Town Farm) on city-owned land that uses sustainable food production techniques to grow thousands of pounds of fresh produce each year. Ultimately, DBCFSN has used farming as a strategy of resistance against forces that have left much of Detroit food insecure, and in the process it has mobilized citizens, built community, and increased access to healthy food for citizens (White 2011).

The medical community is also recognizing the benefits of food justice. Hospital farms in the United States are emerging as a way to produce healthy food for hospital staff, patients, and community members independent of traditional grocery procurement. For example, "The Farm" at St. Joseph Mercy Hospital in Ann Arbor, Michigan turned 20 acres of land into a farm and community garden that is improving access to fresh food, nutrition education, and therapy using a people-centered care approach. The project engages community members, fosters education and exploration, provides access to healing therapy, grows produce to promote a healthy diet, and manages production sustainably (The Farm 2017).

6.7 CONCLUSION

The power of the corporate food regime can be depressing for those concerned with a broad vision of food for all and the belief that sovereignty is necessary for lasting security of healthy and nutritious food. As well, those concerned with the sustenance of non-humans may find it difficult to avoid lapsing into anti-humanism, fearing that human well-being depends on undermining the well-being of other species. But these examples show that another world of food is possible—a world of food in which there is abundant justice and just abundance. We cannot have one without the other.

REFERENCES

Ajl, M. 2014. The hypertrophic city versus the planet of fields. In: *Implosions/Explosions: Towards a Study of Planetary Urbanization*, edited by Neil J. Brenner, 2–19. Berlin, Germany: Jovis.

Alexandratos, N, and J. Bruinsma. 2012. World agriculture towards 2030/2050: The 2012 revision. ESA Working Paper No. 12-03. Rome: FAO.

Altieri, Miguel A., Fernando R. Funes-Monzote, and Paulo Petersen. 2012. Agroecologically efficient agricultural systems for smallholder farmers: Contributions to food sovereignty. *Agronomy for Sustainable Development* 32 (1): 1–13. https://doi.org/10.1007/s13593-011-0065-6.

Altieri, Miguel A., Clara I. Nicholls, Alejandro Henao, and Marcos A. Lana. 2015. Agroecology and the design of climate change-resilient farming systems. *Agronomy for Sustainable Development* 35 (3): 869–890. https://doi.org/10.1007/s13593-015-0285-2.

Ashwood, Loka. 2018. *For-Profit Democracy: Why the Government Is Losing the Trust of Rural America*. New Haven, CT and London, UK: Yale University Press.

Bell, Michael M., and Stéphane Bellon. 2018. Generalization without universalization: Towards an agroecology theory. *Agroecology and Sustainable Food Systems* 0 (0): 1–7. https://doi.org/10.1080/21683565.2018.1432003.

Bell, Michael M., Alexandra Lyon, Claudio Gratton, and Randall D. Jackson. 2008. COMMENTARY: The productivity of variability: An agroecological hypothesis. *International Journal of Agricultural Sustainability* 6 (4): 233–35.

Blossner, Monika. 2015. Malnutrition: Quantifying the health impact at national and local levels. World Health Organization, Nutrition for Health and Development Protection of the Human Environment No. 12. Environmental Burden of Disease Series. Geneva, Switzerland: World Health Organization. http://www.who.int/quantifying_ehimpacts/publications/MalnutritionEBD12.pdf.

Chappell, M. Jahi, Hannah Wittman, Christopher M. Bacon, Bruce G. Ferguson, Luis García Barrios, Raúl García Barrios, Daniel Jaffee, et al. 2013. Food sovereignty: An alternative paradigm for poverty reduction and biodiversity conservation in Latin America. *F1000Research* 2 (November). https://doi.org/10.12688/f1000research.2-235.v1.

Doss, Cheryl R. 1999. Twenty-five years of research on women farmers in Africa: Lessons and implications for agricultural research institutions; with an annotated bibliography. 23720. Economics Program Papers. CIMMYT: International Maize and Wheat Improvement Center. https://ideas.repec.org/p/ags/cimmep/23720.html.

Duncan, Colin Adrien MacKinley. 1996. *The Centrality of Agriculture: Between Humankind and the Rest of Nature*. Montreal, QC: McGill-Queen's Press.

EPA. 2012. *Summary Report: Global Anthropogenic Non-CO2 Greenhouse Gas Emissions: 1990–2030*. Washington, DC: Office of Atmospheric Programs Climate Change Division U.S. Environmental Protection Agency. http://www.epa.gov/climatechange/Downloads/EPAactivities/Summary_Global_NonCO2_Projections_Dec2012.pdf.

Fan, Shenggen, and Peter Hazell. 2001. Returns to public investments in the less-favored areas of India and China. *American Journal of Agricultural Economics* 83 (5): 1217–1222.

FAO. 1996. Rome declaration on world food security. Food and Agriculture Organization of the United Nations. World Food Summit. http://www.fao.org/docrep/003/w3613e/w3613e00.HTM.

FAO. 1999. What is happening to agrobiodiversity? FAO Corporate Document Repository. What is agrobioveristy? http://www.fao.org/docrep/007/y5609e/y5609e02.htm.

FAO, IFAD, and WFP. 2015. *The State of Food Insecurity in the World 2015. Meeting the 2015 International Targets: Taking Stock of Uneven Progress*. Rome, Italy: Food and Agriculture Organization of the United Nations.

FAO, WFP, and IFAD. 2004. *The State of Food and Agriculture 2003– 2004*. Rome: Food and Agriculture Organization of the United Nations. http://www.fao.org/docrep/016/i3027e/i3027e.pdf.

Foley, Jonathan A., Navin Ramankutty, Kate A. Brauman, Emily S. Cassidy, James S. Gerber, Matt Johnston, Nathaniel D. Mueller, et al. 2011. Solutions for a cultivated planet. *Nature* 478 (7369): 337–342. https://doi.org/10.1038/nature10452.

Food First News & Views. 2005. *Global Small-Scale Farmers' Movement Developing New Trade Regimes. Food First News & Views*, organizational newsletter, Volume 28, Number 97 2005, p.2.

Friedmann, Harriet. 2005. From colonialism to green capitalism: Social movements and emergence of food regimes. *Research in Rural Sociology and Development* 11 (January): 227–264.

Godfray, H. Charles J., John R. Beddington, Ian R. Crute, Lawrence Haddad, David Lawrence, James F. Muir, Jules Pretty, Sherman Robinson, Sandy M. Thomas, and Camilla Toulmin. 2010. Food security: The challenge of feeding 9 billion people. *Science* 327 (5967): 812–818. https://doi.org/10.1126/science.1185383.

Hall, Kevin D., Juen Guo, Michael Dore, and Carson C. Chow. 2009. The progressive increase of food waste in America and its environmental impact. *PLOS One* 4 (11): e7940. https://doi.org/10.1371/journal.pone.0007940.

Hazell, P. 2003. The impact of agricultural research on the poor: A review of the state of knowledge. In *Agricultural Research and Poverty Reduction: Some Issues and Evidence*, edited by S. Mathur, D. H. Pachico, and A. L. Jones. Economics and Impact Series. Intenational Center for Tropical Agriculture (CIAT). https://cgspace.cgiar.org/handle/10568/54023.

IAASTD. 2009. *Agriculture at a Crossroads: The Global Report*. Washington, DC: International Assessment of Agricultural Knowledge, Science, and Technology for Development.

ILO. 2017. Agriculture; plantations; other rural sectors. International Labour Organization. Agriculture; Plantations; Other Rural Sectors. 2017. http://www.ilo.org/global/industries-and-sectors/agriculture-plantations-other-rural-sectors/lang--en/index.htm.

IPCC. 2014. *Climate change 2014: Impacts, adaptation, and vulnerability. Part A: Global and Sectoral Aspects. Contribution of Working Group II to the Fifth Assessment Report of the Intergovernmental Panel on Climate Change*. Cambridge, UK: Cambridge University Press and New York, NY: IPCC.

Jacques, Peter J., and Jessica Racine Jacques. 2012. Monocropping cultures into ruin: The loss of food varieties and cultural diversity. *Sustainability* 4 (11): 2970–2997. https://doi.org/10.3390/su4112970.

Jarvis, Devra I., Anthony H. D. Brown, Pham Hung Cuong, Luis Collado-Panduro, Luis Latournerie-Moreno, Sanjaya Gyawali, Tesema Tanto, et al. 2008. A global perspective of the richness and evenness of traditional crop-variety diversity maintained by farming communities. *Proceedings of the National Academy of Sciences* 105 (14): 5326–5331. https://doi.org/10.1073/pnas.0800607105.

La Via Campesina. 2000. Bangalore declaration of the via Campesina – via Campesina. *Via Campesina English* (blog). October 6, 2000. https://viacampesina.org/en/bangalore-declaration-of-the-via-campesina/.

La Via Campesina. 2002. Food sovereignty: A right for all political statement of the NGO/CSO forum for food sovereignty. Declaration NGO Forum FAO Summit Rome+5. https://viacampesina.org/en/index.php/main-issues-mainmenu-27/food sovereignty-and-trade-mainmenu-38/398-declaration-ngo-forum-fao-summit-rome5.

Lappe, Frances Moore. 1991. *Diet for a Small Planet*. Anniversary edition. New York, NY: Ballantine Books.

Lobell, David B., and Christopher B. Field. 2007. Global scale climate–crop yield relationships and the impacts of recent warming. *Environmental Research Letters* 2 (1): 014002.

Maredia, M. K., and D. Byerlee. 1999. The global wheat improvement system: Prospects for enhancing efficiency in the presence of spillovers. Report. CIMMYT. http://repository.cimmyt.org/xmlui/handle/10883/992.

Matson, P. A., W. J. Parton, A. G. Power, and M. J. Swift. 1997. Agricultural intensification and ecosystem properties. *Science* 277 (5325): 504–509. https://doi.org/10.1126/science.277.5325.504.

Mcmichael, Philip. 2008. The peasant as 'Canary'? Not too early warnings of global catastrophe. *Development; Houndmills* 51 (4): 504–511. http://dx.doi.org.ezproxy.library.wisc.edu/10.1057/dev.2008.56.

McMichael, Philip. 2014. Historicizing food sovereignty. *The Journal of Peasant Studies* 41 (6): 933–957. https://doi.org/10.1080/03066150.2013.876999.

McMichael, Philip, and Mindi Schneider. 2011. Food security politics and the millennium development goals. *Third World Quarterly* 32 (1): 119–139. https://doi.org/10.1080/01436597.2011.543818.

Méndez, V. Ernesto, Christopher M. Bacon, Roseann Cohen, and Stephen R. Gliessman, eds. 2015. *Agroecology: A Transdisciplinary, Participatory and Action-Oriented Approach*. 1 edition. Boca Raton, FL: CRC Press.

Micheletti, Michele. 2003. Why political consumerism? In *Political Virtue and Shopping*, 1–36. New York: Palgrave Macmillan. https://doi.org/10.1057/9781403973764_1.

Morris, Michael L., H. J. Dubin, and Thaneswar Pokhrel. 1994. Returns to wheat breeding research in Nepal. *Agricultural Economics* 10 (3): 269–282. https://doi.org/10.1016/0169-5150(94)90028-0.

Navdanya. 2017. Navdanya. http://www.navdanya.org/site/.

OHCHR. 2017. Special rapporteur on the right to food. United Nations. Special Rapporteur on the Right to Food. http://www.ohchr.org/EN/Issues/Food/Pages/FoodIndex.aspx.

Patel, Raj. 2012. *Stuffed and Starved: The Hidden Battle for the World Food System*. 2 Rev Exp edition. Brooklyn, NY: Melville House.

Patel, Rajeev C. 2012. Food sovereignty: Power, gender, and the right to food. *PLOS Medicine* 9 (6): e1001223. https://doi.org/10.1371/journal.pmed.1001223.

Patria, Hayu Dyah. 2013. Uncultivated biodiversity in women's hand: How to create food sovereignty. *Asian Journal of Women's Studies; Seoul* 19 (2): 148–161, 178.

Pingali, Prabhu L. 2012. Green revolution: Impacts, limits, and the path ahead. *Proceedings of the National Academy of Sciences of the United States of America* 109 (31): 12302–12308. https://doi.org/10.1073/pnas.0912953109.

Pionetti, Carine. 2005. *Sowing Autonomy: Gender and Seed Politics in Semi Arid India*. London: International Institute for Environment and Development (IIED). http://pubs.iied.org/14502IIED/.

Pokharel, Pramesh. 2013. Constitutionalization of the struggle for food sovereignty in Nepal: Success, prospects and challenges. In: *La Via Campesina's Open Book: Celebrating 20 Years of Struggle and Hope*, edited by Henry Saragih. Jakarta, Indonesia: La Via Campesina.

Porter, Stephen D., David S. Reay, Peter Higgins, and Elizabeth Bomberg. 2016. A half-century of production-phase greenhouse gas emissions from food loss & waste in the global food supply chain. *Science of the Total Environment* 571 (November): 721–729. https://doi.org/10.1016/j.scitotenv.2016.07.041.

Rosset, Peter, and Maria Elena Martínez-Torres. 2012. Rural social movements and agroecology: Context, theory, and process. *Ecology and Society* 17 (3). https://doi.org/10.5751/ES-05000-170317.

Schuller, Mark. 2008. Haiti's food riots: An early-warning sign of the world food crisis. *International Socialist Review* (59). http://www.isreview.org/issues/59/rep-haiti.shtml.

Scott, James C. 1985. Weapons of the Weak: Everyday Forms of Peasant Resistance. New Haven, CT: Yale University Press.

Sen, Amartya. 2013. *Poverty and Famines: An Essay on Entitlement and Deprivation*. Oxford, UK: Oxford University Press.

Stevenson, J., D. Byerlee, N. Villoria, T. Kelley, and M. Maredia. 2011. Measuring the environmental impacts of agricultural research: Theory and applications to CGIAR research. Independent Science and Partnership Council Secretariat.

The Farm. 2017. St. Joseph Mercy Ann Arbor Hospital. http://www.stjoesannarbor.org/thefarm.

The Ron Finley Project. 2018. Ron Finley. http://ronfinley.com/the-ron-finley-project/.

Tilman, David, Kenneth G. Cassman, Pamela A. Matson, Rosamond Naylor, and Stephen Polasky. 2002. Agricultural sustainability and intensive production practices. *Nature*. Special Features. August 8, 2002. https://doi.org/10.1038/nature01014.

UNDESA. 2015. World population projected to reach 9.7 billion by 2050. United Nations Department of Economic and Social Affairs. https://www.un.org/development/desa/en/news/population/2015-report.html.

Vigouroux, Yves, Adeline Barnaud, Nora Scarcelli, and Anne-Céline Thuillet. 2011. Biodiversity, evolution and adaptation of cultivated crops. *Comptes Rendus Biologies*, Biodiversity in face of human activities/La biodiversite face aux activites humaines 334 (5): 450–457. https://doi.org/10.1016/j.crvi.2011.03.003.

Weis, Tony. 2007. *The Global Food Economy: The Battle for the Future of Farming*. London, UK and New York, NY: Zed Books.

White, Monica M. 2011. D-Town farm: African American resistance to food insecurity and the transformation of Detroit. *Environmental Practice* 13 (4): 406–417. https://doi.org/10.1017/S1466046611000408.

Wik, M, P Pingali, and S Broca. 2008. *Background Paper for the World Development Reports 2008: Global Agricultural Performance: Past Trends and Future Prospects*. Washington, DC: World Bank.

Windfuhr, Michael, and Jennie Jonsen. 2005. *Food Sovereignty: Towards Democracy in Localized Food Systems*. Rugby, Warwickshire, UK: ITDG Publishing.

Wise, Marshall, Katherine Calvin, Allison Thomson, Leon Clarke, Benjamin Bond-Lamberty, Ronald Sands, Steven J. Smith, Anthony Janetos, and James Edmonds. 2009. Implications of limiting CO2 concentrations for land use and energy. *Science* 324 (5931): 1183–1186. https://doi.org/10.1126/science.1168475.

Wittman, Hannah. 2009. Reworking the metabolic rift: La Vía Campesina, agrarian citizenship, and food sovereignty. *The Journal of Peasant Studies* 36 (4): 805–826. https://doi.org/10.1080/03066150903353991.

World Bank. 2007. *World Development Report 2008 : Agriculture for Development*. Washington, DC: World Bank.

7 The Industrialized Food System and Food Insecurity

Jasia Steinmetz

CONTENTS

7.1 INTRODUCTION

When early humans were evolving, the adequacy of foods that were foraged or hunted determined food security. Hunger triggered the search for food within the cornucopia in the surrounding areas. Early humans ate a wide variety of plants and animals, following the abundance of each season. If the food was not poisonous, it was nourishing and nutrient-rich. Food habits developed through observation, trial and error, and knowledge passed through generations. Today, human dietary habits continue to be shaped by our environmental exposure and social learning (Turner and Thompson 2013).

In the past, humans have interacted with and responded to nature. Geologists have noted that there has been a shift in this relationship with humans now dominating aspects of nature that impact the functioning of the Earth as a whole (Malhi 2017). Because humans are significantly changing the Earth, geologists have suggested a new geologic time called The Anthropocene ("new age of man") be recognized (Crutzen 2002). Geological time divides significant changes on the Earth by investigating the Earth's strata caused by forces of nature. The changes embedded in sediment and ice are measured in different ways that provide clues to conditions on the Earth, including climate, land and marine life and atmosphere (Waters et al. 2016). The Anthropocene signals that humans are changing these conditions.

Have we reached the carrying capacity of the Earth for the human population? This has prompted local to global conversations about lifestyle and food habits that humans can maintain to continue to survive and flourish on our planet. Our current food and water systems are contributing to the decline of resources including water, soil, habitat, and biodiversity—all while increasing greenhouse gas emissions (IPES-Food 2017). One measure of the ability of the Earth's resources to support the growing human population is to monitor the adequacy of our food and water systems by considering food security.

7.2   THE RIGHT TO FOOD AND THE RIGHT
TO WATER AND SANITATION

As mentioned in the previous chapter, The United Nations (UN) proclaims that food and water are basic human rights that are to be upheld by all countries. The right to food is the "right of every individual, alone or in community with others, to have physical and economic access at all times to sufficient, adequate and culturally acceptable food that is produced and consumed sustainably, preserving access to food for future generations" (Committee on Economic, Social and Cultural Rights 1999). This right to food includes availability, accessibility, adequacy and sustainability of food for each member of a household. The right to water and sanitation recognizes "the right to safe and clean drinking water and sanitation as a human right that is essential for the full enjoyment of life and all human rights. The right to water is further defined as the right of everyone to sufficient, safe, acceptable and physically accessible and affordable water for personal and domestic uses" (United Nations 2010).

For countries to fulfill these rights, the food system must produce, distribute, and make available wholesome foods and water that support well-being at all stages of the lifecycle. Considerations include the migratory and dynamic behavior of living systems including humans, plants, and animals; the evolution of biomes; and the anthropogenic effects on the Earth and the impacts of climate change. In this Anthropocene era, we must consider the natural boundaries of biomes as the basis of food and water security.

7.3   THE FOUNDATION OF FOOD SYSTEMS:
BIOMES AND NATURAL RESOURCES

Ecosystems are living systems which begin at micro levels and radiate to the higher systems, creating stability at all levels. This relationship between individual or small systems and the larger system and its various ecosystems connects and balances the planet. Thus, the Earth system refers to the interacting physical, chemical, and biological processes that behave as a single, global, self-regulating system (Steffen et al. 2004). A "one size fits all" approach does not apply in the Earth system that is dependent on the health of multiple smaller microbiomes that balance the whole. Major biomes or major communities have a predominant vegetation as well as living beings specifically adapted to that geographic area and may be divided into five types: Aquatic, deserts, forests, grasslands, and tundra (Pullen 2004). These biomes provide our global food and water systems as well as more localized food systems. Water, soil, plants, animals, fish, and biodiversity are unique to each biome.

The ability of each smaller ecosystem to respond to the changing conditions maintains security and sustainability of that ecosystem. The resiliance of complex biological systems, or the capacity to recover quickly from a disturbance, is dependent on redundancy, plasticity, robustness, and stability (Felix and Wagner 2008). Redundancy has simultaneous processes or many components that have the same function. For example, different foods may have similar nutrient profiles that provide for the essential functions of our bodies. Plasticity enables an organism to change when perturbed and leads to evolution as one function may reorganize to serve another purpose. The adaptation of plants to changing water patterns demonstrates plasticity. Robustness is the short-term persistence of an organismal trait under perturbations, while stability is the long-term persistence. Ultimately, our food and water security are dependent on resilient ecosystems.

Knowledge of food and water systems is essential for human survival. Historically, individuals living within unique microbiomes understood ecosystem balance for optimal food production over seasons and passed this biological knowledge to the next generation (Jacome 2009). This was embedded in the local language, customs, spirituality, and daily practices. Historically, food production included diverse crops and animals while seeds saved across seasons resulted in local adaptation to the unique ecosystem. Crop rotations (successive plantings) or intercropping (more than one crop planted in a field at the same time) were used. This provided opportunity for both redundancy and plasticity of the farming system for robustness. For example, in areas of Kenya, early agricultural intercropping of finger millet, sorghum, beans, and sweet potatoes was used to assure a crop would survive varying conditions as each crop has a different tolerance for levels of moisture (Hakansson 1994). These crops evolved to maize, sorghum, finger millet, and pigeon peas for similar staple crops that could withstand the local climate variations (Oniang'o et al. 2003). Successful farmers knew how to harvest and process these foods while those cooking used relevant techniques for preparing and storing. The ability to pass this knowledge from one generation to the next within families and in the community lead to redundancy and plasticity of food system knowledge that assured food security and sustainability.

7.4 FOOD SECURITY

The most basic function of food and water is survival of the human species. However, food is also a commodity that is traded within and across national borders and generates capital. Crops are also used for biofuel. Water is required for manufacturing as is energy. The food-water-energy nexus considers the multiple functions and interrelationships of inputs required by the ecosystem and humans, and this nexus is increasingly challenged in the Anthropocene. Food security reflects the long-term ability of the ecosystem to support human life. As people may voluntarily migrate across nations or involuntarily migrate due to anthropogenic or natural disasters, we consider food security at each of these scales: household, national, global.

Global food security is defined by the UN Food and Agriculture Organization (FAO) as "a situation that exists when all people, at all times, have physical, social and economic access to sufficient, safe and nutritious food that meets their dietary needs and food preferences for an active and healthy life" (FAO 2008). Globally, two measures are used to capture food security: Prevalence of undernourishment and prevalence of severe food insecurity (FAO et al. 2017). In 2016, the prevalence of undernourishment or hunger globally was 815 million people which reflected an 11% increase from the previous year (FAO et al. 2017). Sub-Saharan Africa is the region with the highest prevalence of undernourishment with 22.7% of the population (more than one in five people) in 2016 (FAO et al. 2017). Data from 150 countries, from 2014 through 2016, found that 9.3% (one in ten people) were food insecure—with the highest levels in Africa reaching 27.4% (FAO et al. 2017).

Some countries are facing the double burden of malnutrition—undernourishment and overnourishment—as evidenced by the increasing prevalence of overweight and obesity (FAO et al. 2017). Children are particularly vulnerable to malnourishment within societies. Chronic undernourishment leads to poor growth or stunting (low weight for height) while overnourishment leads to overweight and obesity. From 2000 to 2016, stunting in children under age 5 fell globally from 198 million to 155 million while overweight children under 5 increased from 30 million to 41 million (United Nations 2017).

To support sustainable development in countries that would end poverty, protect the planet, and ensure prosperity for all, the Sustainable Development Goals (SDG) were adopted by nations in 2015 with targets to be achieved by 2030 (United Nations 2015). Several of the SDG encompass food systems and food security:

- Goal 1: End poverty in all its forms;
- Goal 2: End hunger, achieve food security and improved nutrition, and promote sustainable agriculture;
- Goal 3: Ensure healthy lives and promote well-being for all at all ages;
- Goal 6: Ensure availability and sustainable management of water and sanitation for all;
- Goal 7: Ensure access to affordable, reliable, sustainable, and modern energy for all;
- Goal 12: Ensure sustainable consumption and production patterns;
- Goal 13: Take urgent action to combat climate change and its impacts;
- Goal 15: Protect, restore, and promote sustainable use of terrestrial ecosystems, sustainably manage forests, combat desertification, and halt and reverse land degradation and halt biodiversity loss (IFPRI 2014).

Food security is related to ecological, economic, social, and political factors. Ecological disasters such as extended drought or anthropogenic disasters such as political conflict may result in increased food insecurity (FAO 2016a, 2017a). Unfortunately, factors can compound and lead to severe food insecurity, even famine. For example, Yemen ignited into civil war in 2011, followed by ecological and agricultural destruction due to plagues of locusts and flooding from tropical cyclones in 2016 (FAO et al. 2017). By 2017, these factors worsened the economic crisis and resulted in extreme poverty and 60% of the population experiencing severe food insecurity (FAO et al. 2017). Civil war and the lack of healthcare, public works, clean water, and poor sanitation resulting in a cholera outbreak which infected more than one million people (FAO et al. 2017). Illness increases the need for healthy food for recovery.

The food security of the world is dependent on family farming, which produces between 70% and 80% of global food (IYFF+10 World Coordination Committee 2017). Most are smallholder farms with limited resources, especially land (CFS 2013). However, 70% of the people living in poverty have their main source of income and work in farming (IYFF+10 World Coordination Committee 2017). Smallholder farmers, while producing food for their own households and markets, make up the majority of the hungry people and extreme poverty is concentrated in rural areas (FAO 2012a). From the data available in the United States, migrant and seasonal farmworkers have higher food insecurity than the general population in many regions across the country—82% of the workers sampled had food insecurities in the population studied—both in the south and southwest regional areas (Kiehne and Mendoza 2015; Weigel et al. 2007).

Ecological disasters, such as floods or extended drought, can result in severe food production losses resulting in food insecurity for entire populations while displacing farmers (Chau et al. 2015; Lesk et al. 2016). Armed conflicts not only displace populations but also compromise natural resources with the chemical and physical degradation of land, leading to immediate and extended food insecurity (Jensen et al. 2013b; Jensen et al. 2013a). Food insecurity also results from continued diminishment of natural resources in an area such that ecosystems cannot support humanity. For example, the fertilizer runoff from agricultural land into the Mississippi River and accumulating in the Gulf of Mexico has caused an increasing area of eutrophication that does not support fish life (NOAA 2017).

Food security may be positively or negatively impacted by economic policies that favor food production for export over domestic consumption (Clapp 2015; Gadhok 2016). Some may argue there are benefits to these policies (Clapp 2015; Gadhok 2016). For example, food quality or food safety standards international markets may raise these standards for the same crop in the domestic market, adding value to the consumer at home (Gadhok 2016). Food production that moves across national borders may stabilize areas where production is affected by weather or other conditions (Clapp 2015). Food security can also be negatively impacted by rising export crops. Prioritizing export crops would divert resources from farmers that grow traditional or indigenous foods, which tend to be nutritionally superior and locally available (Gadhok 2016). The local availability of a crop may decrease in the exporting country while the import may undermine domestic production, reducing availability for the local population (Clapp 2015).

Countries monitor household food security and report this at the national level. In the United States, food security for a household is defined as access by all members at all times to enough food for an active, healthy life (USDA-ERS 2017a). Food security includes at a minimum the ready availability of nutritionally adequate and safe foods and the assured ability to acquire acceptable foods in socially acceptable ways, e.g., without resorting to emergency food supplies, scavenging, stealing, or other coping strategies (USDA-ERS 2017a).

Food security varies by region or state and within households. For example, a family member such as a mother may skip or reduce meal intake so her children have food. In 2016, 12.3% (15.6 million households) of U.S. households were food insecure, which varied from 8.7% in Hawaii to 18.7% in Mississippi (Coleman-Jensen et al. 2017). Food security differs by location, income, households with children headed by single parents, ethnicity, and urban-rural areas.

7.5 INDUSTRIALIZED FOOD SYSTEM IMPACTS ON FOOD SECURITY

Industrialized food production around the globe has been successful in creating an abundance of calories (IPES 2017). Global food production provides on average 2,400–2,700 calories per day to feed about 12 billion people, which would account for the projected population increases (D'Odorico et al. 2014; FAOSTAT 2012). The calories available in the U.S. food supply rose from 3300 calories per day per capita in the early 1980s to 3900 calories per day by the year 2000 (IOM and NRC 2015). The distribution of calories that leads to accessible foods and the affordability of food influence food security. The prevalence of food insecurity is higher in low-income households as well as rural and urban areas compared to suburban communities (Rabbitt et al. 2017; Global Panel 2017).

Food security must account for the nutritional quality of the food as well as the resilience and sustainability of food and water systems without endangering human safety or health (DeSchutter 2014). The continued and increased industrialization of food and water systems has resulted in both ecosystem damage and human health morbidities (IPES-Food 2017) including: (1) occupational hazards such as pesticide exposure (Elver 2017) and injuries (Lloyd and James 2008; Lovelock et al. 2008) (2) environmental contamination such as nitrogen and phosphate pollution (Tural 2012) (3) antimicrobial resistance (CDC 2013) (4) foodborne diseases (WHO 2015) (5) nutrient deficiencies (Wall et al. 2015) (6) an increased incidence of overweight and obesity (Roberts et al. 2002) (7) the rise in noncommunicable diseases such as heart disease, cancer and diabetes (Kaveeshwar and Cornwall 2014) and (8) and increasing food insecurity (CFS 2016). It is now clear that the consideration of calories alone is insufficient to meet the food security needs of the global population. The following section explores different steps within the industrialized food system that impacts food security.

7.5.1 PRODUCTION

Food production has become the cornerstone of food security in the United States. In providing a stable food supply to maintain a healthy population, the supply-side economic model of providing adequate calories from multiple food groups encouraged small landholder farmers to grow a diverse number of crops and animals. Markets were located and sourced locally and the distance between farmer-to-market-to-consumer was minimized. However, the rise of neoliberal economics and corporate influence, both nationally and internationally, has resulted in a dominant marketplace that restructured the organizing principle of societies (United Nations 2009). Food production is supported by a demand-side economics with retail markets (large multinational grocery stores and fast-food franchises) promoting processed and ultra-processed foods with an extended shelf life that are transported over long distances. Large companies increasingly control more of the market share with highly processed foods more readily available while traditional foods are displaced (FAO et al. 2017). This fosters economies of scale in production—with increased production of a few specialized foods in large quantities that uses more mechanization in planting and harvesting. In other words, the marketplace creates a global food system dependent on very few varieties of crops, animals, poultry, or fish that are produced in large amounts and traded on the commodity market for global distribution. This impacts food security at every level of the food system, from farm to plate.

As mentioned previously, resilience in complex biological systems involves redundancy and plasticity. When disturbed, the biological system will adapt a component to serve many functions. Small landholders produce most of the global food supply and are more likely to have diverse farms to assure a staple food supply (FAO 2014; McKeon 2015). The redundancy of many farmers growing a diverse food supply maintains resiliency in times of perturbations such as climate change, crop failure, or natural disasters. This also maintains redundancy of the nutrients that are present in a variety of foods. For example, each variety of leafy greens may supply varying levels of the same vitamins, minerals, fiber, and phytonutrients, but in unique levels and combinations. This results in a variety of sources of nutrients from similar but not identical vegetables. Any crop failure of one plant does not compromise the source of nutrients as other comparable crops are available.

Agricultural industrialization in North America has resulted in large landholder farmers producing fewer varieties of crops and fewer varieties within crops, prevalent to what the commodity marketplace selects for mechanization and shelf life rather than taste, health, or ecological merit (Rotz and Fraser 2015). The transition to commodity traded foods and the dominance of production for export pushes farmers into an industrialized food production system, based on the large production of one crop that is traded across national boundaries. The increased distance between the sources of production and consumption is a global phenomenon with one-fourth of food produced in the world traded internationally (D'Odorico et al. 2014). In 2010, the United States imported an estimated 10–15% of all food consumed by U.S. households, including more than three-quarters of fresh fruits and vegetables and more than 80% of fresh or frozen fish and seafood (Carnevale 2010).

Disruptions in food production in any area of the world have rippling effects in an industrialized food system. For example, in 2010, natural disasters destroyed almost 25% of the Russian wheat crop and exports halted (Johnstone and Mazo 2011). This caused a panic in the commodity market, driving wheat prices to historically high levels. Countries in the Middle East who depended on Russian wheat imports experienced declines in wheat acquisition and an increase in food insecurity. The food protests that followed contributed to the political unrest known as the Arab Spring.

Diets are becoming globally homogenized, leading to a greater dependency on the 52 major crop commodities that dominate global food supply (Khoury et al. 2014). Seventy-five percent of the food in the world is produced from only 12 plants and five animal species. This lack of biodiversity threatens food security by reducing redundancy and plasticity of the food system and the ability to adapt to further or future disturbances (FAO 2012b). This loss of individual genes and of combinations of genes, such as those found in local ecosystems is called "genetic erosion" (FAO 2017b). The UN Food and Agricultural Organization (FAO) reports that more than 30% (2500 species) of the approximately 8200 animal breeds are at risk of extinction or already extinct (FAO 2017b). Only 30 crops provide 95% of human food-energy needs and just five of them—rice, wheat, maize, millet, and sorghum—provide about 60% (FAO 2017c). The mass extinction of genetic bioavailability creates a ripple effect of species loss to ecosystems.

The sustainability for small- and medium-sized farms is vital for global food security—especially retaining these farmers in low- and middle-income countries. Both production and nutrient diversity diminish with farm size (Herrero et al. 2017). Irrespective of farm size, more diverse farms produce more nutrients (Herrero et al. 2017). For small landholders, competing against prices in the international market has consequences that lead to food insecurity. With the rise of agriculture as trade, small farmers have less resiliency to international price volatility and the impact of trade protectionism that favors developed countries or agribusiness sectors (HLPE 2013; Hopewell 2014). Climate change is expected to increase the vulnerabilities of countries that depend on small landholder agriculture for their food supply and primary occupation (Morton 2007).

This production-centered model to meet international demands based on a few crops has resulted in many agriculture-related impacts including loss of biodiversity, loss of soil, increased water and air pollution, loss of farmer decision-making, loss of seed ownership, and increased costs (Khoury et al. 2014; Rotz and Fraser 2015). The foundational resources for food production are vulnerable and, therefore, food security may be compromised or disappearing.

7.5.2 PROCESSING AND RETAILING

Ideally, consumer choice at the processing and retail level is maximized through a diversity of producers, distributors, and retailers that provide market opportunities for farmers and accessible foods at affordable prices to consumers. Similar to agricultural production, industrialized processing and retailing has undergone globalization and market concentration. Common industrial practices include market consolidation that results in mergers and acquisitions of smaller companies thereby creating a larger company (Wood 2013). This captures more of the market share and facilitates vertical integration when one company owns many aspects of the manufacturing process (Hendrickson et al. 2001). Both practices reduce the numbers of businesses involved in that area. This results in less biodiverse food choices for consumers and less redundancy in essential nutrients, contributing to food insecurity (Hendrickson et al. 2001; Khoury et al. 2014).

Food and agriculture companies grow through major consolidations, mergers, acquisitions, and divestitures, often retaining the product names after new ownership (Laforet 2015). Hence, consumers may not realize that their favorite product is now under the management of a different company or the extent of the market share that a large company controls. The largest ten food and beverage companies in the world held 10% of the world's gross domestic product in 2015: Nestle, PepsiCo, JBS (the world's largest meat—beef, pork, chicken—processor and exporter), Anheuser-Busch InBev, Coca-Cola, Archer Daniels Midland, Tyson Foods, Mondelēz International, Cargill, and Mars (Rowan 2015).

The dependence on food processing is evident in grocery stores. Within the past five years there have been between 17,000 and 21,400 new food products introduced each year with the majority being beverages, snacks, bakery foods, sauces, dressings, and condiment (USDA-ERS 2017b). Food products are industrial formulations of starches, sugars, salt, fats and oils, preservatives, and cosmetic additives (Moodie et al. 2013). These are also called "ultra-processed" foods where food processing occurs beyond what is possible at the household level of canning, freezing, smoking, drying, etc. The increased consumption of ultra-processed food products is associated with obesity and lower micronutrient adequacy of diets (Louzada et al. 2015a, 2015b; Steele et al. 2016, 2017). Ultra-processed foods make up 57.9% of the energy intake in American's diet (Steele et al. 2016)

The retail sector, including global supermarkets, fast-food outlets, and other large food retailers, have consolidated to control the largest portion of sales. These companies have evolved from food distribution to strongly influencing production and consumption behaviors. Supermarkets are increasingly determining what is produced, where, to what standards and price, and the outlets from which food is sold (Burch et al. 2013). These companies influence the food system by deciding the product placement in the store given limited shelf space. Supermarkets have developed their private product line, determining the quality and food safety standards required of farmers and manufacturers (Burch et al. 2013). To maintain low prices, the retailers focus on large suppliers and bypass small producers. The scope and volume of the business including increased business in Asia, Africa, and Latin America leads to the homogenization of the food products offered that are transportable and shelf-stable.

7.5.3 Consumers

The increasing trends of urbanization, globalization, and expanding industrialized food systems resulted in global diets that are transitioning to the Western diet, the dominant diet of Americans (Pingali 2006; Popkin 2006). The increased calories, fat, protein, and weight of foods comes from a small number of mass-produced crops resulting in a higher consumption of refined sugars, refined fats, oils, and meats (Khoury et al. 2014; Tilman and Clark 2014). The predominance of processed and ultra-processed foods marketed by fast-food franchises, convenience stores, grocery stores and large supermarkets shape the demand for these foods (Burch et al. 2013; Stuckler 2012).

With the growth of the industrialized food system supported by a transnational food supply and concentrated retail market, an individual's food security is dependent in part on the availability and access to supermarkets and large grocery stores. A "low access to healthy food area," also called a food desert, is defined by the U.S. Department of Agriculture (USDA) as having limited access to a supermarket, supercenter, or large grocery store (USDA-ERS 2017c). Studies have found that increased fruit and vegetable consumption is linked to the availability and accessibility of supermarkets and grocery stores (Larson et al. 2009; Story et al. 2008).

The United States measures food security from the responses to a series of ten questions and an additional eight questions if the household includes children (USDA-ERS 2017a). The questions capture (1) conditions (worry, weight loss, being hungry) (2) behaviors (reduced or skipped meals, not eating enough), and (3) socioeconomic status. One question, "We couldn't afford to eat balanced meals" pertains to the respondent's perception of meal quality.

Food insecurity, or a lack of adequate amounts of food, is found in 12.3% (15.6 million) of households, whereas 8% or 3.1 million households include children (Coleman-Jensen et al. 2017). Recent data from 2014 reflect a range of food insecurity prevalence in other industrialized countries (FAO 2016b): United Kingdom 10.1%, Italy 8.2%, Spain 7.1%, France 6.9%, Sweden 3.1%, and Switzerland 3.0%. Households that are not poor are more likely to be more food secure and spend more money on food than poor households (Coleman-Jensen et al. 2017). In 2016, the average food-secure households spent 29% more on food than food-insecure households (Coleman-Jensen et al. 2017).

The U.S. Department of Agriculture (USDA) and the U.S. Department of Health and Human Services release Dietary Guidelines every five years based on the available science for healthy lives across the lifespan and diet-related factors in predominant diseases, primarily heart disease, cancer, and diabetes (USDA 2015). These guidelines educate consumers to achieve optimal diets that are adequate in all essential nutrients. Americans are not consuming the foods that meet their nutritional requirements: 80% of Americans did not consume the recommended daily servings of fruit; 90% did not meet vegetable serving recommendations, whereas potatoes account for 25% of all vegetables consumed; nearly 100% did not meet the recommended whole grain servings (USDA 2015). However, 70% exceeded the recommendation for refined grain servings; 80% meet the recommended intake for meat, poultry, and eggs with shortfalls in the plant or dairy protein subgroups; nearly 90% exceed the recommendations for solid fats and added sugars with 100% of children one to eight years old exceeding these recommendations (USDA 2015). In summary, most Americans meet or exceed their calorie intake, but do not achieve a diversity of whole foods to prevent chronic diseases.

Since 1970, the U.S. obesity rate has tripled for adults and children, indicating shifting lifestyles (Fryar et al. 2016a, 2016b). Food consumption studies have indicated that our diets are nutrient-poor (less fruits, vegetables, whole grains, and dairy) and energy-rich (primarily from fats and sugars) (Bentley 2017; Miller et al. 2015). The USDA monitors the food supply, which would indicate if the rise in poor diets is due to decreases in production (Bentley 2017). A comparison between 1970 and 2014 food availability in the United States indicated an increase in the availability of every food group (Bentley 2017). Fruit supply increased 10% with apples, oranges, and bananas the most consumed (Bentley 2017). Vegetable supply increased 17%, with potatoes (half as frozen potatoes), tomatoes (mostly canned), and sweet corn most consumed (Bentley 2017). Dairy supply increased 9% whereas the cheese supply tripled, with an 800% rise in mozzarella cheese during this time period (Bentley 2017). Grain supply increased 28%, primarily in wheat and corn (Bentley 2017). Protein increased 1% with a shift from red meat to chicken (Bentley 2017). Added sugars and a rise in the sweetener supply increased 10% with a 33% drop in refined cane and beet sugars and rise in high fructose corn syrup (Bentley 2017). Added fats and oils availability rose 57% (Bentley 2017). Despite these trends, the U.S. food supply does not produce the quantity of foods to meet the recommendations for a healthy diet (Bentley 2017; Miller et al. 2015). While food availability has increased, these trends indicate limited dietary diversity and quantities along with an increased production of foods harmful to our health. Further insights are offered in Chapter 8.

The purchasing patterns of Americans reflect the influence of the processing and retail markets. Americans are purchasing less unprocessed or slightly processed foods but are purchasing more ultra-processed and ready-to-eat foods (Okrent and Kumcu 2016). Purchases of ingredients that are whole foods or ingredients requiring preparation made up less than a quarter of the average household budget (Okrent and Kumcu 2016). Ready-to-cook meals and snacks account for 26% of the food budget and fast-food and sit-down restaurants constitute half of the household budget (Okrent and Kumcu 2016). In the last decade, the price of basic and complex ingredients grew at a faster pace than ready-to-cook or ready-to-eat foods while the price of meals and snacks at sit-down restaurants slowed resulting in more nutritious diets being more expensive (Monsivais et al. 2010; Okrent and Kumcu 2016). The economies of scale of manufacturing many ultra-processed foods with cheaper ingredients (sugar, fats and oils, sodium) decreases the cost of production for processed foods. Marketing also influences purchasing patterns with ready-to-eat food products and fast foods capturing 57% of total advertising expenditures by food and beverage companies (Okrent and Kumcu 2016). This supports observations of the lopsided promotion of unhealthy foods.

It is also clear that supermarkets, fast-food establishments, and restaurants are directly and indirectly involved in shaping the food environment for consumers, which impacts consumer's food security and health. The burdens of micronutrient deficiency such as vitamins A, C, D, and E, calcium and magnesium, along with hunger, obesity, and the rise of noncommunicable diseases are directly related to the food supply available to consumers within their community (Fulgoni et al. 2011; Global Panel 2017). Ultimately, the retail sector is the predominant source of food for most Americans and increasingly throughout the world.

7.6 CONCLUSION

The global community is at a crossroads of determining the sustainability of the human population on the Earth. The industrialized food system model is not sustainable for the Earth or the global population. Hence, significant political, economic, and cultural changes are urgently needed (IPES-Food 2017). Diets that have increased fruits and vegetables and whole grains while reducing animal products reduces the incidence of chronic disease and greenhouse gas emissions (Hallstrom et al. 2017). These foods must be readily available, accessible, affordable, and desirable for the population to assure food security. Farmers have seen their market options dwindle under the influence of larger processing industries and retail markets that control the food system with an abundance of processed, ultra-processed, ready-to-cook and ready-to-eat food products. Americans spend half of their food budget on fast-food or sit-down restaurants. The Western Diet is also being heavily promoted in other countries. Consumers, advocates, and policy-makers around the world are challenged to shift food systems paradigms to support food security, biodiversity, and improved human health.

REFERENCES

Bentley, J. 2017. *U.S. Trends in Food Availability and a Dietary Assessment of Loss-adjusted Food Availability, 1970–2014*. Economic Information Bulletin Number 166. Washington, DC: USDA Economic Research Service.

Burch, D., J. Dixon, and G. Lawrence. 2013. Introduction to symposium on the changing role of supermarkets in global supply chains: From seedling to supermarket: Agri-food supply chains in transition. *Agriculture and Human Values* 30: 215–224.

Carnevale, C. 2010. The U.S. food and drug administration and imported food safety. In: *Enhancing Food Safety: The Role of the Food and Drug Administration*, edited by R. B. Wallace and M. Oria, Appendix E. Washington, DC: National Academies Press.

CDC. 2013. *Antibiotic Resistance Threats in the United States, 2013*. Atlanta, GA: Center for Disease Control.

Chau, V., N., S. Cassells, and J. Holland. 2015. Economic impact upon agricultural production from extreme flood events in Quang Nam, central Vietnam. *Natural Hazards* 75 (2): 1747–1765.

Clapp, J. 2015. *Food Security and International Trade: Unpacking Disputed Narratives*. Rome, Italy: Food and Agriculture Organization of the United Nations.

Coleman-Jensen, A., M. P. Rabbitt, C. A. Gregory, and A. Singh. 2017. *Household Food Security in the United States in 2016*. Economic Research Report Number 237. Washington, DC: USDA Economic Research Service.

Committee on Economic, Social and Cultural Rights. 1999. CESCR General Comment No. 122: The right to adequate food (Art.11). *United Nations Office of the High Commissioner for Human Rights*. http://www.refworld.org/pdfid/4538838c11.pdf.

CFS. 2013. *Investing in Smallholder Agriculture for Food Security: A Report by the High Level Panel of Experts on Food Security and Nutrition*. Rome: FAO Committee on World Food Security.

CFS. 2016. *Global Strategic Framework for Food Security & Nutrition (GSF)*. Rome, Italy: FAO Committee on World Food Security.

Crutzen, P. 2002. Geology of mankind. *Nature* 415: 23.

D'Odorico, R., J. A. Carr, F. Laio, L. Ridolfi, and S. Vandoni. 2014. Feeding humanity through global food trade. *Earth's Future* 2: 458–469. https://doi:10.1002/2014ER000250.

DeSchutter, O. 2014. Report of the Special Rapporteur on the right to food, Olivier De Schutter. Final Report: The transformative potential of the right to food. *United Nations*. http://www.srfood.org/images/stories/pdf/officialreports/20140310_finalreport_en.pdf.

Elver, H. 2017. Report of the Special Rapporteur on the right to food, UN doc. A/HRC/34/48. Geneva, Switzerland: United Nations Human Rights Council.

FAO. 2008. *Food Security Information for Action: Practical Guides*. Rome: Food and Agricultural Organization of the United Nations.

FAO. 2012a. *The State of Food and Agriculture: Investing in Agriculture*. Rome: Food and Agricultural Organization of the United Nations.

FAO. 2012b. *International Year of Family Farming: Factsheet*. Rome: Food and Agricultural Organization of the United Nations.

FAO. 2014. International year of family farming. *FAO.org*. http://www.fao.org/family-farming-2014/home/what-is-family-farming/en/ (Accessed December 4, 2017).

FAO. 2015. *The State of Food and Agriculture: Social Protection and Agriculture: Breaking the Cycle of Rural Poverty*. Rome: Food and Agriculture Organization of the United Nations.

FAO. 2016a. *The State of Food and Agriculture: Climate Change, Agriculture and Food Security*. Rome, Italy: Food and Agriculture Organization of the United Nations.

FAO. 2016b. *Methods for Estimating Comparable Rates of Food Insecurity Experienced by Adults Throughout the World*. Rome: Food and Agriculture Organization of the United Nations.

FAO. 2017a. *Counting the Cost: Agriculture in Syria After Six Years of Crisis*. Rome: Food and Agriculture Organization of the United Nations.

FAO. 2017b. Animal genetic resources. *FAO.org*. http://www.fao.org/nr/cgrfa/cthemes/animals/en/ (Accessed September 23, 2017).

FAO. 2017c. Plant genetic resources. *FAO.org*. http://www.fao.org/nr/cgrfa/cthemes/plants/en/ (Accessed September 23, 2017).

FAO, IFAD, UNICEF, WFP, and WHO. 2017. *The State of Food Security and Nutrition in the World 2017: Building Resilience for Peace and Food Security*. Rome: Food and Agriculture Organization of the United Nations.

FAOSTAT. 2012. Food and Agriculture Organization. http://faostat.fao.org

Felix, M. A., and A. Wagner. 2008. Robustness and evolution: Concepts, insights and challenges from a developmental model system. *Heredity* 100: 132–140.

Fryar, C. D., M. D. Carroll, and C. L. Ogden. 2016a. *Prevalence of Overweight, Obesity and Extreme Obesity Among Adults Aged 20 and Over: United States, 1960–1962 through 2013–2014*. Atlanta, GA: U.S. Center for Disease Control and Prevention.

Fryar, C. D., M. D. Carroll, and C. L. Ogden. 2016b. *Prevalence of Overweight, Obesity and Extreme Obesity Among Children and Adolescents Aged 2–19: United States, 1960–1962 Through 2013–2014*. Atlanta, GA: U.S. Center for Disease Control and Prevention.

Fulgoni, V. L., D. R. Keast, R. L. Bailey, and J. Dwyer. 2011. Foods, fortificants, and supplements: Where do Americans get their nutrients? *Journal of Nutrition* 141: 1847–1854.

Gadhok, I. 2016. *How Does Agricultural Trade Impact Food Security?* Trade Policy Briefs No.17. Rome: Food and Agriculture Organization of the United Nations.

Global Panel. 2017. *Healthy Diets for All: A Key to Meeting the SDGs*. Policy Brief No. 10. London, UK: Global Panel on Agriculture and Food Systems for Nutrition.

Hakansson, N. T. 1994. Grain, cattle and power: Social processes of intensive cultivation and exchange in precolonial Western Kenya. *Journal of Anthropological Research* 50 (3): 249–276.

Hallstrom, E., Q. Gee, P. Scarborough, and D. A. Cleveland. 2017. A healthier US diet could reduce greenhouse gas emissions from both the food and health care systems. *Climatic Change*. https://doi:10.1007/s10584-017-1912-5.

Hendrickson, M., W. D. Heffernan, P. H. Howard, and J. B. Heffernan. 2001. Consolidation in food retailing and dairy. *British Food Journal* 103 (10): 715–728.

Herrero, M., P. K. Thornton, B. Power, et al. 2017. Farming and the geography of nutrient production for human use: A transdisciplinary analysis. *Lancet Planet Health* 1 (1): e33–42. https://doi.org/10.1016/S2542-5196(17)30007-4.

HLPE. 2013. *Investing in Smallholder Agriculture for Food Security. A Report by the High Level Panel of Experts on Food Security and Nutrition of the Committee on World Food Security*. Rome, Italy: UN Committee on World Food Security.

Hopewell, K. 2014. The transformation of state-business relations in an emerging economy: The case of Brazilian agribusiness. *Critical Perspectives on International Business* 10 (4): 291–306.

IFPRI. 2014. *Global Nutrition Report 2014: Actions and Accountability to Accelerate the World's Progress on Nutrition*. Washington, DC: International Food Policy Research Institute.

IOM (Institute of Medicine) and NRC (National Research Council). 2015. *A Framework for Assessing Effects of the Food System*. Washington, DC: The National Academies Press.

IPES-Food. 2017. Unraveling the Food-Health Nexus: Addressing practices, political economy, and power relations to build healthier food systems. The Global Alliance for the Future of Food and IPES-Food.

IYFF+10 World Coordination Committee. 2017. Decade of family farming: Feeding the world, caring for the earth. Summary concept document. IYFF+10 World Coordination Committee.

Jacome, A. 2009. Mexico traditional agriculture as a foundation for sustainability. Advances in agroecology. In: *The Conversation to Sustainable Agriculture-Principles, Processes, and Practices*, edited by S. R. Gliessman and M. Rosemeyer Boca Raton, FL: CRC Press.

Jensen, D., A. Crawford, R. Whitten, and C. Bruch. 2013a. *Policy Brief 3: Land and Post-Conflict Peacebuilding*. Rome: Environmental Law Institute and UNEP.

Jensen, D., R. Whitten, I. Coyle, and C. Bruch. 2013b. *Policy Brief 2: Assessing and Restoring Natural Resources in Post-conflict Peacebuilding*. Rome: Environmental Law Institute and UNEP.

Johnstone, S., and J. Mazo. 2011. Global warming and the Arab Spring. *Survival* 53: 11–17.

Kaveeshwar, S. A. and Cornwall, J., 2014. The current state of diabetes mellitus in India. *Australasian Medical Journal* 7: 45–48.

Khoury, C. K., A. D. Bjorkman, H. Dempwolf, J. Ramirez-Vellegas, L. Guarino, A. Jarvis, L. H. Rieseberg, and P. C. Struik. 2014. Increasing homogeneity in global food supplies and the implications for food security. *Proceedings of the National Academy of Sciences* 111 (11): 4001–4006.

Kiehne, E., and N. S. Mendoza. 2015. Migrant and seasonal farmworker food insecurity: Prevalence, impact, risk factors, and coping strategies. *Social Work in Public Health* 30 (5): 397–409.

Laforet, S. 2015. Managing brand portfolios: Audit of leading grocery supplier brands 2004 to 2012. *Journal of Strategic Marketing* 23 (1): 72–89.

Larson, N., M. Story, and M. Nelson 2009. Neighborhood environment disparities in access to healthy foods in the US. *American Journal of Preventive Medicine* 36 (1): 74–81.

Lesk, C. P. Powhani, and N. Ramankutty. 2016. Influence of extreme weather disasters on global crop production. *Nature* 529:84–87.

Lloyd, C., and S. James. 2008. Too much pressure? Retailer power and occupational health and safety in the food processing industry. *Work, Employment and Society* 22: 713–730.

Louzada, M. L., L. G. Baraldi, E. Marinez, A. P. Steele, et al. 2015a. Consumption of ultra-processed foods and obesity in Brazilian adolescents and adults. *Preventive Medicine* 81: 9–15.

Louzada, M. L., A. P. Martins, D. S. Canella, et al. 2015b. Impact of ultra-processed foods on micronutrient content in the Brazilian diet. *Revista Saude Publica* 49: 1–8.

Lovelock, K., R. Lilley, D. McBride, S. Milosaviljevic, H. Yates, and C. Cryer. 2008. *Occupational Injury and Disease in Agriculture in North America, Europe and Australasia: A Review of the Literature* [IPRU Report No. ORO77]. Otago, NZ: University of Otago.

Malhi, Y. 2017. The concept of the Anthropocene. *Annual Review of Environment and Resources* 42 (25): 1–28.

McKeon, N. 2015. Global food governance in an era of crisis: Lessons from the United Nations Committee on World Food Security. *Canadian Food Studies* 2 (2): 328–334.

Miller, P. E., J. Reedy, S. I. Kirkpatrick, and S. M. Krebs-Smith. 2015. The United States food supply is not consistent with dietary guidance: Evidence from an evaluation using the Healthy Eating Index-2010. *Journal of the Academy of Nutrition and Dietetics* 115 (1): 95–100.

Monsivais, P., A. Aggarwal, and A. Drewnowski. 2010. Are socio-economic disparities in diet quality explained by diet cost? *Journal of Epidemiology and Community Health* 66: 530–535.

Moodie, R., D., Stuckler, C. Monteiro, et al. 2013. Profits and pandemics: Prevention of harmful effects of tobacco, alcohol, and ultra-processed food and drink industries. *Lancet* 381: 670–679.

Morton, J. F. 2007. The impact of climate change on smallholder and subsistence agriculture. *Proceedings of the National Academy of Sciences of the United States of America* 104 (50): 19680–19685.

NOAA. 2017. NOAA, USGS and partners predict their largest Gulf of Mexico summer 'dead zone' ever. NOAA.org. http://www.noaa.gov/media-release/gulf-of-mexico-dead-zone-is-largest-ever-measured (Accessed September 23, 2017).

Okrent, A. M., and A. Kumcu. 2016. *U.S. Households' Demand for Convenience Foods.* Economic Research Report Number 211. Washington, DC: USDA-Economic Research Service.

Oniang'o, R. K., J. M. Mutuku, and S. J. Malaba. 2003. Contemporary African food habits and their nutritional and health implications. *Asia Pacific Journal of Clinical Nutrition* 12 (3): 231–236.

Pingali, P. 2006. Westernization of Asian diets and the transformation of food systems: Implications for research and policy. *Food Policy* 32: 281–298.

Popkin, B. 2006. Global nutrition dynamics: The world is shifting rapidly toward a diet linked with noncommunicable diseases. *American Journal of Clinical Nutrition* 84: 289–298.

Pullen, S., 2004. The world's biomes Ucmp.berkelety.edu. http://www.ucmp.berkeley.edu/glossary/gloss5/biome/ (Accessed April 17, 2017).

Rabbitt, M. P., A. Coleman-Jensen, and C. A. Gregory. 2017. Understanding the prevalence, severity, and distribution of food insecurity in the United States. USDA-ERS.gov. https://www.ers.usda.gov/amber-waves/2017/september/understanding-the-prevalence-severity-and-distribution-of-food-insecurity-in-the-united-states/ (Accessed October 8, 2017).

Roberts, S. B., M. A. McCrory, and E. Saltzman. 2002. The influence of dietary composition on energy intake and body weight. *Journal of the American College of Nutrition* 21: 140S–145S.

Rotz, S. and E. D. Fraser. 2015. Resilience and the industrial food system: Analyzing the impacts of agricultural industrialization on food system vulnerability. *Journal of Environmental Studies and Sciences* 5: 459–473.

Rowan, C. 2015. The world's top 100 food and beverage companies-2015: Change is the new normal. Foodengineeringmag.com. https://www.foodengineeringmag.com/top-100-food-&-beverage-companies-2015 (Accessed July 10, 2017).

Steele, E. M., L. G. Baraldi, M. L. Louzada, et al. 2016. Ultra-processed foods and added sugars in the US diet: Evidence from a nationally representative cross-sectional study. *BMJ Open* 6. http://bmjopen.bmj.com/content/bmjopen/6/3/e009892.full.pdf

Steele, E. M., B. M. Popkin, B. Swinburn, and C. A. Monteiro. 2017. The share of ultra-processed foods and the overall nutritional quality of diets in the US: Evidence from a nationally representative cross-sectional study. *Population Health Metrics* 15: 6.

Steffen, W., A. Sanderson, P. D. Tyson, et al. 2004. *Global Change and the Earth System: A Planet Under Pressure.* New York, NY: Springer-Verlag Berlin Heidelberg.

Story, M., K. M. Kaphingst, R. Robinson-O'Brien, and K. Glanz. 2008. Creating healthy food and eating environments: Policy and environmental approaches. *Annual Review of Public Health* 29: 253–272.

Stuckler, D., M. McKee, S. Ebrahim, and S. Basu. 2012. Manufacturing epidemics: The role of global producers in increased consumption of unhealthy commodities including processed foods, alcohol and tobacco. *PLoS Med* 9 (6): e1001235.

Tilman, D., and M. Clark. 2014. Global diets link environmental sustainability and human health. *Nature* 515: 518–522.

Turner, B. L., and A. L. Thompson. 2013. Beyond the Paleolithic prescription: Incorporating diversity and flexibility in the study of human diet evolution. *Nutrition Reviews* 71 (8): 501–510.

Turral, H., 2012. *Water Pollution from Agriculture: A Review*. Rome: Food and Agriculture Organization of the United Nations.

United Nations. 2009. *State of the World's Indigenous Peoples*. New York: United Nations

United Nations. 2010. Resolution A/RES/64/292. United Nations General Assembly, July 2010. http://www.un.org/en/ga/search/view_doc.asp?symbol=A/RES/64/292.

United Nations. 2015. Resolution A/RES/70/1. United Nations General Assembly, October 2015. http://www.un.org/ga/search/view_doc.asp?symbol=A/RES/70/1&Lang=E

United Nations. 2017. The sustainable development goals report 2017. https://unstats.un.org/sdgs/files/report/2017/TheSustainableDevelopmentGoalsReport2017.pdf

USDA. 2015. Scientific report of the 2015 Dietary Guidelines Advisory Committee. https://health.gov/dietaryguidelines/2015-scientific-report/PDFs/Scientific-Report-of-the-2015-Dietary-Guidelines-Advisory-Committee.pdf.

USDA-ERS. 2017a. Food security in the U.S.: Measurement. USDA-ERS.gov. https://www.ers.usda.gov/topics/food-nutrition-assistance/food-security-in-the-us/measurement/ (Accessed October 6, 2017).

USDA-ERS. 2017b. New products. USDA.ERS.gov. https://www.ers.usda.gov/topics/food-markets-prices/processing-marketing/new-products/ (Accessed April 10, 2017).

USDA-ERS. 2017c. Food research atlas: Documentation. USDA.ERS.gov. https://www.ers.usda.gov/data-products/food-access-research-atlas/documentation/ (Accessed May 22, 2017).

Wall, D. H., U. N. Nielsen, and J. Six. 2015. Soil biodiversity and human health. *Nature* 538: 69–76.

Waters, C. N., J. Zalasiewicz, C. Summerhayes, et al. 2016. The Anthropocene is functionally and stratigraphically distinct from the Holocene. *Science* 351 (6269): 2622-8-10.

Weigel, M. M., R. X. Armijos, Y. P. Hall, et al. 2007. The household food insecurity and health outcomes of U.S.-Mexico border migrant and seasonal farmworkers. *Journal of Immigrant and Minority Health* 9 (3): 157–169.

WHO. 2015. *WHO Estimates of the Global Burden of Foodborne Diseases*. Rome, Italy: World Health Organization.

Wood, S. 2013. Revisiting the US food retail consolidation wave: Regulation, market power and spatial outcomes. *Journal of Economic Geography* 13: 299–326.

8 The Industrialized Food System and Chronic Disease

Angie Tagtow

CONTENTS

8.1 INTRODUCTION

Food systems are complex and constantly evolving. They consist of numerous food supply chains, a myriad of stakeholders, and are influenced by a multitude of factors. Their scale may range from a backyard garden to global conglomerates. Regardless of scale, their common goal is to get food to consumers. Industrialized food systems are often economically motivated and less focused on environmental, social, or human health gains. They have a profound impact on economic, environmental, social, and human health outcomes.

Further compounding the complexity, the U.S. food system is intricately interwoven to supply chains and systems all over the world. The Institute of Medicine (IOM) offers a visual framework (Table 8.1) that identifies the processes and stakeholders involved in producing, transforming, distributing, consuming, and recycling food (IOM 2015). The framework distinguishes the numerous influences on the food system: domestic and global trade policy; trained labor; technology; culture and society; and consumer knowledge, purchasing, and consumption behaviors. In addition, the

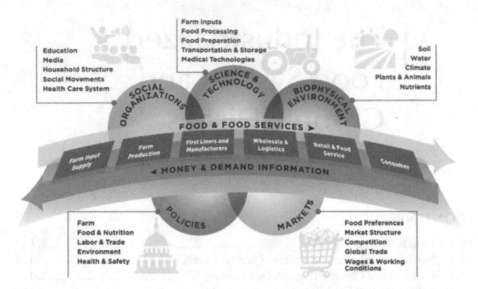

FIGURE 8.1 Links between the food supply chain and the larger biophysical and social/ institutional context. (Institute of Medicine (IOM) and the National Research Council (NRC). 2015. A Framework for Assessing Effects of the Food System . Washington, DC: The National Academies Press.)

framework can assist with evaluating the risks and benefits of food system decisions along with identifying and preventing unintended negative economic, environmental, social, and human health impacts.

What a person eats influences their overall health and well-being. Dietary behaviors and patterns are influenced by a host of social-ecological factors, including the complex system that delivers food from farm to plate. In addition to an individual's knowledge, attitude, and behavior in establishing a healthy dietary pattern, food systems, food policies, and food environments also influence the healthfulness of an individual's diet (U.S. Department of Health and Human Services [USDHHS] and U.S. Department of Agriculture [USDA] 2015).

The quality and adequacy of a dietary pattern is associated with the risk of developing a preventable chronic disease such as cardiovascular disease (CVD), high blood pressure, type 2 diabetes, certain cancers, and poor bone health (Dietary Guidelines Advisory Committee [DGAC] 2015). This chapter examines U.S. food consumption trends, rates of diet-related chronic diseases, the contribution of biodiversity to dietary diversity, and examples of unintended human health consequences of the industrialized food system.

8.2 FOOD CONSUMPTION AND DIETARY QUALITY TRENDS IN THE U.S.

Food consumption trends at the population and individual levels change over time. They are responsive to the changes in the food system and fluctuations in food supply chains. For example, as Americans seek convenience when purchasing food, they eat more food outside of the home. More than $7.31 billion was spent on food eaten outside the home in 2014 (e.g., restaurants, schools, retail stores, and workplace cafeterias). This surpasses the $7.27 billion spent on food eaten at home (Economic Research Service [ERS] 2017a). Historically, total household expenditures on food were greater than total household expenditures on healthcare. However, over the past 15 years, household expenditures on healthcare exceeded expenditures on food eaten inside and outside the home (ERS 2017a).

Measuring food consumption and dietary quality trends requires several data sources. Monitoring the individual health and nutritional status of adults and children is derived from interviews and physical exams of the National Health and Nutrition Examination Survey (NHANES). Findings from NHANES are used to assess risk factors, the prevalence of diet-related chronic diseases (Centers for Disease Control and Prevention [CDC] 2015), and alignment to healthy eating patterns outlined in the *Dietary Guidelines for Americans*. Conversely, the USDA-ERS measures U.S. food consumption trends using food availability data, loss-adjusted food availability data (food spoilage, food waste, etc.), and nutrient availability data as proxies for actual consumption (ERS 2017b). Together, these complimentary data sets assist with constructing a picture of U.S. consumption trends and dietary patterns.

The U.S. government considers a healthy dietary pattern to include a variety of vegetables, fruits (especially whole fruits), grains (at least half of which are whole grains), fat-free or low-fat dairy, a variety of protein foods—with limited saturated fats, *trans* fats, added sugars, and sodium (USDHHS and USDA 2015). The average American falls short of a healthy dietary pattern and rates of chronic disease continue to rise (DGAC 2015). Approximately half of all American adults have one or more preventable chronic disease, many of which are related to unhealthy dietary patterns and lack of physical activity (USDHHS and USDA 2015).

The Healthy Eating Index (HEI) is a measure of average diet quality and adequacy in the U.S. and the extent to which Americans conform to the *Dietary Guidelines for Americans* (Center for Nutrition Policy and Promotion [CNPP] 2017). An average diet quality score is calculated using NHANES food consumption data and mapping it across 12 food components. The total HEI score is the sum of the component scores and has a maximum of 100 points; the higher the score the greater conformance to the *Dietary Guidelines* (CNPP 2017). Overall, average diet quality in the U.S. does not meet recommendations as noted in Figure 8.2.

While Table 8.1 notes slight improvements in the HEI for children ages 2–17, adults age 18–64, and older adults (≥65 years), shortfalls in achieving the recommended healthy dietary pattern are evident (CNPP 2016).

A closer examination of foods and other components of an average American diet reveals that approximately three-fourths of the population has an eating pattern that is low in vegetables, fruits, dairy, and oils as seen in Figure 8.2. More than 50% of the population is meeting or exceeding total grain and total protein foods recommendations, but are not meeting the recommendations for certain subgroups such as whole grain and lean protein (USDHHS and USDA 2015). Most Americans exceed the recommendations for added sugars, saturated fats, and sodium. Figure 8.2 illustrates that as Americans consume a more healthful diet, there will be a shift closer to the center line of the diagram for each food category and component.

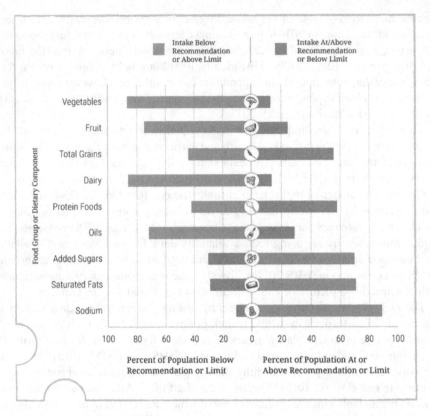

FIGURE 8.2 Dietary intakes compared to recommendations. Percent of the U.S. population aged 1 year and above who are below, at, or above each dietary goal or limit. (United States Department of Health and Human Services (USHHS) and United States Department of Agriculture (USDA) 2015.)

TABLE 8.1
Healthy Eating Index-2010 (HEI) Total Scores for Children 2–17 Years, Adults 18–64 Years, and Older Adults Greater than 65 Years (Mean Score and Standard Error)

Period	Children 2–17	Adults 18–64	Older Adults ≥65 years
	HEI Mean Score (standard error) Maximum = 100		
2005–2006	49.48 (0.66)	53.67 (0.78)	63.50 (0.98)
2007–2008	51.82 (1.14)	54.30 (1.16)	64.12 (1.03)
2009–2010	53.47 (0.77)	57.34 (0.86)	65.90 (0.56)
2011–2012	55.07 (0.72)	58.27 (0.98)	68.29 (1.76)

Source: Adapted from Center for Nutrition Policy and Promotion (CNPP) 2016.

The USDA-ERS's Food Availability Data System (FADS) dates to 1909 and includes food availability data, loss-adjusted food availability data, and nutrient availability data of more than 200 foods (ERS 2017b). Food availability data is a snapshot of the composition of the food system and used as a proxy for food consumption. Since 1970, diets in the U.S. include more food overall and more food across all the major food groups including fruits and vegetables (ERS 2017b). The FADS validates the NHANES findings in that the average U.S. diet falls short of the recommendations of the *Dietary Guidelines*. Specifically, "Americans consume too many foods that are high in added fats and oils, added sugar and sweeteners, and [refined] grains; and they consume too few foods and beverages that are nutrient-dense, such as vegetables, seafood, low-fat dairy products, and fruit" (Bentley 2017).

Further examination of the current U.S. food supply using the HEI-2010 reveals that the foods available through the U.S. food system also fall short of adherence to *Dietary Guidelines* and scores only 55 out of a possible 100 points (Miller et al. 2015). Additionally, the composition of the U.S. food supply does not align with dietary recommendations as outlined below (Bentley 2017; ERS 2017b):

- *Fruit*: Bananas and apples lead fresh fruit per capita availability. Fresh orange availability per person has fallen over the past four decades. However, since 1970, total fruit availability rose 10% from 237.6 pounds per person (fresh-weight equivalent) to 261.4 pounds per person in 2014. Despite the increase, this equates to an average consumption of only 43% of the recommended two cup-equivalent of fruit per the *Dietary Guidelines*.
- *Vegetables*: Potatoes, tomatoes, and iceberg lettuce accounted for over half of the per capita availability of fresh vegetables until the 1990s, but fell to 37% of fresh vegetable availability in 2015. Conversely, the amount of total vegetables available for consumption rose 17% from 327.9 pounds (fresh-weight equivalent) per person in 1970 to 383.6 pounds in 2014. Again, despite the increase, the average consumption totaled 66% of the recommended 2.5 cup-equivalent for vegetables per the *Dietary Guidelines*.
- *Grains*: The *2015–2020 Dietary Guidelines for Americans* recommends at least half of overall grain consumption be in the form of whole grains. The availability of total grains (wheat flour, rice, corn products, oat products, and barley products) increased 28% from 1970 to 2014 (rice was not included after 2010). Americans consumed 12% over the recommended six ounce-equivalent of total grains per day in 2014. However, average intakes of whole grains per NHANES are far below recommended levels across all age-sex groups and average intakes of refined grains are well above recommended limits for most age-sex groups (USDHHS and USDA 2015).
- *Dairy Products*: While the per capita availability of all fluid milk and milk products in the U.S. increased 9% from 1970 to 2014 – a result of the rise in cheese and yogurt – the consumption of fluid milk has decreased causing total pounds of dairy products available to decrease. In 2014, Americans consumed 49% of the recommended three cup-equivalent of dairy per the *Dietary Guidelines*.
- *Protein Foods (nuts, meat, poultry, and seafood)*: From 1970 to 2014, the total amount of protein foods (not including seeds and soy products) available for

consumption increased 1%. Chicken was the largest contributor to the growth by doubling the per capita availability for consumption. Subsequently, there was a decrease in red meat availability (beef, pork, lamb, veal, and mutton). Between 1970 and 2014, the per capita availability of beef and pork declined by 35% and 11%, respectively. Despite the decline in per capita availability, Americans consumed on average 29% over the recommended 5.5 ounce-equivalent of meat, poultry, fish, shellfish, eggs, and nuts per person per day in 2014. Specifically, teen boys and adult men exceeded the recommended intake of meats, poultry, and eggs. The average intake of seafood is low for all age-sex groups, whereas the average intake of nuts, seeds, and soy products are close to recommended levels (USDHHS and USDA 2015).

- *Sodium*: Sodium is ubiquitous in the food supply. Much of the sodium consumed in the U.S. is from processed and packaged foods, which makes it a challenge for individuals to control (DGAC 2015; Food and Drug Administration [FDA] 2016a). While considered a food component to limit in a healthy diet, the per capita availability of sodium in the U.S. food supply has ranged from 1,150 to 1,230 milligrams (mg) per day. Higher sodium intakes over the last decade coincide with the increased consumption of cheese (Hiza and Bente 2011). Excessive sodium intake is associated with increased blood pressure and hypertension, a leading contributor to CVD and numerous morbidities (IOM 2013). On average, Americans ages 2 and older consume 3,463 mg of sodium per day, 1,463 mg more than the recommended amount (2,000 mg) for a healthy dietary pattern (DGAC 2015). An additional nutrient of concern is potassium. Potassium is essential for heart and muscle function, and is often found in vegetables, fruits, whole grains, and dairy (USDHHS and USDA 2015). American diets fall short of meeting the recommendation for potassium further increasing the risk of developing a chronic disease (USDHHS and USDA 2015).

- *Added Sugars and Sweeteners*: Another dietary component of concern is added sugars. Between 1970 and 1999, the use of high fructose corn syrup in food and beverages sharply increased while beet and cane sugar use decreased. Since 1999, there has been a decrease in the per capita availability of high fructose corn syrup, while cane and beet sugar availability has increased. The *Dietary Guidelines* suggest that calories from added sugars and sweeteners not exceed 10% of daily calories or 200 calories per day (12.5 teaspoons for a 2,000-calorie/day diet) (USDHHS and USDA 2015). On average, Americans consumed 366 calories (roughly 23 teaspoons) of added sugars and sweeteners daily in 2014; that was 83% over the recommended 12.5 teaspoons per day. Intakes as a percent of calories are particularly high among children, adolescents, and young adults (DGAC 2015).

- *Added Fats and Oils*: Between 1970 and 2010 (data for fats and oils is only available to 2010), the availability of both added fats (saturated) and oils (unsaturated) in the food supply increased by 57%, to an average of 82.2 pounds per person. This was the result of increased availability of salad and cooking oils while the availability of butter remained constant. The *2015–2020 Dietary Guidelines* recommends a dietary pattern that includes less than 10% of calories per day from saturated fat (approximately 22 grams (g) for 2,000 cal diet) and 27 g per day of "healthy oils" such as olive or canola (USDHHS and USDA 2015). However, less than 29% of Americans consume a diet with less than 10% of calories from saturated fat (DGAC 2015) and average intakes of "healthy oils" are slightly below the *Dietary Guidelines for Americans* recommendations for all age-sex groups (USDHHS and USDA 2015).

- *Calories*: Overconsuming calories leads to a less healthful dietary pattern and contributes to the increased risks of overweight, obesity, and other diet-related chronic diseases. From 1970 to 2010, the average daily per capita calories from the U.S. food supply increased more than 22% to 2,476 calories as seen in Table 8.2. The largest gain in available calories came from a 66% increase in added fats, oils, and dairy fats, followed by a 42% increase in available calories from flour and cereal products. Added sugars and sweeteners peaked at 415 calories in 2000 (almost a 20% increase from 1970), but declined to 360 average daily per capita calories in 2015. The average daily per capita calories available from fruit saw a modest increase of 22%, however, the calories available from vegetables saw a decline of 2%.

8.3 DIET-RELATED CHRONIC DISEASE TRENDS IN THE U.S.

Noncommunicable diseases (NCDs), or chronic diseases, exist for extended periods of time and are often the result of behavioral, environmental, physiological, or genetic factors (World Health Organization [WHO] 2017a). Unhealthy diets, alcohol consumption, tobacco use, and physical inactivity are associated with an increased risk of mortality. Globally, more than 40 million people die each year—often prematurely—of NCDs (WHO 2017a) that could have been prevented through healthy lifestyle behaviors. Impoverished populations and communities of color have higher rates of NCDs because of an increased use of tobacco, unhealthy eating patterns, as well as limited access to healthful food or healthcare (WHO 2017a).

Many of the leading NCDs in the U.S.—diseases of the heart, malignant neoplasms (cancer), cerebrovascular diseases (stroke), and diabetes—are linked to diet. Between 1980 and 2015, overall deaths in the U.S. rose by 36.3%, as did deaths from malignant neoplasms (43.1%) and diabetes mellitus (128.2%). There was a 16.7% decrease in deaths from heart and cerebrovascular diseases (17.6%) over 35 years, although heart disease still remains the number one killer in the U.S. as noted in Table 8.3 (National Center for Health Statistics [NCHS] 2017).

Mortality and the morbidities associated with chronic diseases could be substantially reduced with preventive measures (WHO 2017a). In the U.S., about 117 million people, or 50% of the population, have one or more chronic conditions because of unhealthy behaviors (Ward et al. 2014). Individuals with multiple chronic conditions compound the burden of disease through decreased activities of daily living; increased absenteeism; increased prescription costs and healthcare spending—and ultimately, lowered life expectancy (Gerteis et al. 2014). Four of the top ten most prevalent chronic conditions among U.S. adults ages 18 and older are directly linked

TABLE 8.2

Average Daily Per Capita Calories from the U.S. Food Availability, Adjusted for Spoilage and Other Waste

Year	Meat, Eggs, and Nuts	Dairy	Fruit	Vegetables	Flour and Cereal Products[a]	Added Fats and Oils and Dairy Fats	Sugar and Sweeteners (Added)	Total
1970	506	234	67	129	409	346	333	2,024
1975	492	224	72	127	415	351	318	1,999
1980	494	219	77	123	437	372	335	2,058
1985	516	231	81	130	475	424	352	2,210
1990	499	223	81	132	540	411	369	2,255
1995	510	219	85	140	566	434	401	2,355
2000[b]	533	221	88	141	596	545	415	2,540
2005	545	223	86	132	571	586	396	2,538
2010	525	221	82	126	581	575	367	2,476
2015	529	219	82	131	524	NA	360	NA
Percent change 1970 to 2010	3.8%	-5.6%	22.4%	-2.3%	42.1%	66.2%	10.2%	22.3%

Source: Adapted from Economic Research Service (ERS) 2017b; Calculated by ERS/USDA based on data from various sources (see https://www.ers.usda.gov/data-products/food-availability-per-capita-data-system/loss-adjusted-food-availability-documentation/). Data last updated Feb. 1, 2017.

Note: Due to the termination of select Current Industrial Reports by the Census Bureau, data on durum flour cannot be updated beyond 2010. The absence of data on durum flour is not critical to the Food Availability Data System since data are still available at a higher level of aggregation (i.e., wheat flour). Annual data and per capita estimates for rice are unavailable beyond 2010 due to a large and unexplained decline in the implied total domestic and residual use estimate. Residual use accounts for all unreported losses in the milling, transporting, and marketing of rice, and also offsets any statistical error in another supply and use account. Due to the termination of select Current Industrial Reports (CIR) by the Census Bureau, data on some added fats and oils could not be updated beyond 2010 in the Food Availability Data System. This means that certain summary estimates—such as per capita daily amounts of calories and food pattern equivalents (or servings)—cannot be calculated beyond 2010 for the added fats & oils group. Additionally, the summary estimates or totals across all food groups cannot be calculated beyond 2010.

NA = Not available.

a Does not include rice after 2010.

b In 2000, the number of firms reporting vegetable oil production to the Census Bureau increased, and this contributed to the spike in the data for salad and cooking oils, shortening, and aggregated numbers that use these estimates, such as total vegetable fats and oils, total added fats and oils, and total calories from added fats and oils and from all foods.

TABLE 8.3
Leading Causes of Death in the U.S., 1980 and 2015

	1980		2015	
	Cause of Death	# Deaths	Cause of Death	# Deaths
Rank	All causes	1,989,841	All causes	2,712,630
1	Diseases of heart	761,085	Diseases of heart	633,842
2	Malignant neoplasms	416,509	Malignant neoplasms	595,930
3	Cerebrovascular diseases	170,225	Chronic lower respiratory diseases[a,b]	155,041
4	Unintentional injuries	105,781	Unintentional injuries	146,571
5	Chronic obstructive pulmonary diseases[a]	56,050	Cerebrovascular diseases	140,323
6	Pneumonia and influenza[b]	54,619	Alzheimer's disease	110,561
7	Diabetes Mellitus	34,851	Diabetes mellitus[c]	79,535
8	Chronic liver disease and cirrhosis	30,583	Influenza and pneumonia2	57,062
9	Atherosclerosis	29,449	Nephritis, nephrotic syndrome and nephrosis[c]	49,959
10	Suicide	26,869	Suicide	44,193

Source: Adapted from NCHS, *Health, United States, 2016: With Chartbook on Long-term Trends in Health*. U.S. Health and Human Services, Centers for Disease Control and Prevention, Hyattsville, MD, 2017, Table 19.

[a] Between 1998 and 1999, the cause of death title for Chronic obstructive pulmonary diseases in the International Classification of Diseases, 9th Revision (ICD–9) was renamed to Chronic lower respiratory diseases (CLRD) in ICD–10.

[b] Starting with 1999 data, the rules for selecting CLRD and Pneumonia as the underlying cause of death changed, resulting in an increase in the number of deaths for CLRD and a decrease in the number of deaths for pneumonia. Therefore, trend data for these two causes of death should be interpreted with caution.

[c] Starting with 2011 data, the rules for selecting renal failure as the underlying cause of death were changed, affecting the number of deaths in the nephritis, nephrotic syndrome, and nephrosis and diabetes categories. These changes directly affect deaths with mention of renal failure and other associated conditions, such as diabetes mellitus with renal complications. The result is a decrease in the number of deaths for nephritis, nephrotic syndrome, and nephrosis and an increase in the number of deaths for diabetes mellitus. Therefore, trend data for these two causes of death should be interpreted with caution. For more information, see Technical Notes in Deaths: Final data for 2011, available from: http://www.cdc.gov/nchs/data/nvsr/nvsr63/nvsr63_03.pdf.

to diet: Hypertension (26.7%) is immediately followed by hyperlipidemia (21.9%); diabetes (9.5%) is the sixth and coronary artery disease (5.3%) is ninth (Gerteis et al. 2014). According to the Agency for Healthcare Research and Quality (AHRQ), individuals with one chronic condition spend almost 2.5 times more on healthcare expenditures as compared to those without any chronic conditions; those with three chronic conditions spend almost six times more on healthcare (Gerteis et al. 2014). Chronic disease rates generally increase with age. However traditional adult-onset chronic diseases such as type 2 diabetes, are increasing in prevalence among children (DGAC 2015).

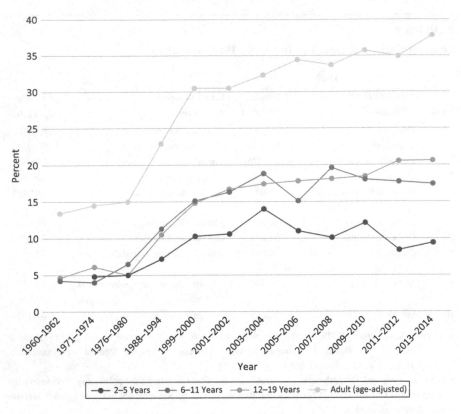

FIGURE 8.3 Percent of U.S. adults aged 20 and over 1 and children ages 2 to 19 with obesity 1960–2014. (Adapted from National Center for Health Statistics (NCHS) 2017, Table 53; Fryar et al. 2012; NCHS 2008.)

Comprehensive public health interventions to combat diet-related chronic diseases requires a thorough assessment of chronic conditions including the following:

- *Overweight and Obesity*: Overweight in adults is defined as a Body Mass Index (BMI) greater than or equal to 25–29 while obesity in adults is defined as a BMI greater than or equal to 30 (NCHS 2008). Overweight and obesity are often precursors to diet-related diseases such as type 2 diabetes, hypertension, CVD, and some cancers. The consumption of excess calories and a lack of physical activity are major factors leading to weight gain. Almost 80% of U.S. adults and adolescents do not meet the minimum recommendations for physical activity (USDHHS 2017). Seventy-three percent of students are not physically active for at least 60 min a day and more than two-thirds of students, grades 9–12, are in front of a screen (television, computer, etc.) for three or more hours per day (NCHS 2017, Table 52). Overweight and obesity rates for adults and children in the U.S. have risen significantly (Figure 8.3) and are higher for racial and ethnic minorities, households with limited resources, and communities of color (DGAC 2015). In 2014, 70.7% of adults—almost three in four adults in the U.S.—were overweight or obese. This represents a 28% increase since 1988 (NCHS 2017, Table 53) and nearly 40% of adults are considered obese (NCHS 2017, Table 53). Obese adults spend 42% more on direct healthcare costs as compared to adults with a healthy BMI (Finkelstein et al. 2009). Despite a 10.5% increase in obesity among youth ages 12–19, obesity rates among all children have begun to level off as noted in Figure 8.3 (NCHS 2017, Table 53; Fryar et al. 2012).

- *CVD*: Deaths from cardiovascular and cerebrovascular diseases account for about one-third of deaths in the U.S. as noted in Table 8.3. The American Heart Association (AHA) estimates that 92.1 million U.S. adults (i.e., about 30%) have CVD and it is projected that 43.9% of U.S. adults will exhibit some form of CVD by 2030 (AHA 2017). CVD is more prevalent in Hispanics and Native Americans as compared to non-Hispanic whites (DGAC 2015). Hypercholesterolemia and hypertension are risk factors for CVD. In 2014, 29.3% of adults in the U.S. had hypercholesterolemia, an increase from 21.5% in 1988 (NCHS 2017, Table 53). In 2014, 33.5% of U.S. adults had hypertension, an increase from 24.1% in 1988 (NCHS 2017, Table 53). That number increases to almost 50% of African-American adults with hypertension. Additionally, one in ten children have high blood pressure (FDA 2016a).

- *Diabetes*: In 2014, 12.7% of adults in the U.S. had type 2 diabetes (diagnosed and undiagnosed), an increase from 8.3% in 1988 (NCHS 2017, Table 53). Between 2001 and 2009, rates of type 2 diabetes in youth ages 10–19 years increased 30.5% and impacts about one of every 2,000 youth (DGAC 2015). The projected number of youth with type 2 diabetes is expected to quadruple (Imperatore et al. 2012) and one in three U.S. adults (CDC 2010) could have diabetes by 2050 if current trends continue.

- *Cancer*: Cancer, or malignant neoplasms, are the second leading cause of death in the U.S. (Table 8.3) and globally. According to the WHO, cancer claimed 8.8 million lives in 2015, of which more than 600,000 were in the U.S. Nearly one in five deaths in the U.S. and one in six deaths worldwide are caused by cancer (NCHS 2017, Table 19; WHO 2017b). It is predicted that the number of new cases of cancer will rise about 70% worldwide over the next 20 years (WHO 2017b). Diet-related cancers include colorectal, breast, and prostate. Colorectal cancer is the second leading cause of cancer death in the U.S., followed by breast cancer (NCHS 2017, Table 19). Prostate cancer is the fifth leading cause of cancer death in the U.S. (Howlander et al. 2017). One-third of deaths from cancer are a result of neglected modifiable dietary behaviors including poor dietary patterns, low fruit and vegetable consumption, a high BMI, lack of physical activity, and excessive alcohol and tobacco use. Eliminating these risk factors and adopting healthy behaviors could reduce cancer risk by 30–50% (WHO 2017b).

8.3.1 DIET-RELATED CHRONIC DISEASE AND HEALTHCARE EXPENDITURES

The cost of diet-related chronic disease and unhealthy behaviors account for most healthcare costs in the U.S. In 2015, more than $3.2 trillion was spent on healthcare

TABLE 8.4

Gross Domestic Product (GDP) and National Health and Prescription Drug Expenditures in the U.S., 1980 and 2015

	1980	2015
	Amount, in billions	
GDP	$2,863	$18,037
National Health Expenditures	$255.3	$3,206.6
National Health Expenditures as Percent of GDP	8.9%	17.8%
Prescription Drug Expenditures	$12.0	$324.6
Prescription Drug Expenditures as Percent of GDP	0.4%	1.8%

Source: Adapted from NCHS, *Health, United States, 2016: With Chartbook on Long-term Trends in Health.* U.S. Health and Human Services, Centers for Disease Control and Prevention, Hyattsville, MD, 2017, Tables 93 and 94.

in the U.S. (NCHS 2017). This represents an increase of more than 1,155% in 35 years and accounted for more than 17% of the Gross Domestic Product (GDP) (NCHS 2017, Table 93) (Table 8.4). Healthcare costs attributed to CVD were $316.1 billion (AHA 2017); diabetes $245 billion (American Diabetes Association 2015); cancer $157 billion (NCI 2017a); and obesity is between $147 billion and $210 billion (Finkelstein et al. 2009; Cawley and Meyerhoefer 2012). Individuals with diet-related chronic diseases not only have higher healthcare costs but also higher prescription drug expenses. In 2015, more than $324 billion was spent on prescription drugs, which represents a 2,605% increase since 1980 as demonstrated in Table 8.4 (NCHS 2017, Table 94) (Table 8.4).

In the last five decades, technological and pharmaceutical advances have contributed to decreasing rates of mortality and increasing life expectancy in the U.S. These advances have also brought a substantial increase in healthcare expenditures. However, modest dietary modifications can have an enormous impact on decreasing healthcare expenditures. For example, if everyone in the U.S. were to consume just one additional serving (1/2 cup) of vegetables or fruits per day, it is estimated it would save more than $2.7 trillion in healthcare expenditures (O'Hara 2013).

8.4 HUMAN HEALTH CONSEQUENCES OF THE INDUSTRIAL FOOD SYSTEM

The industrialized food system in the U.S. produces a high volume of food for human and animal consumption. It also uses technology to increase efficiencies and minimize food safety risks, producing food that is relatively inexpensive while serving as a major force in the global economy. The rapid evolution of both the U.S. and global food systems has resulted in intensively cultivating fewer varieties of agricultural products, resulting in a plethora of processed foods while delivering more food calories per person. Yet, economic and geographic inequalities limit access to healthy food for many populations as delineated in Chapters 6 and 7. Again, using the 2015 IOM food system framework (Figure 8.1) to evaluate the risks and benefits of food system decisions can minimize future unintended consequences, especially on human health.

The science of understanding the food systems' impact on human health offers an expansive breadth of research that is examining the human health benefits and risks associated with the production, processing, packaging, distributing, purchasing, and consumption of food. Debates about the science, policies, ethics, economic, environmental, social, and health impacts of important issues such as pesticides, genetic engineering, cloning, growth hormones, additives, preservatives, food marketing, and food delivery will continue. While not an exhaustive assessment, the following examples are food system decisions that negatively impact human health.

8.4.1 BIODIVERSITY, DIET DIVERSITY, NUTRIENT DENSITY, AND FOOD PRODUCTION

Scientists agree that biodiversity is quintessential to the Earth's ecosystem as it underpins environmental and human health. Both biodiversity and agrobiodiversity are fundamental to supporting diversified food production and optimal nutrient output, creating a foundation for healthy and sustainable dietary patterns (Berti and Jones 2013; Hunter and Fanzo 2013; Frison 2011). Theoretically, there is a positive relationship between agricultural biodiversity and dietary diversity, and it would be logical to equate that if farmers grew only one or two crops, there would be little dietary diversity. The reliance on just a few crops in a food system would not deliver the diverse food and nutrients needed for a healthy dietary pattern and likely would lead to micronutrient deficiencies and malnutrition as discussed in Chapter 7.

The U.S. food supply offers an overwhelming number of options for consumers with an average of 40,000 food products in a grocery store (Food Marketing Institute 2017) with approximately 21,000 new food and beverage products entering the market each year (ERS 2017c). These new products are often processed and packaged using ingredients from all over the world. Hence, a paradox exists. As the number of food and beverage products available to consumers has risen substantially, the diversity of agricultural products (agrobiodiversity) has declined in U.S. and globally in the last 100 years.

The U.S. Agricultural Census has tracked farming data for more than 150 years, specifically farm demographics, crop and livestock data, and economic indicators. In the last 100 years, the total number of farms in the U.S. has decreased by 63%. In 1900, each farm in the U.S. provided food for 13 people, whereas in 2012 each farm provided food for 149 people as shown in Table 8.5. In addition to the decrease in farms and increased reliance on farms to support a growing population, the overall diversity of agricultural crop species has declined in the U.S. although there is variation between and within regions (Aguilar et al. 2015).

Further examination reveals that the U.S. agriculture system does not supply enough of the right types of foods to support healthy dietary patterns and relies heavily on imported fruits and vegetables. If Americans were to eat according to dietary recommendations (based on the *2005 Dietary Guidelines for Americans*), the U.S. agricultural system would need to harvest an additional 7.4 million acres in fruits, vegetables, and whole grain crops, and produce an additional 111 billion pounds of milk and milk products (Buzby et al. 2006).

TABLE 8.5

Changes in U.S. Farms, Acres in Farms, and Ratios of Farms and Acres in Farms Per Population for 1900, 1954, and 2012

	U.S. Agricultural Census		
	1900[a]	1954[b]	2012[c]
Number of Farms	5,739,657	4,782,416	2,109,303
Number of Acres in Farms	841,201,546	1,158,191,511	914,527,657
U.S. Population[d]	76,308,387	163,025,854	313,914,040
Ratio of Farms per Population	1:13	1:34	1:149
Ratio of Acres in Farms per Population	100:9	100:14	100:34

[a] U.S. Department of the Interior, 1902.
[b] U.S. Department of Commerce, 1954.
[c] National Agricultural Statistical Services, 2014.
[d] U.S. Census, www.census.gov.

There have been substantial innovations in agricultural food production in the last century that produces food more quickly, inexpensively, and uniformly that can also endure extended transit times. These innovations over time may have led to lower nutrient concentrations. USDA researchers evaluated changes in nutrient content for 43 garden crops (mostly vegetables) between 1950 and 1999 (Davis et al. 2004). They found that all 43 foods had declined in protein, calcium, phosphorus, iron, riboflavin, and ascorbic acid. They concluded this might be the result of hybridization to garner greater yields or to obtain certain desirable attributes such as appearance (Davis et al. 2004). A similar evaluation was conducted in the United Kingdom using the government's *Composition of Foods* data from 1930 to 1980 (Mayer 1997). The UK found reductions in calcium, magnesium, copper, sodium, iron, and potassium in 20 vegetables and 20 fruits. In addition, the vegetables and fruits had an increase in water content and a decrease in dry matter producing a dilution effect (Mayer 1997). Some researchers argue that comparing historical food composition tables and standards for measuring micronutrients in foods are not reliable and does not account for changes in genetic varieties, geographic origin, season, degree of ripeness, variation in sampling, and analytical and statistical methods (Marles 2017). However, researchers do agree that additional data is needed—especially considering increasing atmospheric CO_2 levels and climate change. Certain grains and legumes may increase in carbohydrate content while decreasing in protein, zinc, and iron content. (Myers et al. 2014).

Globally, agrobiodiversity is in a critical state. According to the Food and Agriculture Organization (FAO), 75% of edible plant genetic diversity has been displaced if not lost. Thirty percent of livestock breeds are close to extinction, and many fish population are extinct due to overfishing (FAO 2004). Today, more than 75% of the world's food is generated from 12 plants and five animal species (FAO 2004). Approximately two-thirds of the global diet consists of rice, maize, and wheat (FAO 2004).

Numerous influences, such as climate change and destructive weather events, changing market forces, cost of inputs, trade and agriculture policies, availability of technology, and consumer demand has limited the diversity of agricultural crops and has created a homogenous food supply (Aguilar et al. 2015). This evolution of the industrial food system has increased vulnerabilities across food supply chains resulting in decreased resilience and increased domestic and global food insecurity as noted in Chapter 9. With an increasing global population, there is an urgent need to adjust food and agriculture policies and to redesign food systems, agricultural lands, and farming practices to produce the quality and quantity of foods needed to support healthy dietary patterns for all.

8.4.2 GLYPHOSATE AND FOOD PRODUCTION

Pesticides are chemicals used to protect crops against insects, fungi, weeds, and other pests. They are also used to control the vectors of tropical diseases, such as mosquitoes (WHO 2017c; WHO 2016c). Globally, more than 1,000 pesticides—in the form of fungicides, herbicides, and insecticides—are used to protect food crops from pests (WHO 2017). Glyphosate, a broad-spectrum herbicide, is the most widely used pesticide in the U.S. (United State Geological Survey [USGS] 2017) and throughout the world (International Agency for Research on Cancer (IARC) 2016). According to the National Pesticide Information Center, there are more than 750 products in the U.S. that contain glyphosate (Henderson et al. 2010). Glyphosate is registered in more than 130 countries (IARC 2016) with an anticipated sales of $8.79 billion in 2019 (Transparency Market Research 2014). Glyphosate is widely used in food production, commercial applications such as golf courses and industrial areas, residential lawns and gardens, and in waterways to control invasive plant species (Henderson et al. 2010).

Glyphosate is the most common herbicide used in food production. It kills most plants and grasses by being absorbed through the leaves and preventing the plant from producing specific proteins needed for growth (Henderson et al. 2010). Glyphosate tightly binds to soil and may take up to six months for bacteria in the soil to break it down (Henderson et al. 2010). It can be found in ground and surface water systems (U.S. Environmental Protection Agency [USEPA] 2017; Schribner et al. 2007).

Several crops in the U.S., specifically corn, soybeans, cotton, canola, and sugar beets have been genetically engineered (ERS 2017d) to resist applications of glyphosate. Glyphosate was first sold commercially in the U.S. in 1974 (Benbrook 2016) and between 1992 and 2015, there was a 1,375% increase in glyphosate use with more than 275 million pounds applied to crops in 2015 (USGS 2017). This increase is the result of the adoption of genetically engineered glyphosate-resistant crops (Schribner et al. 2007) and the decline in the price of glyphosate (Benbrook 2016). The U.S. Geological Survey's Pesticide National Synthesis Project tracks annual pesticide use for more than 500 different pesticides and their potential for adverse effects on aquatic life and drinking water supplies. The rates of agricultural glyphosate applications throughout the U.S. are noted in Figure 8.4 with the highest concentrations in the upper Midwest and along the Mississippi River Valley (USGS 2017). In 2015, most states had areas with annual glyphosate applications of more than 88 pounds of glyphosate per square mile (USGS 2017). This is in contrast to states such as Illinois,

Iowa, Kansas, Minnesota, North Dakota, South Dakota, and Wisconsin that had 75–100% of their respective states applying glyphosate at application rates greater than 88 pounds per square mile (Figure 8.4) (USGS 2017). Other pesticides such as 2,4-D, atrazine, dicamba, and many others have similar patterns of concentrated application across the U.S. While agricultural regions may use a variety of pesticides, the collective impacts of agriculture and non-agriculture pesticide application loads on both the natural environment and human health have not been addressed.

Several federal agencies oversee the regulation and monitoring of pesticides, including glyphosate. The USEPA Office of Pesticide Programs is responsible for regulating pesticides per the 1996 *Federal Insecticide, Fungicide, and Rodenticide Act* (7 U.S.C. §136 et seq. (1996). The USEPA must ensure that pesticides will not cause "unreasonable adverse effects on the environment, including: (1) any unreasonable risk to man or the environment, taking into account the economic, social, and environmental costs and benefits of the use of any pesticide, or (2) a human dietary risk from residues that result from a use of a pesticide in or on any food inconsistent with the standard under section 408 of the *Federal Food, Drug, and Cosmetic Act*" (Office of Pesticide Programs 2000). The USDA's Pesticide Data Program conducts "sampling, testing, and reporting of pesticide residues on agricultural commodities in the U.S. food supply, with an emphasis on those commodities highly consumed by infants and children" (Agricultural Marketing Service (AMS) 2016). Lastly, the U.S. FDA administers the Pesticide Residue Monitoring Program that monitors pesticide

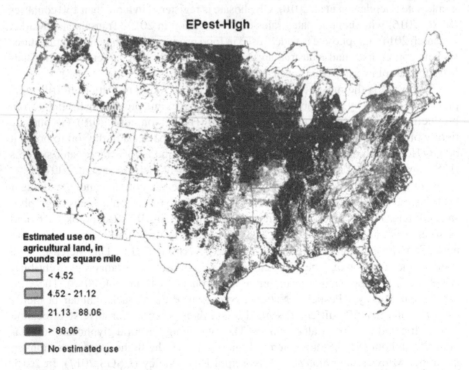

EPest-High

Estimated use on
agricultural land, in
pounds per square mile

- < 4.52
- 4.52 - 21.12
- 21.13 - 88.06
- > 88.06
- No estimated use

FIGURE 8.4 Estimated U.S. agricultural use of glyphosate, 2015. (U.S. Geological Survey, Pesticide National Synthesis Project, 2017.)

residue on foods imported into the U.S. and the domestic food supply as outlined in the *Federal Food, Drug, and Cosmetic Act* (FDA 2017a).

The long-term use of pesticides, including glyphosate, in global food production has resulted in both ecosystem and human health impacts. Researchers continue to evaluate the ecological impact of pesticides in soil, water, and air and they have identified at least 220 plant species that have become tolerant or resistant to one or more pesticides (Heap 2014). The recurrent use of glyphosate in weed management practices has resulted in glyphosate-resistant weeds (Beckie 2011; Benbrook 2016). This ecosystem response has led food producers to use greater concentrations of pesticides, sequenced applications, and pesticide "cocktails" that include a mixture of pesticides to control weeds and pests (Beckie 2011; Heap 2014).

Most foods consumed in the U.S. are grown with the use of pesticides, therefore, pesticide residue is likely present on the surfaces or inside these foods (USEPA 2017). Dietary exposure to glyphosate may be from fruits or vegetables that have not been thoroughly washed or from some vegetables that may take up glyphosate through the soil (Henderson et al. 2010). Intake may also occur if hands are not thoroughly washed after the application of glyphosate or by touching plants that are still wet with spray (Henderson et al. 2010). Regular dietary exposure to glyphosate in adults and children is a major concern because of the unknown immediate and long-term health impacts (National Research Council 1993). However, exposure thresholds or 'tolerances' set by the government are estimates at best as controlled trials to determine the human health impacts of pesticide exposure would be unethical.

According to the FDA, the levels of pesticide residues in the U.S. food supply are generally in compliance with the EPA's permitted pesticide tolerances (Bates et al. 2014). In 2014, FDA found no pesticide residues in 71% of domestic ($n = 1,458$) and 53% of imported human food samples ($n = 4,814$). More than one percent of domestic food samples and almost 12 percent of imported food samples had pesticide residues that were above compliance levels. A majority (75.7 percent) of the imported samples were fruits and vegetables (Bates et al. 2014). Residues from 212 different pesticides were detected in the 2014 samples but at trace levels of 0.1 parts per million (PPM) or less (Bates et al. 2014). However, glyphosate was not one of the pesticides analyzed by FDA in 2014 (Bates et al. 2014, Appendix A). Historically, glyphosate has been considered to be of low acute toxicity (Benbrook 2016). However, the adverse human health effects of glyphosate exposure continue to be debated. Despite this, animal and human studies have associated glyphosate exposure to cancer (e.g., non-Hodgkin lymphoma, multiple myeloma, leukemia), developmental and reproductive disorders, endocrine disruption, immune and neurological anomalies, and kidney and liver failure (Benbrook 2016; WHO(c) 2016c; Henderson et al 2010; De Roos et al. 2005).

In 1985, the USEPA originally classified glyphosate as possibly carcinogenic to humans as did the IARC but changed the classification to a Group E non-carcinogen in 1991 (USEPA 1993, IARC 2016). Subsequently, the EPA revised their Reregistration Eligibility Decision (RED) for glyphosate and increased the oral Reference Dose (RfD) to ≤ 2.0 mg per kilogram of body weight per day (mg/kg bodyweight/d) (USEPA 1993). The EPA will review the registration of glyphosate, as well as every registered pesticide, every 15 years (USEPA 2009).

Farm families and pesticide applicators are specifically vulnerable to pesticide exposure and potential adverse health effects. Acquavella and colleagues (2004) evaluated urinary glyphosate in 48 farm families and found that 60% of the farmers, 4% of spouses, and 12% of children had detectable levels of glyphosate in their urine the day glyphosate was applied on the farm. Concentrations of urinary glyphosate were highest among farmers who did not wear gloves while working with glyphosate. However, urinary concentrations did decrease to non-detectable levels for all farmers within 72 hours post-application (Acquavella et al. 2004). A similar study examining urinary concentrations of organophosphate pesticides in children found a significantly reduced urinary concentration of organophosphates when children switched from a non-organic diet to an all organic diet (Lu et al. 2006).

In 2015, the IARC conducted a scientific review to understand glyphosate and cancer risk. The 92-page monograph summarizes the *sufficient* evidence of carcinogenicity of glyphosate in animal studies and the *limited* evidence of carcinogenicity of glyphosate in humans, although they identified a positive association between glyphosate and non-Hodgkin lymphoma. The IARC classified glyphosate as a Group 2A carcinogenic (IARC 2015). Despite criticism, the IARC stands behind its research.

The emerging scientific evidence of environmental and human health impacts of glyphosate have prompted some scientists to request more frequent health risk assessments as well as reductions in the glyphosate thresholds in both the U.S. and European Union in an effort to reduce risk of toxicity and further resistance (Benbrook 2016, Antoniou et al. 2012). Longitudinal research is essential to monitor the frequency and levels of glyphosate residue in domestic and imported food as well as their subsequent impact on human health and the natural environment.

8.4.3 ANTIMICROBIALS AND FOOD PRODUCTION

Discovered in the 1920s, antimicrobials, or antibiotics, became a powerful tool to stop infections caused by bacteria in humans. When penicillin became available in the 1940s, the likelihood of stopping a life-threatening infection increased; surgical procedures became safer; and life expectancy increased. Although additional classes of antibiotics were discovered over the next 30 years, no new classes of antibiotics have been developed since the 1970s (Aminov 2010).

In 2014, U.S. healthcare providers prescribed more than 266 million outpatient antibiotic prescriptions (CDC 2014) with approximately 30% of the antibiotics prescribed in the outpatient setting deemed unnecessary (Fleming-Dutra et al. 2016). Perhaps lesser known is that over 70% of the antibiotics sold in the U.S. are used in animals that are destined for the food supply (FDA 2016b). The use of antibiotics in animal agriculture treats clinical diseases, enhances growth, and prevents disease outbreaks. There is a higher probability of disease outbreaks in intensive livestock and aquaculture operations with a high density of animals in confined spaces. Livestock and fish in these operations require aggressive prophylactic strategies to prevent infection through the use of antibiotics (Landers et al. 2012; Meek et al. 2015) that are provided in feed or water (FDA 2016b). More than 34.2 million pounds of antibiotics were administered to livestock in the U.S. in 2015 (Table 8.6). According to the FDA, domestic sales of medically important antimicrobials approved for use

TABLE 8.6

Medically Important Antimicrobial Drugs Approved for Use in Food-Producing Animals Actively Marketed 2009–2015 Domestic Sales and Distribution Data Reported by Drug Class

Drug Class	2009 Annual Totals (kg)[a]	2010 Annual Totals (kg)[a]	2011 Annual Totals (kg)[a]	2012 Annual Totals (kg)[a]	2013 Annual Totals (kg)[a]	2014 Annual Totals (kg)[a]	2015 Annual Totals (kg)[a]	Percent Change 2009–2015
Aminoglycosides[b]	222,117	211,790	214,895	277,854	267,734	304,160	344,120	54%
Cephalosporins[b]	20,145	24,588	26,611	27,654	28,337	31,722	32,341	61%
Lincosamides[b]	93,330	154,653	190,101	218,140	236,450	233,681	182,543	96%
Macrolides[b]	562,062	553,229	582,836	616,274	563,251	621,769	627,770	12%
Penicillins[b]	691,644	884,419	885,304	965,196	828,721	885,975	936,669	35%
Sulfas[b]	505,880	517,128	383,105	493,514	383,469	452,224	380,186	-25%
Tetracyclines[b]	5,260,995	5,602,281	5,652,855	5,954,361	6,514,779	6,604,199	6,880,465	31%
Not Independently Reported[c,d]	329,391	281,221	319,991	344,428	370,551	345,609	317,885	-3%
Subtotal	7,686,564	8,229,309	8,255,697	8,897,420	9,193,293	9,479,339	9,701,979	26%
Not Currently Medically Important[e]	4,900,893	5,057,788	5,313,340	5,725,327	5,591,752	5,882,221	5,874,997	20%
Total	12,587,457	13,287,097	13,569,037	14,622,747	14,785,045	15,361,560	15,576,976	24%

Source: Adapted from FDA, *Summary Report on Antimicrobials Sold or Distributed for Use in Food-Producing Animals.* U.S. Department of Health and Human Services, Washington, DC, 2016b, Table 10.

a kg = kilogram of active ingredient. Antimicrobials reported in International Units (IU) were converted to kg.

b Includes antimicrobial drug applications that are approved and labeled for use in both food-producing animals (e.g., cattle and swine) and nonfood-producing animals (e.g., dogs and cats).

c Guidance for Industry #213 states that all antimicrobial drugs and their associated classes listed in Appendix A of FDA's Guidance for Industry #152 are considered "medically important" in human medical therapy

d Antimicrobial classes for which there were fewer than three distinct sponsors actively marketing products domestically are not independently reported.

e Refers to any microbial class not currently listed in Appendix A of FDA's Guidance for Industry #152.

in food producing animals increased by 26% from 2009 through 2015 (FDA 2016b) with tetracycline as the leading class of antimicrobials provided to food-producing animals (FDA 2016b) (Table 8.6).

A consequence of the extensive use of antibiotics in humans and livestock has led to antimicrobial resistance. Antimicrobial resistance is a result of microorganisms' adaptive ability to survive and multiply due to the routine prophylactic use of antibiotics, rendering many antibiotic therapies ineffective. The resistant bacteria may spread from animal products (Brower et al. 2017) or fresh produce through contaminated water or soil; prepared food through contaminated surfaces; and the contamination of waterways, air, and manure (CDC 2013). The CDC estimates that one in five antimicrobial-resistant infections in the U.S. are caused by bacteria from food and animals (CDC 2013).

The science and surveillance confirms that the extent of antimicrobial resistance infections is directly correlated with the amount of antibiotics used in animal agriculture and human medicine (Goosens et al. 2005). Antimicrobial resistance is not a new phenomenon, as practitioners early as 1954 documented an increased prevalence of antibiotic-resistant staphylococci in a Philadelphia hospital (Bondi et al. 1954). Today, antimicrobial resistance is a critical global public health threat. It is estimated that the costs due to antimicrobial resistance will amount to $100 trillion by 2050 (O'Neill 2016). Eliminating the non-therapeutic use of antibiotics in animal agriculture and aquaculture and the judicious use of antimicrobials in human medicine will reduce antimicrobial resistance and the likelihood of emerging multidrug-resistance strains (DANMAP 2015; Dorado-Carcia et al. 2015).

8.4.4 *TRANS* FATS AND FOOD PROCESSING

Trans fats, or *trans* fatty acids, are created when hydrogen atoms are added to liquid oils, a process known as hydrogenation, and the liquid oils turn into solid fats (FDA 2017b). These partially hydrogenated oils (PHO), or *trans* fats, naturally occur in meat and dairy products, but are most often manufactured ingredients for processed and packaged food products. The most common *trans* fats used by food manufacturers are partially hydrogenated cottonseed oil and partially hydrogenated soybean oil. *Trans* fats are less expensive compared to butter or lard and they increase flavor stability and shelf life in processed foods. The most common foods that contain *trans* fat are margarine and vegetable shortening, but they may also be found in baked goods, frostings, pies, crackers, cookies, chips, snack foods, frozen pizza, and salad dressings.

The three most recent editions of the *Dietary Guidelines* have recommended that Americans limit their consumption of *trans* fat due to the association between the consumption of trans fat and elevated low-density lipoproteins (LDL) cholesterol, which increases risk for CVD (USDHHS and USDA 2015; USDA and USDHHS 2010; USDHHS and USDA 2005). Because of the cardiovascular health risks associated with *trans* fat (IOM 2002), the U.S. FDA required food manufacturers to include *trans* fat content on the Nutrition Facts Label of packaged foods (FDA 2003). In 2015, the FDA announced that *trans* fats are no longer Generally Recognized as Safe (GRAS) under any condition in food products (FDA 2015) and required food manufacturers to phase out trans fat in their products by June 2018 (FDA 2016c). The WHO also recommended significantly reducing or eliminating *trans* fats from the food supply (Uauy et al. 2009).

The impact of these federal actions has resulted in the decreased use of *trans* fat in the global food supply; reduced consumption of *trans* fats altogether (Restrepo 2017)—and a projected healthcare savings (FDA 2015). Many European countries have phased out *trans* fats in their food systems (WHO 2015). Farmers and vegetable oil producers have begun to produce healthier oils. Food processors have reformulated many products, and in 2015 more than 86% of *trans* fats in foods and beverages were removed (Grocery Manufacturers Association [GMA] 2015). Researchers studying blood plasma levels of *trans* fat found American adults reduced their intake of *trans* fats by more than 52% between 1999 and 2010 (Restrepo 2017). The study also found that there were positive outcomes on blood pressure, LDL and HDL cholesterol, and triglycerides (Restrepo 2017) which could further decrease the economic and disease burden of CVD. The FDA estimates the expected health gains of of removing *trans* fat from the food supply is $130 billion over 20 years (FDA 2015).

8.4.5 BISPHENOL A (BPA) AND FOOD PACKAGING

While Chapter 5 delineated the impact of disposable plastics on the natural environment and biodiversity, there are also numerous synthetic compounds used in food and beverage containers. In the last several decades, there has been growing concern of how these compounds may interact with foods and impact human health. Researchers are examining how packaging materials may migrate or leach into food; how they are metabolized and/or bio-accumulate in the body—and their potential risk of physiological impacts.

An example of such a compound is BPA. Since the 1960s, BPA has been used as a chemical to manufacture polycarbonate—a hard, clear plastic most commonly used in beverage bottles—and as a protective lining inside metal food and beverage cans and also jar caps. BPA is also common in kitchenware and household storage containers. Exposure to BPA can come in the form of ingestion, inhalation, and through the skin (FDA 2016d). When ingested, BPA is metabolized in the liver and most is excreted in the urine. BPA is ubiquitous across products in the home, workplace, and schools where regular exposure may lead to bio-accumulation. This is of greater concern to infants and children due to the potential impact of BPA on the early stages of growth and development (Nachman et al. 2014).

Studies have found that individuals who consume a diet consisting of canned and packaged foods have higher levels of BPA metabolites in their blood, urine, and breast milk as compared to those whose diets consist of fresh, non-packaged foods (Rudel et al. 2011; Halden 2010). Children and adolescents have higher urinary levels of BPA compared to adults (Halden 2010). Researchers have determined that BPA disrupts the functionality of estrogen receptors and may be linked to female and male infertility, early puberty, breast and prostate cancer, polycystic ovary syndrome, and other reproductive disruptions (Konieczna et al. 2015; Halden 2010).

The FDA must approve the use of any substances that may migrate from packaging into food, and be identified as an indirect food additive or food contact substance

(FDA 2016d). The FDA's food contact regulations and notification program assesses the likely migration from the packaging material to assure that any migration to food occurs at safe levels. Following a review of 300 studies published between 2009 and 2013, the FDA concluded that BPA is quickly metabolized once ingested and does not accumulate in blood or tissues, including fetal tissues (FDA 2014). However, the EPA addressed the variability and limitations across studies, and concluded that more high-quality controlled studies are warranted (FDA 2014).

8.4.6   RED AND PROCESSED MEAT AND FOOD CONSUMPTION

As previously mentioned, most Americans fall short of consuming a diet that aligns with the *Dietary Guidelines for Americans* (Figure 8.2). Of the protein subgroups, Americans consume at or above recommended levels of meat, fish, and poultry, especially adolescent boys and men (USDHHS and USDA 2015). Meat, fish, and poultry provide protein and essential nutrients such as iron to the diet. However, they also contribute saturated fat and sodium to the diet. According to Daniel et al. (2011), total meat consumption has continued to rise in the U.S. and globally. Although there has been an increase in poultry consumption and a decrease in beef consumption (ERS 2017b), 58% of the total meat consumed in the U.S. is red meat and 22% is processed meat (Daniel et al. 2011). Red meat includes beef, pork, lamb, veal, goat, and non-bird game such as venison, bison, and elk (USDHHS and USDA 2015). Processed meat includes meat, poultry, or seafood products preserved by smoking, curing, or salting, or addition of chemical preservatives (e.g., bacon, sausage, hot dogs, sandwich meat, packaged ham, pepperoni, and salami) (DGAC 2015).

Dietary patterns that have higher intakes of red and processed meats increase the risk of obesity, diabetes, CVD, and certain cancers (DGAC 2015; Micha et al. 2010). Additional evidence suggests an increased risk of age-related cognitive impairment and depression as well (DGAC 2015). Because of the related burden of chronic disease, the 2015 DGAC recommended a healthy dietary pattern low in red and processed meats (DGAC 2015). According to the National Cancer Institute, colorectal cancer is the fourth most common cancer diagnosed in the U.S. (NCI 2017b) and the second leading cause of cancer death in the U.S. (NCHS 2017). In 2014, there were 38.3 new cases of colon and rectal cancer per 100,000 people with 14.1 deaths per 100,000 people.

In 2015, the IARC reviewed the association between the consumption of processed and red meat and cancer. They classified processed meat as a Group 1 human carcinogen based on sufficient evidence that the consumption of processed meat causes colorectal cancer in humans. The IARC further concluded that the "consumption of red meat as probably carcinogenic to humans (Group 2A), based on limited evidence that the consumption of red meat causes cancer in humans and strong mechanistic evidence supporting a carcinogenic effect" (IARC 2015a; IARC 2015b).

8.5   CONCLUSION

The science of food systems and chronic disease offers a multitude of opportunities to understand the risks to human health. This is in addition to an equally complex set of indicators to measure the ecological, social, and economic health impacts of food systems. The nutritional quality of U.S. diets falls short of the *Dietary Guidelines for Americans* and directly contributes to the epidemic rates of chronic disease in both adults and children alike—not to mention their subsequent healthcare costs. This is further compounded by the widening gap between the increasing homogeneity of agriculture and the food and nutrients needed for a healthy dietary pattern. When decisions are made across food supply chains—from food production to food consumption—the intended and unintended consequences must be critically examined and rectified.

REFERENCES

Acquavella, J., B. Alexander, J. Mandel, C. Gustin, B. Baker, P. Chapman, and M. Bleeke. 2004. Glyphosate biomonitoring for farmers and their families: Results from the farm family Exposure study. *Environ Health Perspective* 112 (3): 321–326.

Agricultural Marketing Service (AMS). Pesticide data program. Last modified on November 10, 2016. https://www.ams.usda.gov/datasets/pdp (Accessed September 12, 2017).

Aguilar, J., G. Gramig, J. Hendrickson, D. Archer, F. Forcella, and M. Liebig. 2015. Crop species diversity changes in the United States: 1978–2012. *PLoS One* 10 (8): e0136580. https://doi.org/10.1371/journal.pone.0136580 (Accessed August 14, 2018).

American Diabetes Association (ADA). 2015. The economic costs of diabetes in the U.S. in 2012. Last modified June 22, 2015. http://www.diabetes.org/advocacy/news-events/cost-of-diabetes.html (Accessed July 18, 2017).

American Heart Association (AHA). 2017. Heart disease and stroke statistics – 2017 update. A Report from the American Heart Association, 2017. *Circulation* 135: e146–e603. http://circ.ahajournals.org/content/135/10/e146 (Accessed August 16, 2017).

Aminov, R. 2010. A brief history of the antibiotic era: Lessons learned and challenges for the future. *Frontiers in Microbiology* 1: 1–7.

Antoniou, M., M. Habib, C. Howard, R. Jennings, C. Leifert, R. Nodari, C. Robinson, and J. Fagan. 2012. Teratogenic effects of glyphosate-based herbicides: Divergence of regulatory decisions from scientific evidence. *Journal of Environmental and Analytical Toxicology* S4: 1–13. doi:10.4172/2161-0525.S4-006.

Bates, L., T. Councell, M. Kelly, S. Purnell, L. Robin, C. Liang, M. Wehr, C. Sack, X. Zhao, K. Atkinson, and R. Lovell. 2014. *Pesticide Residue Monitoring Program Fiscal Year 2014 Pesticide Report*. Washington, DC: U.S. Food and Drug Administration. https://www.fda.gov/downloads/Food/FoodborneIllnessContaminants/Pesticides/UCM546325.pdf (Accessed September 12, 2018).

Beckie, H. 2011. Herbicide-resistant weed management: Focus on glyphosate. *Pest Management Science* 67(9):1037–1048.

Benbrook, C. 2016. Trends in glyphosate herbicide use in the United States and globally. *Environmental Sciences Europe* 28 (1): 1–15. https://www.ncbi.nlm.nih.gov/pmc/articles/PMC5044953/pdf/12302_2016_Article_70.pdf (Accessed September 12, 2017).

Bentley, J. 2017. *U.S. Trends in Food Availability and a Dietary Assessment of Loss-Adjusted Food Availability, 1970–2014*, EIB-166. Washington, DC: U.S. Department of Agriculture, Economic Research Service. https://www.ers.usda.gov/webdocs/publications/82220/eib-166.pdf?v=42762 (Accessed August 14, 2017).

Berti, P., and A. Jones. 2013. Biodiversity's contribution to dietary diversity. Magnitude, meaning and measurement. In *Diversifying Food and Diets, Using Agricultural Biodiversity to Improve Nutrition and Health*, edited by Jessica Fanzo, Danny Hunter, Teresa Borelli, and Federico Mattei, 190–191. New York, NY: Routledge.

Bondi, A., F. Pfaff, E. Free, and R. Swerlick. 1954. Public health aspects of the development of antibiotic-resistance staphylococci. *American Journal of Public Health* 44:
789–793.

Brower, C., et al. 2017. The prevalence of extended-spectrum beta-lactamase-producing multi-
drug-resistance *Escherichia coli* in poultry chickens and variation according to farming
practice in Punjab India. *Environmental Health Perspectives* 25: 077015-1–077015-10.

Buzby, J., H. Farah Wells, and G. Vocke. 2006. *Possible Implications for U.S. Agriculture
from Adoption of Select Dietary Guidelines*. Washington, DC: U.S. Department of
Agriculture, Economic Research Service.

Cawley, J. and C. Meyerhoefer. 2012. The medical care costs of obesity: An instrumental
variables approach. *Journal of Health Economics* 31 (1): 219–230.

Centers for Disease Control and Prevention (CDC). 2010. CDC newsroom press release.
Number of Americans with diabetes projected to double or triple by 2050. Last
modified October 22, 2010. https://www.cdc.gov/media/pressrel/2010/r101022.html
(Accessed September 11, 2017).

Centers for Disease Control and Prevention (CDC). 2013. *Antibiotic Resistant Threats in the
United States, 2013*. Washington, DC: U.S. Health and Human Services. https://www.
cdc.gov/drugresistance/pdf/ar-threats-2013-508.pdf (Accessed July 14, 2017).

Centers for Disease Control and Prevention (CDC). 2014. *Outpatient Antibiotic
Prescriptions—United States, 2014*. Washington, DC: U.S. Health and Human
Services.   http://www.cdc.gov/getsmart/community/pdfs/annual-reportsummary_
2014.pdf (Accessed July 14, 2017).

Centers for Disease Control and Prevention (CDC). 2015. About the national health and nutrition examination survey. Last modified November 6, 2015. https://www.cdc.gov/nchs/
nhanes/about_nhanes.htm (Accessed August 14, 2017).

Center for Nutrition Policy and Promotion (CNPP). Healthy eating index. Last modified November
2016. https://www.cnpp.usda.gov/healthyeatingindex (Accessed August 15, 2017).

Daniel, C., A. Cross, C. Koebnick, and R. Sinha. 2011. Trends in meat consumption in the
USA. *Public Health Nutrition* 14 (4): 575–583.

DANMAP 2015. *Use of Antimicrobial Agents and Occurrence of Antimicrobial Resistance
in Bacteria from Food Animals, Food and Humans in Denmark*. ISSN 1600-2032.
http://www.danmap.org/~/media/Projekt%20sites/Danmap/DANMAP%20reports/
DANMAP%20%202015/DANMAP%202015.ashx (Accessed September 11, 2017).

Davis, D., M. Epp, and H. Riordan. 2004. Changes in USDA food composition data for
43 garden crops, 1950 to 1999. *Journal of the American College of Nutrition* 23 (6):
669–682.

De Roos, A., A. Blair, J. Rusiecki, J. Hoppin, M. Svec, M. Dosemeci, D. Sandler, and M.
Alavanja. 2005. Cancer incidence among glyphosate-exposed pesticide applicators in
the Agricultural Health Study. *Environmental Health Perspective* 113 (1): 49–54.

Dietary Guidelines Advisory Committee (DGAC). 2015. *Scientific Report of the 2015
Dietary Guidelines Advisory Committee. Advisory Report to the Secretary of Health
and Human Services and the Secretary of Agriculture*. Washington, DC: Government
Printing Office.

Dorado-García, A., H. Graveland, M. Bos, K. Verstappen, B. Van Cleef, J. Kluytmans, J.
Wagenaar, and D. Heederik. 2015. Effects of reducing antimicrobial use and applying a cleaning and disinfection program in veal calf farming: Experiences from an
intervention study to control livestock-associated MRSA. *PLoS ONE* 10 (8): e0135826.
doi:10.1371/journal. pone.0135826.

Economic Research Service (ERS). 2017a. Food expenditures. *Data Products*. Last modified August 8, 2017a. https://www.ers.usda.gov/data-products/food-expenditures.aspx
(Accessed July 17, 2017).

Economic Research Service (ERS). 2017b. Food availability (per capita) data system. Interactive charts and highlights. *Data Products*. Last modified July 26, 2017b. https://www.ers.usda.gov/data-products/food-availability-per-capita-data-system/interactive-charts-and-highlights/#selected (Accessed August 1, 2017).

Economic Research Service (ERS). 2017c. New products. Food Markets Prices. Last modified April 5, 2017c. https://www.ers.usda.gov/topics/food-markets-prices/processing-marketing/new-products/ (Accessed August 18, 2017).

Economic Research Service (ERS). 2017d Biotechnology overview. *Farm Practices Management*. Last modified July 12, 2017. https://www.ers.usda.gov/topics/farm-practices-management/biotechnology/ (Accessed September 12, 2017).

Finkelstein, E., J. Trogdon, J. Cohen, and W. Dietz. 2009. Annual medical spending attributable to obesity: Payer- and service-specific estimates. *Health Affairs* 28 (5): w822–831.

Fleming-Dutra, K., A. L. Hersh, D. J. Shapiro, M. Bartoces, E. A. Enns, T. M. File, J. A. Finkelstein et al. 2016. Prevalence of inappropriate antibiotic prescriptions among US ambulatory care visits, 2010–2011. *JAMA* 315 (17): 1864–1873.

Food and Agriculture Organization (FAO). 2004. What is happening to agrobiodiversity? ftp://ftp.fao.org/docrep/fao/007/y5609e/y5609e00.pdf (Accessed August 18, 2017).

Food and Drug Administration (FDA). 2003. Food labeling: Trans. 68 FR 41433. 21 CFR 101. *Federal Register*. Docket Number: 94P-0036, July 11, 2003. https://www.federalregister.gov/documents/2003/07/11/03-17525/food-labeling-trans (Accessed August 14, 2017).

Food and Drug Administration (FDA). 2014. *Memorandum. Final Report for the Review of Literature and Data on BPA*. June 6, 2014. https://www.fda.gov/downloads/Food/IngredientsPackagingLabeling/FoodAdditivesIngredients/UCM424011.pdf (Accessed August 9, 2017).

Food and Drug Administration (FDA). 2015. Final determination regarding partially hydrogenated oils. 80 FR 34650. *Federal Register*. Docket Number: FDA-2013-N-1317. Last modified June 17, 2015. https://www.federalregister.gov/documents/2015/06/17/2015-14883/final-determination-regarding-partially-hydrogenated-oils (Accessed August 14, 2017).

Food and Drug Administration (FDA). 2016a. Sodium reduction. Food Additive Ingredients. Last modified October 7, 2016a. https://www.fda.gov/food/ingredientspackaginglabeling/foodadditivesingredients/ucm253316.htm (Accessed August 15, 2017).

Food and Drug Administration (FDA). 2016b. *Summary Report on Antimicrobials Sold or Distributed for Use in Food-Producing Animals*. Washington, DC: U.S. Department of Health and Human Services.

Food and Drug Administration (FDA). 2016c. Food labeling: Revision of the nutrition and supplemental facts labels. 21 CFR Part 101. *Federal Register*. Docket Number: FDA-2012-N-1210. Last modified May 27, 2016c. https://www.gpo.gov/fdsys/pkg/FR-2016-05-27/pdf/2016-11867.pdf (Accessed August 14, 2017).

Food and Drug Administration (FDA). 2016d. Bispehnol A (BPA): Use in food contact application, 2014. Public Health Focus. Last modified February 5, 2016d. https://www.fda.gov/newsevents/publichealthfocus/ucm064437.htm (Accessed August 9, 2017).

Food and Drug Administration (FDA). 2017a. Pesticide residue monitoring program. Foodborne Illness Contaminants. Last modified September 11, 2017a. https://www.fda.gov/Food/FoodborneIllnessContaminants/Pesticides/ucm200679.htm (Accessed September 12, 2017).

Food and Drug Administration (FDA). 2017b. Trans fat. Food. Last modified May 10, 2017b. https://www.fda.gov/food/ucm292278.htm (Accessed September 11, 2017).

Food Marketing Institute (FMI). 2017. Supermarket facts. Our Research. https://www.fmi.org/our-research/supermarket-facts (Accessed August 18, 2017).

Frison, E., J. Cherfas, and T. Hodgkin. 2011. Agricultural biodiversity is essential for a sustainable improvement in food and nutrition security. *Sustainability* 3 (1): 238–253.

Fryar, C., M. Carroll, and C. Ogden. 2012. *Prevalence of Obesity Among Children and Adolescents: United States, Trends 1963–1965 Through 2009–2010*. Washington, DC: U.S. Health and Human Services, National Center for Health Statistics.

Gerteis, J., D. Izrael, D. Deitz, L. LeRoy, R. Ricciardi, T. Miller, and J. Basu. *Multiple Chronic Conditions Chartbook*. AHRQ Publications No, Q14-0038. Rockville, MD: US Health and Human Services, Agency for Healthcare Research and Quality, 2014. https://www. ahrq.gov/sites/default/files/wysiwyg/professionals/prevention-chronic-care/decision/ mcc/mccchartbook.pdf (Accessed July 18, 2017).

Goossens, H., M. Ferech, R. Vander Stichele, M. Elseviers, and ESAC Project Group. 2005. Outpatient antibiotic use in Europe and association with resistance: A cross-national database study. *Lancet* 365, 579–587.

Grocery Manufacturers Association (GMA). 2015. GMA petitions FDA to approve low-level uses of partially hydrogenated oils. News Release. August 5, 2015. http://www.gma-online.org/news-events/newsroom/gma-petitions-fda-to-approve-low-level-uses-of-partially-hydrogenated-oils/ (Accessed August 18, 2017).

Halden, R. 2010. Plastics and health risks. *Annual Review of Public Health* 31: 179–194.

Heap, IM. 2014. Global perspective of herbicide-resistant weeds. *Pest Management Science* 70: 1306–1315.

Henderson, A. M., Gervais, J. A., Luukinen, B., Buhl, K., and Stone, D. 2010. Glyphosate General Fact Sheet; National Pesticide Information Center, Oregon State University Extension Services. Reviewed 2015. http://npic.orst.edu/factsheets/glyphogen. html.

Hiza, H., and L. Bente. 2011. *Nutrient Content of the U.S. Food Supply: Developments Between 2000 and 2006*. Home Economics Research Report No. 59. Washington, DC: U.S. Department of Agriculture, Center for Nutrition Policy and Promotion. https:// www.cnpp.usda.gov/sites/default/files/nutrient_content_of_the_us_food_supply/ Final_FoodSupplyReport_2006.pdf (Accessed August 15, 2018).

Howlader, N., A.M. Noone, M. Krapcho D. Miller, K. Bishop, C.L. Kosary, M. Yu, J. Ruhl, et al. (eds.). 2017. *SEER Cancer Statistics Review, 1975–2014*. Bethesda, MD: US Health and Human Services, National Cancer Institute. Last modified April 2017. https:// seer.cancer.gov/csr/1975_2014/ (Accessed August 14, 2017).

Hunter, D. and J. Fanzo. 2013. Introduction. In *Diversifying Food and Diets, Using Agricultural Biodiversity to Improve Nutrition and Health*, edited by Jessica Fanzo, Danny Hunter, Teresa Borelli, Federico Mattei, 1–5. New York, NY: Routledge.

Imperatore, G., J. Boyle, R. Thompson, D. Case, D. Dabelea, R. Hamman, J. Lawrence, et al. 2012. Projections of Type 1 and Type 2 diabetes burden in the U.S. population aged <20 years through 2050. *Diabetes Care* 35 (12): 2515–2520. http://care.diabetesjournals. org/content/35/12/2515.short (Accessed July 18, 2017).

Institute of Medicine (IOM) and the National Research Council (NRC). 2015. *A Framework for Assessing Effects of the Food System*. Washington, DC: The National Academies Press.

IOM of the National Academies. 2002. *Dietary Reference Intakes for Energy, Carbohydrate, Fiber, Fat, Fatty Acids, Cholesterol, Protein, and Amino Acids*. Washington, DC: Food and Nutrition Board.

IOM of the National Academies. 2013. *Sodium Intake in Populations: Assessment of Evidence*, edited by Brian Strom, Ann Yaktine, and Maria Oria. Washington, DC: The National Academies Press. http://www.nap.edu/openbook.php?record_id=18311 (Accessed August 14, 2017).

International Agency for Research on Cancer (IARC) Monograph Working Group. 2015a. Carcinogenicity of consumption of red and processed meat. *The Lancet* 16:1599–1160. http://www.thelancet.com/journals/lanonc/article/PIIS1470-2045(15)00444-1/fulltext (Accessed August 9, 2017).

IARC. 2015b. IARC monographs evaluate consumption of red meat and processed meat. Press Release. October 2015b. https://www.iarc.fr/en/media-centre/pr/2015/pdfs/ pr240_E.pdf (Accessed August 9, 2017).

IARC. 2016. *IARC Monographs on the Evaluation of Carcinogenic Risk to Humans. Some Organophosphate Insecticides and Herbicides. Glyphosate.* Lyon, France: World Health Organization. Last modified August 11, 2016. http://monographs.iarc.fr/ENG/ Monographs/vol112/mono112-10.pdf (Accessed September 12, 2017).

Konieczna, A., A. Rutkowska, and D. Rachon. 2015. Health risk of exposure to bisphenol A (BPA). *National Institute Public Health* 66 (1): 5–11.

Landers, T., B. Cohen, T. Wittum, and E. Larson. 2012. A review of antibiotic use in food animals: Perspective, policy and potential. *Public Health Reports* 127: 4–22.

Lu, C., K. Toepel, R. Irish, R. Fenske, D. Barr, and R. Bravo. 2006. Organic diets significantly lower children's dietary exposure to organophosphorus pesticides. *Environmental Health Perspective* 114 (2): 260–263.

Marles, R. 2017. Mineral nutrient composition of vegetables, fruits and grains: The context of reports of apparent historical declines. *Journal of Food Composition and Analysis* 56: 93–103.

Mayer, A. 1997. Historical changes in the mineral content of fruits and vegetables. *British Food Journal* 99 (6): 207–211.

Meek, R., V. Hrushi, and L. Piddock. 2015. Nonmedical uses of antibiotics: Time to restrict their use? *PLOS*. https://doi.org/10.1371/journal.pbio.1002266.

Micha, R., S. Wallace, and D. Mozzaffarian.2010. Red and processed meat consumption and risk of incident coronary heart disease, stroke, and diabetes: A systematic review and meta-analysis. *Circulation* 121 (21): 2271–2283.

Miller, P., J. Reedy, S. Kirkpatrick, and S. Krebs-Smith. 2015. The United States food supply is not consistent with dietary guidance: Evidence from an evaluation using the healthy eating index-2010. *Journal of the Academy of Nutrition and Dietetics* 115 (1): 95–100.

Myers, S, et al. 2014. Increasing CO_2 threatens human nutrition. *Nature* 510: 139–142.

Nachman, R.M., J. Hartle, P. Lees, and J. Groopman. 2014. Early life metabolism of Bisphenol A: A systematic review of the literature. *Current Environmental Health Reports* 1 (1): 90–100.

National Agricultural Statistics Service (NASS). 2012 *Census of Agriculture: United States Summary and State Data. Volume 1.* Washington, DC: U.S. Department of Agriculture, 2014. https://www.agcensus.usda.gov/Publications/2012/Full_Report/ Volume_1,_Chapter_1_US/usv1.pdf (Accessed August 18, 2017).

National Cancer Institute (NCI). 2017a. Cancer prevalence and cost of care projections. http:// costprojections.cancer.gov/ (Accessed July 18, 2017).

National Cancer Institute (NCI). 2017b. Surveillance, epidemiology, and end results program. Cancer stat facts: Colon and rectum cancer. https://seer.cancer.gov/statfacts/html/col-orect.html (Accessed August 9, 2017).

National Cancer Institute (NCI). 2017c. Colon and rectum cancer. Number and new cases and deaths per 1000,000 people (all races, males and females), age-adjusted. https://seer. cancer.gov/statfacts/html/ld/colorect.html (Accessed August 9, 2017c).

National Center for Health Statistics (NCHS). 2008. *Prevalence of Overweight, Obesity and Extreme Obesity Among Adults: United States, Trends 1976–80 through 2005–2006.* Hyattsville, MD: U.S. Health and Human Services, Centers for Disease Control and Prevention.

NCHS. 2017. *Health, United States, 2016: With Chartbook on Long-term Trends in Health.* Hyattsville, MD: U.S. Health and Human Services, Centers for Disease Control and Prevention. https://www.cdc.gov/nchs/data/hus/hus16.pdf#019 (Accessed July 25, 2017).

National Research Council (NRC). 1993. *Pesticides in the Diets of Infants and Children.* Washington, DC: National Academy Press.

Office of Pesticide Programs (OPP). 2000. *Available Information on Assessing Exposure from Pesticides in Food.* Washington, DC: U.S. Environmental Protection Agency. https://www.regulations.gov/document?D=EPA-HQ-OPP-2007-0780-0001 (Accessed September 12, 2017).

O'Hara, J.K. 2013. *The $11 Trillion Reward. How Simple Dietary Changes Can Save Lives and Money, and How We Get There.* Washington, DC: Union of Concerned Scientists.

O'Neill, J. 2016. *Tackling Drug-Resistant Infections Globally: Final Report and Recommendations 2016.* United Kingdom: Wellcome Trust, and HM Government.

Restrepo, B. 2017. Further decline of *trans* fatty acids levels among US adults between 1999–2000 and 2009–2010. *American Journal of Public Health* 107 (1): 156–158.

Rudel, R., J. Gray, C. Engel, T. Rawsthorne, R. Dodson, J. Ackerman, J. Rizzo, J. Nudelman, and J. Brody. 2011. Food packaging and Bisphenol A and Bis(2-Ethyhexyl) Phthalate exposure: Findings from a dietary intervention. *Environmental Health Perspectives* 119 (7): 914–920.

Scribner, E., W. Battaglin, R Gillion, and M. Meyer. 2007. *Concentrations of Glyphosate, its Degradation Product, Aminomethylphosphonic Acid, and Glufosinate in Ground- and Surface-water, Rainfall, and Soil Samples Collected in the United States, 2001-06.* Washington, DC: U.S. Geological Survey Scientific Investigations Report.

Transparency Market Research. 2014. Glyphosate market for genetically modified and conventional crops – Industry analysis, size, share, growth, trends and forecast 2013–2019. *Glyphosate Market.* Last modified February 11, 2014. http://www.transparencymarket-research.com/glyphosate-market.html (Accessed September 12, 2017).

Uauy, R., A. Aro, R. Clarke, R. Chafoorunissa, M. L'Abbe, D. Mozzaffarian, M. Skeaff, S. Stender, and M. Tavella. 2009. WHO scientific update on *trans* fatty acids: Summary and conclusions. *European Journal of Clinical Nutrition* 63:S68–S75.

United States Geological Survey (USGS). Pesticide national synthesis project. Estimated annual agriculture pesticide use - Glyphosate. Last modified September 11, 2017. https://water.usgs.gov/nawqa/pnsp/usage/maps/show_map.php?year=2015&map=GLYPHOSATE&hilo=L&disp=Glyphosate (Accessed September 12, 2017).

U.S. Department of Agriculture (USDA) and U.S. Department of Health and Human Services (USDHHS). 2010. *Dietary Guidelines for Americans, 2010.* 7th Edition, Washington, DC: U.S. Government Printing Office.

U.S. Department of Commerce (USDC). 1954. *United States Census of Agriculture. Volume II General Report.* Washington, DC: U.S. Department of Commerce. http://usda.mannlib.cornell.edu/usda/AgCensusImages/1954/02/01/1954-02-01.pdf (Accessed August 18, 2017).

U.S. Department of Health and Human Services (USDHHS). Healthy People 2020: Physical Activity. https://www.healthypeople.gov/2020/topics-objectives/topic/physical-activity (Accessed July 24, 2017).

U.S. Department of Health and Human Services (USDHHS) and U.S. Department of Agriculture (USDA). 2005. *Dietary Guidelines for Americans.* 6th Edition, Washington, DC: U.S. Government Printing Office.

U.S. Department of Health and Human Services (USDHHS) and U.S. Department of Agriculture (USDA). December 2015. *2015–2020 Dietary Guidelines for Americans.* 8th edition. Washington, DC: Government Printing Office.

U.S. Department of the Interior (USDI). 1902. *Agriculture. Part 1. Farms, Livestock, and Animal Products. Twelfth Census of the United States, Taken in the Year 1900.* Washington, DC: Census Office. http://usda.mannlib.cornell.edu/usda/AgCensusImag es/1900/05/01/1835/33398096v5.pdf (Accessed August 18, 2017).

U.S. Environmental Protection Agency (USEPA). 1993. *Re-registration Eligibility Decision (RED) Glyphosate. EPA-738-R-93-014.* Washington, DC: U.S. Environmental Protection Agencyhttps://archive.epa.gov/pesticides/reregistration/web/pdf/glyphosate. pdf (Accessed September 12, 2017).

U.S. Environmental Protection Agency (USEPA). 2009. *Glyphosate Final Work Plan (FWP) Registration Review Case No. 0178.* Washington, DC: U.S. Environmental Protection Agencyhttps://www.regulations.gov/document?D=EPA-HQ-OPP-2009-0361-0042 (Accessed September 12, 2017).

U.S. Environmental Protection Agency (USEPA). 2017. Assessing human health risk from pesticide. Pesticide Science and Assessing Pesticide Risks. Last modified August 31, 2017. https://www.epa.gov/pesticide-science-and-assessing-pesticide-risks/assessing-human-health-risk-pesticides (Accessed September 12, 2017).

Ward, B., J. Schiller, and R. Goodman. 2014. Multiple chronic conditions among US adults: A 2012 update. *Preventing Chronic Disease* 11: E62.

World Health Organization (WHO). 2015. Eliminating trans fats in Europe. Last modified September 21, 2015. http://www.euro.who.int/en/health-topics/disease-prevention/nutrition/news/news/2015/09/eliminating-trans-fats-in-europe (Accessed August 19, 2017).

WHO. 2016a. Obesity and overweight fact sheet. Media Centre Fact Sheets. Last modified June 2016a. http://www.who.int/mediacentre/factsheets/fs311/en/ (Accessed July 27, 2017).

WHO. 2016b. Antimicrobial resistance. *Media Centre Fact Sheets.* Last modified September 2016b. http://www.who.int/mediacentre/factsheets/fs194/en/ (Accessed July 14, 2017).

WHO. 2016c. Food safety: Frequently asked questions. *Food Safety.* Last modified May 27, 2016c. http://www.who.int/foodsafety/faq/en/ (Accessed September 12, 2017).

WHO. 2017a. Noncommunicable diseases. *Fact Sheets.* Last modified June 2017a. http://www.who.int/mediacentre/factsheets/fs355/en/ (Accessed July 18, 2017).

WHO. 2017b. Cancer fact sheet. *Media Centre Fact Sheet.* Last modified February 2017b. http://www.who.int/mediacentre/factsheets/fs297/en/ (Accessed July 27, 2017).

WHO. 2017c. Media centre. Pesticide residue in food. *Media Centre Fact Sheets.* Last modified July 2017c. http://www.who.int/mediacentre/factsheets/pesticide-residues-food/en/ (Accessed September 12, 2017).

9 Popular Foods and Biodiversity Loss

Jessica Jones-Hughes, Mildred L. Alvarado,
Cristina Liberati, Carly Kadlec, Tobias Lunt, Dary
Goodrich, Leif Rawson-Ahern, and Ravdeep Jaidka

CONTENTS

9.1 INTRODUCTION

When the first signs of domesticated agriculture began to sprout around 12,000 years ago, there was a deep and wide abandonment of hunting and gathering traditions as communities experienced the benefit of planned, efficient, and intensive food production. The simple technique of seeding and harvesting plants to augment wild-growing food marks one of the most significant transformations in the evolution of human culture, triggering the Neolithic age, with the creation of permanent cities and civilizations, and spurring immense population growth (Ember 2014; National Geographic 2016; Barker 2006). The change from hunting and gathering to domesticated agriculture also shifted biodiversity dramatically (Zimmerer et al. 2016).

139

Habitat change is the most important driver of biodiversity, and during the Neolithic age the Earth first experienced a conversion of forests and biodiverse areas to cropland. Through this shift that began in the Neolithic age and has continued into present day, it is estimated that an extraordinary array of plant and animal species that once lived on the planet are now extinct (Miller et al. 2012).

Today, there are few hunting and gathering communities left. The majority of communities, even in the most remote villages—take part in an interconnected global food system. An extensive network of shipping and transit technologies allow us to enjoy even the most perishable fruits and vegetables thousands of miles from their original home (National Geographic 2016). Historically, the biodiversity of food systems varied greatly from one region to another. Today, five cereal crops provide 60% of human energy intake worldwide (FAO 2017).

While we have access to a larger network of food than ever before, we are also more physically and culturally disconnected from the foods that nourish us daily. In the U.S., for example, the sight of grocery store aisles lined with inexpensive, packaged food is more familiar than fields, forests, or farms. The rapid loss of agricultural knowledge over the last 100 years has led to a severing of the link between the consumers of food and the people, places, and growing practices that produce it (Lowder et al. 2016). As the human population has become more disconnected from food and where it comes from, large companies have taken control and crafted a consolidated model of food production and distribution. As the food system continues to consolidate, a few companies have come to control most of the supply of food on the grocery shelf. The research by Philip Howard at Michigan State University illustrates the consolidation in the food system; for instance, 85% of all soybean production is controlled by four multinational corporations (James et al. 2012).

Alongside the consolidation of food purveyors has come a dwindling in the number of animal and plant species. Plant genetic diversity has decreased in part due to farmers worldwide who have abandoned their multiple local varieties and replaced them with genetically uniform, high-yielding varieties (FAO 2017). In addition, the replacement of small-scale farms with large, monoculture farms has greatly accelerated. Over the last 100 years, the amount of arable land in agriculture production has remained constant, yet the number of individual farms has diminished (USDA 2012).

Small-scale farmers are key allies in the preservation of biodiversity and agro-biodiversity globally (Zimmerer et al. 2016; FAO 2017). The pressure that farmers face to adapt to an inexpensive, efficient food system means that small holders are unable to sustain their farms and livelihoods when competing with large-scale farms (Lowder et al. 2016). As of 2016, 84% of the world's farmers are small holders, but together they operate only 12% of the world's agricultural land (Lowder et al. 2016). The replacement of small-scale farms by large-scale agriculture in most commodities has meant immense environmental degradation and loss of biodiversity (Lowder et al. 2016; State of the World 2011; Zimmerer et al. 2016). "Improving food security, reducing poverty and improving sustainability over the coming decades will be inextricably linked to the development of strategies that are relevant and appropriate to small-scale farmers" (FAO 2017).

This chapter will illustrate some of the challenges in the modern day agricultural system through the lens of several popular foods—bananas, cacao, coffee, sugar, palm oil, and tea—and an "emerging food"—avocados. These foods illuminate the detrimental impact of the current food system to biodiversity. In order to mitigate the loss of biodiversity and the ongoing consolidation of land, global agricultural systems must change. To be successful in the revitalization of the natural environment, we must preserve, nurture, and expand the integration of biodiversity through small-scale food production.

9.2 BANANA PRODUCTION

Bananas are the most consumed fruit in the world, followed by apples (FAOSTAT 2017). According to the Food Agricultural Organization (2014), world banana production reached 114 million tons, with India as the largest banana-producing country in the world at 29.8 million tons and China as the second largest producing country at 11.7 million tons (FAOSTAT 2017). In 2014, the U.S. was the world's largest banana importer, importing 4.5 million tons—a 10% increase from 2010. In 2013, the exported banana reached 20 million tons with Ecuador being the largest exporter in the world at 5.3 million tons (FAOSTAT 2017). Costa Rica, Colombia, Guatemala, and Honduras are some of the largest exporters from the Latin American region. Central America was the second largest exporting region in the world, followed by Colombia. Hence, more than 50% of the world's exported banana came from some of the poorest countries in Latin America. The banana industry depends on those countries whose environmental regulations, social conditions, and economic infrastructures are highly vulnerable to manipulation. Bananas must be grown in an area where temperatures range from 18.5°–35.5°C (65.3°–95.9°F). Humid tropical areas are ideal locations to obtain this temperature or microclimate.

Only one type of banana species is grown and traded internationally now: the Cavendish. Prior to that, the fungal root infection Panama disease devastated the previously prevalent Gros Michel variety of banana (Koeppel 2008). The Cavendish was created to resist Panama disease caused by strains of a soil fungus called *Fusarium oxysporum f. sp.cubense (Foc)*. Because bananas generally exist in a plantation style monoculture agricultural systems, the plants are highly susceptible to pests, fungi, and diseases. As a result, large amounts of insecticides, fungicides, and other pesticides are applied in order to maintain plant health and protect them from potential threats. As pests and diseases grow stronger and more resistant to pesticides, even more harmful pesticides must be applied. Pesticides can also contaminate waterways and groundwater as well as entire ecosystems and are concerning with regard to human health (Martinelli and Filoso 2008).

Some Asian banana-producing countries such as Indonesia, Malaysia, and the Philippines are now suffering from the disease and, as a result, the Cavendish is disappearing in those countries (Koeppel 2008). While Panama disease has not yet been documented in Latin American countries, the banana leaf disease Sigatoka Negra is a serious phytopathological problem threatening the crop (Koeppel 2008).

Monoculture agricultural systems are a way of producing large volumes of product at the lowest possible cost. These systems weigh heavily on the use of natural resources in low-income communities and countries, since these areas have the climate, soil conditions, and cheap labor necessary to produce high volumes of food at a low cost. Large multinational corporations are planting bananas on extensive amounts of land in Central and South America.

Latin American countries are characterized by their cultural diversity and the food produced is determined by the culture and the tropical weather. For example, maize is the staple food in Mexico and Central America as the potato is in the Andean countries. Across cultures, there is a genuine desire to work the land and produce food. While Latin America exports more than 12 million tons of bananas to the global marketplace, it has come at the price of: (1) Devastating the ancestral agricultural system along with economic deprivation to banana workers, (2) environmental degradation, and (3) the destruction of human life due to conflict (El Heraldo 2014). There are still thousands of small-scale banana producers who care for the land with their ancestral practices daily and work cooperatively for the good of the local and global community. Although bananas are not native to Latin American countries, small-scale and community-level banana production can contribute to well-being and ecological care by using local knowledge of the biological and geological processes that are involved in food production. When small-scale farmers grow hundreds of cultivars, the ensuing biodiversity functions as a rampart against disease (Butler 2013).

9.3 CHOCOLATE AND BIODIVERSITY LOSS: THE ENVIRONMENTAL IMPACT OF CACAO PRODUCTION

While it may not always be the first ingredient listed in a chocolate bar, cacao is the most important. Cacao comes from cacao trees, of which the scientific name, *Theobroma cacao*, is often translated to 'food of the gods' (World Cocoa Foundation 2017). The fruit on cacao trees presents in an array of colors from bright green to dark reddish purple, and grows on the branches as well as from the trunk of the tree. The oblong cacao pod contains an average of 40 seeds, each encased in a sweet pulp that is commonly known as *baba* in Latin America. At harvest time, the seeds and *baba* are removed by hand and collected into large piles or boxes. The mixture is then fermented and dried before being bagged for storage and sale.

As seen on the map in Figure 9.1, cacao is grown in countries that fall within 20° of the equator, with 90% still being grown on small family farms (Equal Exchange).

The average size of these farms is 5–10 acres. This crop provides a livelihood for up to 50 million people across the globe (Schmitz et al. 2015). However, cacao farming is a livelihood that is not economically sustainable for the cacao farmer and leaves them impoverished. Most of these farmers live on less than $2 per day (Houston et al. 2012). While cacao may be their primary source of income, they often grow other crops to supplement their income as it is only harvested one or two times per year. One can commonly find bananas, citrus, mangos, avocados, coconuts, and other tropical fruits on a cacao farm.

Traditional or rustic cacao farms often have used shade trees in their farming practices, but the modernization of cacao farming and the use of select genetic varieties has led to a reduction in canopy cover in certain regions. With traditional/rustic agricultural methods, the ground on a cacao farm will be littered generously with

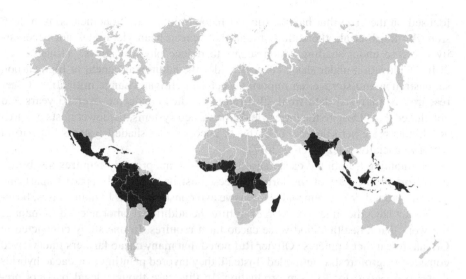

FIGURE 9.1   The Cacao Belt: Countries where cacao is grown are shown in a darker shade and are generally located on or near the equator. Created by Cristina Liberati, MALD, Equal Exchange.

fallen leaves from the trees. The understory provides a warm, moist environment for the insects that pollinate the cacao along with nurturing all aspects of biodiversity. Other animals, particularly birds, rodents, monkeys, and even sloths frequently inhabit the farms.

There is significant overlap between the world's biodiversity hotspots and the production areas for cacao. The birthplace of *Theobroma cacao* is the Amazon, which is the largest tropical rainforest in the world. A farm can never provide the ecosystem services that a primary forest—especially rainforest—is able to provide. However, where agriculture is replacing primary forest, cacao and its sister crop coffee may be best suited to minimize the damage to the environment. "Research conducted in Latin America indicates that the capacity of cocoa plantations to conserve birds, ants, and other wildlife is greater than in any other anthropogenic land use systems," notes Richard Asare of the University of Copenhagen's Center for Forest, Landscape and Planning (2006).

Not all cacao farms are created equal, however, when it comes to biodiversity. As was noted previously, traditional or rustic farms tend to maintain polyculture and agroforestry systems and, by default, preserve biodiversity. A study done in West Africa found that certain types of native trees "happen to be among the most preferred species of farmers due to their economic and traditional values." (Asare 2006). Farmers tended to keep these trees on their properties, despite the fact that governments in the region conducted active campaigns to remove them in order to mitigate pests and diseases affecting cacao production.

Sunlight is often the best treatment to prevent the spread of these pests and diseases in cacao. Modern agribusiness practices often prescribe the reduction or removal of tree cover to increase productivity, creating largely monoculture farms focused on the crop that has the highest income potential. Nonetheless, in a 2016 study by Rajab et al., the authors found that "cacao bean yield does not necessarily decrease under shading which seems to reduce physical stress," (Rajab et al. 2016). Cultivation under shade cover provides the additional benefit of high carbon sequestration and storage, an important factor in climate change mitigation. Other researchers analyzed data from 23 different studies conducted over 26 years and concluded that "Despite the lower yields for shaded systems, the lower costs per area and higher price per kilogram of coffee or cocoa causes shaded systems to perform better financially." (Jezeer et al. 2017).

Maintaining traditional cacao agroforestry systems properly requires a substantial effort on the part of the farmer. Trees must be adequately spaced apart and expertly pruned. Weed removal is intensive and constant work. In many cases, farmers do not have the time or resources to hire the additional labor needed to manage the work that a healthy, biodiverse cacao farm requires. In one study conducted in Ghana, researcher Francoise Olivier Ruf noted that many cacao farmers interviewed considered agroforestry outmoded. Instead, they favored planting new cacao hybrids that are designed for full-sun production. In this case though, legal barriers prevented farmers from participating in legal timber markets (Ruf 2011).

The costs of cacao agroforestry can be offset in some cases by the income that certain timber trees can offer (Somarriba et al. 2017). Farmers at one cooperative in Peru are taking advantage of intercropping high value timber trees to diversify their incomes and to invest in their retirement as noted in the forthcoming story about Julio López Dávila. This type of large and long-term investment is still inaccessible for many small-scale farmers, despite the fact that some of the varieties of timber trees are mature and ready to harvest in as little as six years.

In addition to the benefit of carbon sequestration, the prevention of deforestation on cacao farms provides the ecosystem services of preserving animal habitat, and in some cases saving entire species. The Quevedo region of Ecuador is home to the brown-headed spider monkey. Scientists estimate that only 250 of these animals remain in the wild and they thrive in the rainforest of this region (Fulton 2017). This also happens to be an area that produces cacao, and farmers have been cutting down rainforest to plant cacao. Samuel von Rutte, originally from Switzerland, moved to Ecuador decades ago to farm cacao in Quevedo. He began working with farmers willing to stop cutting down forests and instead market their cacao to buyers who would pay a premium for eco-friendly, high-quality beans. The efforts paid off. Farmers have more than tripled the price for their product and in 2016 the Tesoro Escondido Spider Monkey Reserve was established on 1,100 hectares in the area (Fulton 2017). Farmers are more optimistic about their futures as well.

In stark contrast to the situation in Ecuador, illegal cacao farming in Cote d'Ivoire has led to the loss of all primate species in more than a dozen national parks and reserves (Zielinski 2015). Years of violence in the region has led many refugees from neighboring countries to settle in the country in formerly protected areas. Migrants have turned to cacao production for income, and hunted the animals in those areas for food. "The illegal farms in the region are an extreme example of the loss of biodiversity that has occurred worldwide due to land conversion." (Zielinski 2015).

Biodiversity loss will continue to occur without the use of truly sustainable farming practices as the world's appetite for chocolate increases. Industrial production of cacao favors full sun and clearcut plots, yet alternatives that are less destructive exist. While there are compromises to be made, chocolate makers and consumers can demand products that preserve the dignity of the people and the natural environments that produce cacao. More training and education for farmers will help them enact sustainable options as well.

One such example is Julio López Dávila, a member of the Cooperativa Agraria Cacaotera Acopagro (ACOPAGRO) since 2013. When he joined he was producing about 500 kilos of cacao per hectare. "I didn't know anything until I became a member," he remarked in one interview (López 2015). As a benefit of joining the cooperative, he began to receive technical assistance. He was also able to take advantage of additional training and support offered through a collaboration between ACOPAGRO and Equal Exchange's U.S. Agency for International Development (also known as USAID) Cooperative Development Program. He has increased his production by 60% in the course of three years. He now produces 800 kilos of cacao per hectare, and also grows citrus fruits, bamboo passion fruit, and produces his own compost. Julio gives credit to the technical assistance he received for his progress, though much of his success can be attributed to his own dedication and ingenuity.

The cooperative that Julio joined also leveraged funding from a nonprofit called PurProject to help Julio and other farmers invest in timber trees (PureProject 2016). This form of strategic agroforestry that combines the benefits of reforestation with increased cash crop production may provide a promising roadmap for biodiversity conservation. This initiative combines the support of his family, the cooperative, the nonprofit sector, and commercial partners. There is an African proverb that says, "If you want to go fast, go alone; but if you want to go far, go together."

9.4 COFFEE AND BIODIVERSITY

To discuss biodiversity and coffee requires acknowledging the depth and breadth of this subject. Biodiversity in coffee ranges from a discussion of the genetic diversity of the identified coffee germplasm to the impact of coffee farm structures on micro- and macro-fauna—and everything in between. There is no single lens through which to evaluate coffee and biodiversity, which multiplies the potential coffee has to contribute—both positively and negatively—to biodiversity conservation. Due to the number of ways in which coffee and biodiversity interact, as well as coffee's global importance as a lead cash crop in the tropics (specifically in Latin America), coffee holds a unique position as a commodity crop with the potential to positively impact biodiversity conservation (McCarthur 2016).

There is a growing consensus among conservation and biodiversity scholars that conservation aims will not be achieved solely through protected areas management due to the relatively small total area reserved for conservation (Garcia 2009). Over the past decade, conservation researchers have begun to identify the untapped and unmeasured potential of coffee farmers to contribute to conserving biodiversity, and now call for them to be included as direct stakeholders in the design and implementation of agroforestry-centric conservation efforts (Garcia 2009). Coffee holds this potential to contribute to biodiversity in agroforestry systems due to the multiplicity of ways the crop intersects with biodiversity and geography in the most ecologically diverse landscapes in the world (Mougel 1999).

Globally, 70%–80% of coffee is produced by smallholder farmers with plots that average less than 10 hectares/farm (International Coffee Organization 2016). The more widely grown Arabica species grows well under shade trees in either a mono-culture or polyculture system in the tropical belt (National Coffee Association n.d.). Studies on biodiversity and coffee have evaluated the different agricultural system designs used in coffee cultivation and their relative impact on biodiversity. In a study from Mexico, Moguel and Toledo quantify through an exhaustive literature review the impact of different coffee production systems on the biodiversity of five groups of organisms: Plants, arthropods, birds, amphibians, and reptiles (Moguel 1999). Their research affirms that the value of shaded coffee farms is primarily derived from preserving habitat in areas that have been heavily deforested (Moguel 1999). Research on polyculture agroforestry coffee farms demonstrates that preventing deforestation positively contributes to biodiversity (Moguel 1999).

The fluctuations of the global commodity price leave farmers precariously exposed to risk. Over the past decade, the composite commodity price of coffee has averaged $1.37/lb, and since the first quarter of 2015 the composite price has been lower while the cost of production has consistently increased over the same period (International Coffee Organization 2016). With limited economic power and a lack of economic recognition of the biodiversity benefits of a traditional polyculture sys-tem, farmers are not incentivized or encouraged to promote conservation through their farm systems in the commodity-based trade system. These subsistence coffee farmers have struggled for decades to bring their crop to market, cover their costs of production with commodity pricing, and gain access to technical assistance or markets that support their long-term economic prosperity.

Despite the growth of fair-trade and organic certification systems as a way to recognize and reward the social and environmental benefits of small-farmer grown coffee, these certification systems do not provide necessary technical assistance or sufficient financial rewards to promote the widespread adoption (or return to) polyc-ulture agroforestry systems. Farmer-led conservation through farm management has not been widely recognized or measured by the coffee industry.

Biodiversity conservation has not historically been rewarded by the global commodity market as inherent to the value of coffee and yet, biodiversity on cof-fee farms can provide incredible value to ecosystems around the world. The con-servation of threatened habitat, protection of genetic diversity of the wild crop, carbon capture, and other positive environmental externalities are just a few of the headline impacts of biodiversity conservation efforts in coffee (A. Mendez Lopez and E. Ruiz, personal communication, June 24, 2017). Looking towards the future, producer and consumers along the supply chain will have to develop ways to encourage, measure, and reward biodiversity conservation. There also must be a greater investment in scientific research to examine and experiment with questions of biodiversity and coffee (A. Mendez Lopez and E. Ruiz, personal communica-tion, June 24, 2017).

9.4.1 CASE STUDY: SMALL COFFEE FARMER COOPERATIVE IN CHIAPAS, MEXICO

A small farmer coffee cooperative in Chiapas, Mexico, presents an interesting case study of how coffee, community, and biodiversity interact. After a major hurricane hit the Yucatán peninsula in the mid-2000s, the Comon Yaj Noptic Cooperative worked together with the non-profit organization Pronatura to study the bird species that migrate to Chiapas from North America. Farmer members of the cooperative and community members learned the scientific names of the migratory species and monitored their designated areas monthly to report the trends in migratory species presence over a five year period (A. Mendez Lopez and E. Ruiz, personal communication, June 24, 2017). This project relied on local knowledge of the land and bird species to monitor biodiversity and the impact of climate change on habitat availability for migratory species. Impacts of this study included increasing local employment, increasing awareness and preservation of a biologic corridor, successfully using community-based participatory research, and designing climate change impact studies (A. Mendez Lopez and E. Ruiz, personal communication, June 24, 2017).

This program improved the economic circumstances of the participants. One outcome of the project included an eco-tourism project to host international birding enthusiasts in the El Triunfo Biosphere Reserve (A. Mendez Lopez and E. Ruiz, personal communication, June 24, 2017). This particular project combined community-centered development, conservation, and economic empowerment at a farmer-cooperative level and resulted in biological monitoring of bird species over a period of six years in the biosphere's buffer zone (Mendez López 2015). The farmer-bird monitors recorded the presence of migratory and year-round species in the buffer zone and the species recorded ranged from critically endangered species to populations that are not threatened.

9.5 PALM OIL PRODUCTION AND BIODIVERSITY LOSS

Palm oil is deeply intertwined in a consumer's everyday life. Palm oil is included in about half of all packaged products sold in supermarkets and is widely used in cosmetics, detergents, and processed foods (World Wildlife Fund 2017). The vast majority of palm oil is produced in Malaysia and Indonesia, with some production in South America and West Africa (Carrasco et al. 2014). A high-yielding and profitable crop rich in saturated fats, palm oil is the most widely consumed and traded vegetable oil on the planet, with production nearly doubling between 2004–2014, driven largely by growing export markets (FAO 2017). This "palm oil revolution" has been supported by vast expansion of planted areas, including conversion of forest into cropland, with devastating effects for tropical ecosystems. Substantial biodiversity loss has resulted from palm expansion into some of the most sensitive regions, which also serve as key carbon sinks to mitigate climate change (Vijay et al. 2016). Further, palm oil production often follows land clearing via forest and peatland burning, which destroys habitat key to biodiversity, emits highly significant quantities of greenhouse gases, and may have long-term impacts to public health through the inhalation of harmful particulate matter (Chisholm et al. 2016).

Palm oil is usually planted as a monocrop, in large swaths centered around the high-capacity processing plants necessitated by the crop's short shelf life after harvest. Unlike other tropical perennial crops, there is little opportunity for productive polyculture with palm oil. There is also concern that even if yields per plant improve, palm oil-induced deforestation may increase (Carrasco et al. 2014). Forests remain vulnerable in tropical palm oil-producing areas around the globe, increasing the risk of extinction of mammal and birds.

While palm oil plantations have demonstrated harmful effects on ecosystems, the social dynamics of the crop are complex. Palm oil investment in Asia was initially driven by government subsidies and private investment, including vertically integrated agribusinesses—a pattern of development that can potentially be detrimental to smallholder farmers (Key et al. 1999). Smallholders have since followed these initial investments into palm oil and now largely drive the expansion of the crop, and currently account for 35%–40% of production in Indonesia, the world's top producer (ISPOC 2012). At odds with the ecological damage caused by its cultivation, there is evidence that smallholders in Asia have benefited substantially from the expansion of palm oil production thanks to higher incomes and resultant improvements to nutritional status; however, these benefits elude the poorest of the poor, widening inequality within local communities (Euler et al. 2017).

In order for palm oil to be produced sustainably without impacting biodiversity, it is essential that the poorest and most vulnerable are included in the benefits and development of sustainable agriculture as described in the Sustainable Development Goals. Another promising step is the formation of the Roundtable on Sustainable Palm Oil, designed to answer consumer concerns about palm oil production and improve practices in the sector—alongside a moratorium on new land concessions that reduces the expansion of palm oil into forests, although much more work remains to be done. This will require transparency and recognition of control and power in this industry, alongside a better understanding of the unintended local consequences of the voluntary sustainability standards (Oosterveer et al. 2014).

9.5.1 SEEKING PALM OIL SOLUTIONS

Indonesia, the site of the worst deforestation due to palm oil, offers a window into how to move forward with solutions. Over the past ten years, increased consumer awareness has levied heavy pressure on food processors to avoid palm oil that destroys tropical forests. As a result, the Indonesian government has issued moratoria on forest and peatland clearing, as well as a moratorium on the licensing of new palm oil concessions (Government of Indonesia 2011). Additionally, major producers have voluntarily adopted No Deforestation, No Peat, and No Exploitation (NDPE) policies (Sen 2017). Since its formation in 2004, the Roundtable on Sustainable Palm Oil (RSPO) has expanded its certification scheme for sustainable oil production rapidly, and boasts a stated commitment to the advancement of smallholder livelihoods (Webber et al. 2015). Nevertheless, significant gaps in monitoring and enforcement of these schemes remain (Vijay et al. 2016; Carrasco et al. 2016; Marin-Burgos et al. 2015).

Despite early successes, however, much work remains to be done to ensure conservation and humanitarian goals are met in tandem. Ironically, large firms active in Indonesia are increasingly seeking land concessions to farm palm oil in West Africa—the original home of the crop—expanding business while avoiding the deforestation controversy in Indonesia (Wich et al. 2014). Regulation, monitoring, enforcement, and conservation-based market initiatives will all have to work together in order to stop deforestation (Vijay et al. 2016). Furthermore, rigorous and well-planned regulation and the complete cessation of burning to clear lands can simultaneously enhance biodiversity while also mitigating greenhouse gas emissions (Austin et al. 2015). While no silver bullet exists, continued consumer pressure is a linchpin for solving the problems of the palm oil boom.

9.6 SUGARCANE AND BIODIVERSITY

Sugar is something most of us love, many of us crave, and some even call it an addiction. It has become ubiquitous in many cultures around the globe, influenced by the Western Diet. Once reserved as centerpiece for celebrations, it is now found in much more than baked treats. Sugar is in many foods we eat daily, from breakfast cereal to hamburger buns and ketchup. Because sugar has become part of our everyday lives, it has the largest production volume of any commodity crop (Odegard et al. 2015). This fact alone means that the sugar we eat comes with a large environmental price tag.

Though it is hard to tell from the white, processed sugar we purchase in the grocery aisle, sugar is produced from two different crops: sugarcane and sugar beets. Eighty percent of the world's sugar is produced from sugarcane and 20% comes from sugar beets (International Sugar Organization 2016). In the U.S about 45% comes from sugarcane and 55% from sugar beets (USDA 2017). Sugarcane is a perennial grass in the genus *Saccharum* and the family *Poaceae*, along with crops like wheat, rice, maize, and sorghum. Sugarcane flourishes in hot, tropical environments in over 100 countries around the world, but none matches Brazil, which is by far the leader in global sugarcane production (International Sugar Organization 2016). Sugarcane grows up to 20 feet tall and is cultivated as a monoculture. In the U.S., sugarcane is grown industrially in Louisiana, Florida, Texas, and Hawaii (USDA 2017). Sugar beets are root crops grown in more temperate climates throughout the world with commercial production found in 11 states in the U.S. located in the Northwest, the Mid-West, the Great Plains, and Great Lakes (USDA 2017). Both sugarcane and sugar beets contain sucrose, which is extracted from the plants during the first stage of processing at sugar mills. The liquid sucrose is then purified, concentrated, and crystalized to create the sugar we consume. Sugars sold in the U.S. are typically refined white or brown sugars (often white sugars with molasses added back), but there are many different types of sugar produced through variations in the production process. It should be noted that since genetically engineered sugar beets were first allowed in the market in 2005, by the 2009/2010 crop year they comprised 95% of U.S. sugar beet production (USDA 2018).

While the environmental impact of sugarcane is similar in many ways to other agricultural products given the massive worldwide demand for sugar, some believe that sugarcane has had the largest environmental impact of any crop (Clay 2004). In the major sugar-producing countries between 1960 and 2007, sugarcane production increased by over 250%. The land area required to meet this increased production grew over 200% (Fischer 2008). When considering the environmental impacts of sugarcane, the recent growth in production has also been driven by the booming biofuels industry, which uses large volumes of sugarcane (Hess et al. 2016). This combined demand has led to dramatic increases in land used for sugarcane farming.

Sugarcane is predominantly harvested in two ways: By hand with machetes, or with large industrial machines. Small-scale farmers use machetes while industrial farms use machinery to harvest the cane that is faster and cheaper. The environmental impacts can vary widely depending on the type of production and its location. In addition to the biodiversity loss ensued with land transformation altogether, sugarcane is associated with many environmental issues including soil degradation, water and air pollution, and biodiversity loss.

9.6.1 Soil Degradation

The conventional/industrialized system of sugarcane production can lead to high levels of soil degradation due to extended periods of soil exposure and soil compaction. Sugarcane farming leaves the soil bare when the field is initially converted to sugarcane—between the annual harvest and regrowth cycle—and when fields are replanted with cane every five to six years. Under these barren conditions, there can be high rates of topsoil loss from winds and rain. Estimates of soil erosion loss vary between 15 to >500 tons/hectare/year (Cheesman 2004). In many places, sugarcane is planted on marginal or sloped terrain without proper terracing or soil management, which exacerbates the soil loss. Soil degradation also occurs on mechanized farms due to compaction of the soil from heavy machinery, leading to long-term changes in the physical properties of the soil structure (Martinelli and Filoso 2008). This loss of topsoil and soil compaction can lead to lower levels of organic matter and nutrients in the soil, impacting both soil health and the soil's ability to support microorganisms, as well as contributing to lower yields (Meyer 2011).

Soil degradation not only impacts the overall health of the land but can also lead to soil loss that can damage aquatic ecosystems (Meyer 2011). Water pollution from sugarcane can be caused by two main issues: Soil erosion and pesticide/ fertilizer runoff. Due the higher levels of soil erosion associated with sugarcane production, large quantities of silt and sediment can enter local watersheds causing downstream damage to the water system (Martinelli and Filoso 2008).

If not managed using best practices, not only will soil end up in local water systems, but pesticides and fertilizers will also be removed during the runoff. This impacts the health of both freshwater and marine ecosystems. One of the most critical examples of this problem is the widespread coral bleaching occurring in recent years on the Great Barrier Reef, the largest living body on Earth (New York Times 2016). While there are various threats to the Great Barrier Reef, agricultural runoff, including from sugarcane farming, is seen as a major concern for the reef (Queensland Government 2017). Sugarcane is an important crop for the state of Queensland, Australia, where a large land area bordering the ocean is under cultivation. It has been documented that nitrogen and phosphorous runoff from sugarcane farms contributes disproportionately higher amounts of these nutrients than other agricultural activities (Baker 2003). Runoff from sugarcane farms plays a role in the decline of the overall water quality throughout the Great Barrier Reef, threatening both the coral as well as the many other species of fish and animals in the reef ecosystem. Valuing the global importance of the Great Barrier Reef and realizing the destruction it may face, the Australian government has created the "Reef 2050 Water Quality Improvement Plan" to measure and reduce threats to the reef, including working with sugarcane farmers to combat the potential for run off into the marine environment (Australian Government 2017).

9.6.2 SUGARCANE AND AIR POLLUTION

Air pollution is another major concern with sugarcane production. A traditional practice in conventional cane fields is to burn fields annually before harvest. While this makes harvesting easier, it leads to higher levels of carbon monoxide and ozone around cane fields, negatively effecting the health of the environment, the laborers, and the local community (World Wildlife Fund 2005). This practice also leads to further soil degradation and erosion (Fischer et al. 2008).

9.6.3 SUGACANE AND BIODIVERSITY LOSS

Given its widespread production throughout the tropics and because sugarcane is a monoculture, it arguably has had a larger impact on biodiversity than any other agricultural product (Cheesman 2004). Several of the most critical challenges to biodiversity have been habitat loss and pollution. While the expansion of land use for sugarcane has slowed in recent years, the centuries-long historical growth of the sugarcane industry has led to large-scale habitat loss throughout the tropics. Some countries now devote up to 50% of their agricultural lands to sugarcane production, which required the clearing of huge areas of natural vegetation to grow this crop (Clay 2004). Sugarcane has displaced flora and fauna, forcing them out of their natural habitat. Given the scale of the industry, this displacement can affect entire regions, such as the Caribbean, which is no longer a region of significant biodiversity in large part due to cane production (Clay 2004).

In many cases, sugarcane farms have expanded into biologically diverse, unique, and critical ecosystems such as wetlands and riparian zones. These lands, bordering both river and marine environments, both serve as a habitat for animals while buffering and protecting these ecosystems. Though much of the recent expansion of sugar production in Brazil has not taken place near the Amazon, it has occurred in the Cerrado region, known to be a biologically important area of the country (Fischer 2008). Due to sugarcane production and cattle ranching, 75% of the riparian vegetation has been lost in this area (Fischer 2008). In the U.S., over 200,000 hectares of the Florida Everglades, the largest subtropical ecosystem in the U.S., have been converted to sugarcane production. Draining large areas of the Everglades for human activities including agricultural land for sugar has led to a 90% decline in wading bird populations (Cheesman 2004).

Downstream pollution from sugarcane farms can lead to myriad threats to biodiversity in river and marine ecosystems. Farm pollution can have a dramatic impact on nutrient levels in ecosystems creating large algal blooms or creating the right environment for the detrimental growth of certain species. Beyond the coral bleaching of the Great Barrier Reef, another threat to the coral is the crown-of-thorns starfish (Australian Government 2017). Under normal conditions, this starfish plays a balanced role in this ecosystem. However, during times of flooding that cause excess nitrogen runoff from farms, the crown-of-thorns population spikes. The overpopulation of this starfish has caused widespread destruction of hard corals throughout the reef (Fraser 2017).

The upshot is that sugar production is not always sweet. With wide-ranging and often devastating implications for our environment, conventional production methods of sugarcane is far from sustainable. However, due to consumer demands and market pressures, the sugar industry is starting to change. Government regulations, industry adopted practices, and sustainable certifications such as organic and fair trade are pushing the industry to create more environmentally friendly practices (Meyer et al. 2011). While there is much still to be done, change has begun.

9.6.4 CASE STUDY: PARAGUAY LEADING THE ORGANIC SUGAR REVOLUTION

It is hard for many nations to compete in the sugar industry that is dominated by large volume producers like Brazil and India. This is especially true for a small, landlocked countries like Paraguay that lacks the resources to invest in its national sugar industry on the scale of its neighbor, Brazil. In 1994, one of Paraguay's sugar mills realized there was an opportunity for a new market in Europe: Organic sugar produced with more environmentally friendly practices and without synthetic inputs. The mill made the switch to organic and soon other sugar mills in Paraguay as well as the government took note and began to invest in organic sugar production for the niche but growing organic sugar market. Since the mid-1990s, Paraguay has led the organic sugarcane revolution and remains the largest producer of organic sugar in the world. This success has allowed them to maintain an industry that supports thousands of small-scale farmers while also creating a more sustainable farming system that creates long-term benefits for the environment.

While still a monoculture, organic sugarcane production uses various farm management techniques aimed at alleviating some of the worst environmental impacts of conventional production. Organic farming is often focused on building and maintaining the health of the soil rather than solely managing the health of the crop. On organic farms in Paraguay, instead of using synthetic fertilizers to add nitrogen, farmers will instead use "green manure," which is the practice of growing nitrogen fixing plants in the field (Schumman 200). In addition to building soil health, growing these additional plants on the farm reduces nitrogen runoff and soil erosion, and provides a natural form of weed control. Additional information on green manure is found in the vignette in Chapter 10. Another major visible difference between organic and conventional cane production is that organic producers do not burn their fields, thus decreasing air pollutants and making the fields more habitable for animals and insects. Organic farming often comes with higher costs, but it is important for consumers to value the true labor costs and the high level of environmental and social returns derived from this alternative production method. Shifting to organic production on a large scale has allowed Paraguay to incorporate regenerative practices while also giving consumers a choice to purchase organic sugar on the grocery store shelf.

9.7 TEA AND BIODIVERSITY LOSS

Tea is one of the oldest and most widely consumed beverages in the world, and is second only to water in terms of global beverage consumption (Chang 2015). Tea is also one of the most important cash crops, providing income for millions of people around the world (Chang 2015). The scientific name for tea is *Camellia sinensis*, and it should not be confused with herbal infusions, which are known as tisanes. The new growth of the tea plant, usually two leaves and a bud, are traditionally plucked by hand and undergo a variety of processing steps to create the finished product. The tea leaves must be processed within hours of harvesting. The processing steps vary according to each style of tea. Black tea, for example, undergoes *withering* to reduce the moisture in the leaves; *rolling* to bruise the leaves and release enzymes; *oxidizing* so black tea leaves develop a dark rich brown color; and finally *drying* followed by *sorting* by size and grade (Equal Exchange 2017). Green tea, on the other hand, is steamed or fired to prevent the leaves from oxidizing. The steaming or firing is what allows the leaves to retain the light green color (Equal Exchange 2017).

The tea plant is best suited to a mid-elevation terrain in tropical or sub-tropical climates, with temperatures ranging from 10° – 30°C (50° – 86°F). Tea is heavily reliant on natural rainfall and is very sensitive to climatic variation. While tea is grown in more than fifty countries, almost 80% of the global tea supply comes from just four countries: China, India, Kenya, and Sri Lanka (Chang 2015). Tea cultivation varies greatly from country to country, with a mix of large-scale plantations established under colonialism and small-scale farmers who mostly sell freshly harvested tea leaves to bought leaf factories (Chang 2015). In India, the second largest producer of tea, approximately 70% of the 1.2 million tons of tea produced annually comes from colonial era plantations, while the remaining 30% comes from smallholder farms of 10 hectares of land or less.

India's plantations pay workers around $2 per day depending on the region in addition to non-cash compensation in the form of housing, food rations, primary schooling for children, daycare, and medical services (Chang 2015). In India, these services are required by the Plantation Labor Act of 1951 (PLA). However, the delivery of these services is inconsistent and unreliable (Human Rights Institute 2014). Women, who make up 70% of the tea plantation workforce in India, are disproportionately affected (FIAN International 2016). Similarly, the farm gate price paid to small-scale tea farmers for freshly harvested green leaves falls below the cost of production when including the labor of the farmer. This creates a difficult and unsustainable livelihood for many small farmers who lack access to producer co-operatives (FIAN International 2016).

Tea plantations have a significant impact on the natural landscape. In the example of India, tea plantations cover an estimated 1100 km² of land that was primary forest when the land was cleared for tea more than a century ago (Osuri 2010). Ongoing deforestation is common around plantations, as wood is a common source of fuel and for cooking. Tea plantations are open monocropped expanses with sparsely interspersed shade trees, usually *Grevillea robusta,* also known as the silver oak, which has a dual purpose for timber (Sidhu 2015). This monocropped landscape leads to further forest and habitat fragmentation and as a result, plantations are significantly different from the surrounding forests (Osuri 2010). Due to its specific agro-climatic requirements, tea also has a high vulnerability to changes in climate and weather patterns (Chang 2015). New diseases and pests have emerged with greater frequency in recent years, and a 2016 study from Assam, India, found a correlation between tea yield decline and average temperature rise, particularly if above 35°C (95°F) (Duncan 2016).

Inorganic agro-chemicals are widely used in tea cultivation, impacting soil microflora and crop yields. Starting in the 1980's, inputs of agro-chemicals almost doubled yields, but these gains have since plateaued. Since inorganic fertilizers do not improve or restore soil quality, soil degradation from centuries of expansive monocropping has created nutrient deficient soil, leading to erosion and lower water-holding ability, soil acidification, reduced organic matter, nutrient leaching, and loss of crucial soil biota. Depleted soil is typically addressed through the use of additional external fertilizer inputs, both organic and inorganic, while the decreased water-holding ability of the soil has led to a greater need for irrigation—all of which are increasing the cost of production. Additional research identified a strong correlation between earthworm population and green leaf yields and strongly suggests that earthworms fare much better under organic cultivation (Senapati 2014; Senapati et al. 2002).

As with cacao, tea is heavily cultivated in hotspots of biodiversity such as the Western Ghats in southern India. The Western Ghats is a UNESCO World Heritage site and is considered one of the world's eight hotspots of biodiversity (UNESCO 2017). The Western Ghats is also where 18% of India's tea production occurs (Daniels 2003). There is a growing awareness of the need to create more hospitable environments for wildlife through land management of human-modified agricultural land (Kumara 2004). This is also true for abandoned plantations, which tend to be nutrient-poor and particularly vulnerable to invasive species after decades or centuries of monocropping.

As the research shows, the tea sector influences biodiversity and is influenced by biodiversity in a multitude of ways. The long-term monocropping of tea on plantations has led to biodiversity-poor, nutrient deficient ecosystems. However, positive changes can be made through intercropping, nitrogen-fixing cover crops, vermiculture, and organic composting. Land management strategies to help sustain the movement of wildlife through tea plantations will help to achieve sustainable biodiversity in the human-modified landscapes of tea (Osuri 2010). Additionally, the increase of small tea farmers in recent years indicates a potential opportunity to shift away from plantations and towards small farming, with benefits to be gained for biodiversity preservation. Small growers tend to retain greater biodiversity when producing tea, both through retention of the forest and through intercropping of cash crops and subsistence crops in close proximity (Das 2015). Small-scale home gardens tend to support and provide sanctuary for species diversity through "sustainable agroforestry systems that are repositories of species and genetic diversity" (Das 2015). However, low green leaf prices, a lack of small farmer organizations (such as co-operatives) in the tea sector, and continued lack of access to share in the additional profits of factory processing represent systemic barriers for small tea farmers throughout the world.

9.7.1 CASE STUDY: POTONG TEA GARDEN—DARJEELING, INDIA

The infrastructure of India's tea industry dates back to mid-1800s, during the height of colonialism when a vast system of tea plantations was established. These plantations emphasized monocropping and exploitative labor practices to maximize profits (Bhowmik 2011). Today, monocropping is still the common practice and workers continue to endure low cash wages and other abuses from their plantation employers who control most aspects of life on plantations, such as housing and access to other services like basic education, health services, and food rations (Human Rights Institute 2014).

The Potong Tea Garden, a longtime partner of the alternative trade organization Equal Exchange, is challenging the status quo of the plantation system. Potong began as a colonial plantation but today is collectively run by the farmers. This groundbreaking model was established in partnership with Tea Promoters of India (TPI), a family-owned and operated tea company with several tea gardens of their own in Darjeeling, Dooars, and Assam. TPI has been working for decades with small-scale tea producers like Potong and provides vital processing, administrative, organizational development, and agricultural support. Potong's 343 farmer members democratically control their tea garden, a model that is unheard of in the tea industry.

Potong and TPI have also been working to revitalize the tea garden after 150 years of monocropped cultivation. Their efforts include rehabilitating the soil by reintroducing micronutrients through vermicomposting and companion planting with native and non-native species including leguminous plants, grasses, and other green crops to bind soil, reduce erosion, maintain moisture, and manage pests. Other activities include planting shade trees to protect against extreme sun, and introducing banana trees to revive natural water sources within the tea garden. These efforts have fostered greater biodiversity and resilience for the tea garden ecosystem, creating a safer working environment for farmers through organic agriculture practices (G. Mohan, Personal Communication, April 3, 2017). Potong and TPI have observed a resurgence of wildlife in the area including rabbit, deer, pangolin, porcupine, and larger predators such as boar and the occasional leopard (G. Mohan, Personal Communication, April 3, 2017).

9.8 EMERGING FOODS: AVOCADOS AND BIODIVERSITY LOSS

While avocados have recently become a staple in American kitchens and restaurants, the fruit is ripe with history. *Persea americana*, the scientific name for the avocado, is believed to have originated in the state of Puebla, Mexico, approximately 12,000 years ago (Galindo-Tovar et al. 2007). From there, the fruit spread to Central and South America, continuing on to the Caribbean islands and the U.S. Avocado trees were first planted in Florida in 1833 and then in California in 1856

(Boriss et al. 2017). Today, avocados have a global reach. Some of the major avocado-producing countries are Mexico, Dominican Republic, Peru, Indonesia, Colombia, Chile, Kenya, and the U.S. In 2014, Mexico alone represented 30% of the global avocado production (FAO 2017). In that same year, the U.S. ranked 7th in the world, producing approximately 3% of the global production (FAO 2017).

When considering avocados, the most striking statistic lies in its soaring demand. Global avocado consumption is growing about 3% every year (Mulderij 2016). In the U.S., avocados have transitioned from an exotic fruit to a staple grocery item. In 1980, the average American consumed less than a pound of avocados a year. By 2012, this figure jumped to five pounds (Kruskal 2016). Avocado consumption began to soar in the 1990s, aided by a change in U.S. policy lifting import restrictions from Mexico, nutritional claims labeling avocado as a healthy fat, and a series of successful marketing campaigns (Khazan 2015). Ever since, demand has grown exponentially. With demand soaring at a breakneck pace year after year, supply cannot be matched in a sustainable way. The emergence of avocados as a popular food has had unintended outcomes, even impacting the countries producing avocados.

Eighty percent (80%) of the avocados consumed in the U.S. come from Michoacán, Mexico, the only Mexican state permitted by the U.S. government to export avocados to the U.S. up until 2016 (Perez and Durisin 2017). To keep pace with the rising demand for avocados in the U.S., farmers in Mexico are clearing forests in order to plant more avocado trees. Demand is booming and the fruit yields lucrative prices in the U.S., giving farmers an economic incentive to clear forests as a means to make some quick cash.

Between 1974 and 2011, approximately 110,000 acres of forest in Michoacán's central highlands were turned into avocado orchards, according to a study by the National Autonomous University of Mexico (Burnett 2016). Experts state that deforestation continues to accelerate. According to Jaime Navía, president of Grupo Interdisciplinario de Tecnología Rural Apropiada (GIRA), a nonprofit based in Michoacán promoting sustainable rural development, approximately 65,000 acres—the majority forest cover—have been converted to avocado orchards since that study. These are staggering numbers that shine a light on the scale of the deforestation.

Michoacán is also the winter home of monarch butterflies (USDA Forest Service n.d.). Every winter, monarch butterflies start their migratory journey from Canada and the U.S. to the pine and oak forests of Michoacán, covering over 2,500 miles in their trek. The orange and black spotted butterflies are attracted to the warmer temperatures of the Michoacán forests and spend their winter months in the Monarch Butterfly Biosphere Reserve, a 135,000 acre protected area (UNESCO).

As farmers in Michoacán clear forests to pave way for avocado orchards, they are inevitably clearing forests that act as the winter habitat of monarch butterflies, thus imperiling the migratory pattern and the fate of this species. In fact, the fate of monarch butterflies is already in jeopardy. Their status as an endangered species is currently under review, which means this destruction of habitat is further threatening the species (U.S. Fish and Wildlife Service 2017). Thus, the consequences of the avocado boom offer an example of how accelerating demand can distort the natural environment upon which a multitude of biodiversity depends upon.

9.8.1   CASE STUDY: PRAGOR AVOCADO FARMING
COOPERATIVE, MICHOACÁN, MEXICO

Michoacán, Mexico, is the avocado capital of the world. The rich volcanic soils and the unique microclimate lend itself to some of the highest quality avocados. While avocado production in Michoacán continues to boom due to rising demand in the U.S., production entails clearing forests to make room for avocado orchards.

Within this changing landscape stands Pragor, a small farmer cooperative in Michoacán. Pragor farmers are pioneers in organic and fair trade avocados in Mexico. They are small-scale farmers, with an average farm size of 10 hectares. They shifted to organic production over a decade ago as a means to take care of the environment and their communities (S. Romero, personal communication, November 17, 2016). Distressed by the deforestation, they have undertaken several measures to ensure that Pragor members are not contributing to deforestation.

First, the cooperative has strict criteria for enrolling new members into the cooperative. One of the criteria is that farmers must have been growing avocados organically for a minimum of six years. Since the newer avocado orchards are a result of deforestation, this measure ensures that any members of the cooperative have not contributed to deforestation. Second, the cooperative has begun a reforestation project using their Fairtrade Premium dollars (S. Romero, personal communication, November 17, 2016). Working in conjunction with the federal government, avocado growers and other members of the community are given pine seedlings as a means to encourage reforestation. Additionally, the cooperative continuously ensures that their members are not contributing to deforestation and are actively involved in reforestation efforts. Pragor members make up a small percentage of the avocado industry; they are 25 out of 22,000 registered avocado farmers in Michoacán (APEAM 2017). Ultimately, this group of small farmers is emerging as a model for sustainable avocado production in the region and is offering U.S. consumers a choice to consume ethically produced avocados.

9.9   CONCLUSION

Through the lens of several popular foods, Chapter 9 offers a glimpse into the challenges of the modern day agricultural system. While this chapter has only scratched the surface on the impact of these particular foods on biodiversity loss, they share a story that is often replicated as new foods emerge along with increased global demand (James et al. 2012). At the same time, the case studies portrayed in this chapter provide inspiration into the impact that a different type of food system can cultivate globally. To be successful in the revitalization and maintenance of biodiversity, the authors of this chapter ask each reader to support small-scale farmers globally. Each of us has the power to take action by rethinking our individual food purchases, activism, policy change, and by supporting organizations and farmers that are successfully working toward the preservation and expansion of biodiversity through small-scale food production. Immediate action is needed.

REFERENCES

Asare, R. 2006. *A Review on Cacao Agroforestry as a Means for Biodiversity Conservation.* University of Copenhagen. http://www.bio.miami.edu/horvitz/bil235/cacao/cacao06/ms/ms%20Cacao/cocoa%2520review.pdf

Asociación de Productores y Empacadores Exportadores de Aguacate de Mexico APEAM. 2017. http://www.apeamac.com/que-es-apeam/ (Accessed October 3, 2017).

Austin, K. G., S. K. Prasad, L. U Dean, F. Stolle, and J. Vincent. 2015. Reconciling oil palm expansion and climate change mitigation in Kalimantan, Indonesia. *PLOS One* 10 (5): e0127963. doi:10.1371/journal.pone.0127963.

Australian Government. 2011–2017. http://www.reefplan.qld.gov.au/ (Accessed August 22, 2017).

Australian Government. http://www.environment.gov.au/marine/gbr/case-studies/sugar-cane farming (Accessed August 22, 2017).

Australian Government, Great Barrier Reef Marine Park Authority. 2017. http://www.gbrmpa.gov.au/about-the-reef/animals/crown-of-thorns-starfish (Accessed 22, 2017).

Baker, G. 2006. *The Agriculture Revolution in Prehistory: Why Did Foragers Become Farmers?* Oxford, UK: Oxford University Press.

Baker, J. 2003. A report on the study of land-sourced pollutants and their impacts on water quality in and adjacent to the Great Barrier Reef. Report prepared for Intergovernmental Steering Committee, GBR Water Quality Action Plan.

Bhowmik, Sharit K. 2011 Ethnicity and isolation: Marginalization of tea plantation workers. *Race/Ethnicity: Multidisciplinary Global Contexts* 4(2): 235–253.

Boriss, H., H. Brunke, and M. Kreith. 2017. Avocados. Agricultural Marketing Resource Center. http://www.agmrc.org/commodities-products/fruits/avocados/ (accessed May 10, 2017).

Burnett, V. 2016. Avocados imperil monarch butterflies' winter home in Mexico. *The New York Times.* https://www.nytimes.com/2016/11/18/world/americas/ambition-of-avocado-imperils-monarch-butterflies-winter-home.html (Accessed May 10, 2017).

Butler, D. 2013. Fungus threatens top banana, December 2013. http://www.nature.com/news/fungus-threatens-top-banana-1.14336.

Carrasco, L. R., C. Larrosa, E. J. Milner-Gulland, and D. P. Edwards. 2014. A double-edged sword for tropical forests. *Science* 346 (6205): 38–40.

Chang, Kaison. 2015a. *World Tea Production and Trade Current and Future Development.* Report. Rome: Food and Agricultural Organization of the United Nations.

Chang, Kaison. 2015b. *Socio-Economic Implications of Climate Change for Tea Producing Countries.* Report. Rome: Food and Agricultural Organization of the United Nations.

Chang, Kaison. 2015c. *Contribution of Tea Production and Exports to Food Security, Rural Development and Smallholder Welfare in Selected Producing Countries.* Report. Rome, Italy: Food and Agricultural Organization of the United Nations.

Cheesman, O. 2004. *Environmental Impacts of Sugar Production: The Cultivation and Processing of Sugarcane and Sugar Beet.* Oxfordshire, UK: CABI Publishing.

Chisholm RA, L.S. Wijedasa, T. Swinfield. 2016. The need for long-term remedies for Indonesia's forest fires. *Conservation Biology* 30 (1): 5–6.

Clay, J. 2004. *World Agriculture and the Environment: A Commodity-By-Commodity Guide to Impacts and Practices.* Washington, DC: Island Press.

Ember, C. 2014. Hunter-gatherers. In: *Explaining Human Culture: Human Relations Area Files,* edited by C. R. Ember. http://hraf.yale.edu/ehc/summaries/hunter-gatherers, (Accessed on July 15, 2017).

Daniels, R.J. Ranjit. 2003. Impact of tea cultivation on anurans in the Western Ghats. *Current Science* 85 (10): 1415–1422.

Das, Tapasi, and Ashesh Kumar Das. 2015. Conservation of plant diversity in rural homegardens with cultural and geographical variation in three districts of Barak Valley, Northeast India. *Economic Botany* 69 (1): 57–71.

Duncan, J. M. A., S. D. Saikia, N. Gupta, and E. M. Biggs. 2016. Observing climate impacts on tea yield in Assam, India. *Applied Geography* 77: 64–71.

El Heraldo. 2014. Nuevo asesinato por conflictos de tierras en Honduras. April 4. http://www.elheraldo.hn/sucesos/623019-219/nuevo-asesinato-por-conflictos-de-tierras-en-honduras.

Equal Exchange Website: Equalexchange.coop (Accessed May 10, 2017).

Euler, M., V. Krishna, S. Schwarze, H. Siregar, and M Qaim. 2017. Oil palm adoption, household welfare, and nutrition among smallholder farmers in Indonesia. *World Development* 93 (May): 219–35. doi:10.1016/j.worlddev.2016.12.019.

FIAN International. 2016. *A Life without Dignity – The Price of Your Cup of Tea*. Report, Heidelberg: Global Network for the Right to Food and Nutrition.

Fischer, G., E. Teixeira, E. T. Hizsnyik, and H. v. Velthuizen. 2008. Chapter 2 Land use dynamics and sugarcane production. In *Sugarcane Ethanol: Contributions to Climate Change Mitigation and the Environment*, edited by P. Zuurbler and J. v. d. Vooren, 29–62. The Netherlands: Wageningen Academic Publishers.

Food and Agriculture Organization of the United Nations. 2017. FAOSTAT statistics database. http://www.fao.org/faostat/en/#data/QC (Accessed May 10, 2017).

Fraser, G., K. Rohde, and M. Silburn. 2017. Fertiliser management effects on dissolved inorganic nitrogen in runoff from Australian sugarcane farms. *Environmental Monitoring and Assessment* 189 (8): 409.

Fulton, A. 2017. *Save the Monkeys, Save the Trees, Sell the Chocolate*. National Public Radio. January 30, 2017. http://www.npr.org/sections/thesalt/2017/01/30/511630381/save-the-monkeys-save-the-trees-sell-the-chocolate.

Galindo-Tovar, M. E., A.M. Arzate-Fernandez, N. Ogata-Aguilar, and I. Landero-Torres. 2007. The Avocado (Persea Americana, Lauraceae) crop in Mesoamerica: 10,000 years of history. *Harvard Papers in Botany* 12 (2): 325–334.

Garcia, C., A. B. Honil, G Jaboury, D. N Cheryl, M. N. Konerira, et al. 2009. Biodiversity conservation in agricultural landscapes: Challenges and opportunities of coffee agroforests in the Western Ghats, India. *Conservation Biology*.

Government of Indonesia. 2011. Presidential Instruction No. 10/2011 Moratorium on granting of new li- censes and improvement of natural primary forest and peatland governance. Jakarta, Indonesia.

Hess, T.M., J. Sumberg, T. Biggs, et al. 2016. A sweet deal? Sugarcane, water and agricultural transformation in Sub-Saharan Africa. *Global Environmental Change* 39, 181–194.

Houston, H. and T. Wyer 2012. *Why Sustainable Cocoa Farming Matters for Rural Development*. Center for Strategic and International Studies. https://www.csis.org/analysis/why-sustainable-cocoa-farming-matters-rural-development

Human Rights Institute. *The More Things Change… The World Bank, Tata and the Enduring Abuses on India's Tea Plantations*. Report. New York, NY: Columbia Law School, 2014.

International Coffee Organization. 2016. *Assessing the Economic Sustainability of Coffee Growing Study*. London: International Coffee Organization.

International Sugar Organization. 2016. https://www.isosugar.org/sugarsector/sugar. (Accessed August 22, 2017).

ISPOC (2012). *Indonesian Sustainable Palm Oil System: Indonesian Palm Oil in Numbers 2012*. Jakarta, Indonesia: Indonesian Sustainable Palm Oil Commission.

Jamoo, H. S., M. Hendrickson and P. Howard. 2012. Networks power and dependency in the agrifood industry. Department of Agricultural & Applied Economics Working Paper. February 1, 2012. SSRN: https://ssrn.com/abstract=2004496orhttp://dx.doi.org/10.2139/ssrn.2004496.

Jezeer, R., P. Verweij, M. Santos, and R. Boot. 2017. Shaded coffee and cocoa – double dividend for biodiversity and small-scale farmers. *Ecological Economics* 140: 136–145. http://www.sciencedirect.com/science/article/pii/S0921800915302512.

Koeppel, D. 2008. *Banana, the Fate of the Fruit that Changed the World*. USA: Pengiun Group.

Key, N., and D. Runsten. 1999. Contract farming, smallholders, and rural development in Latin America: The organization of agroprocessing firms and the scale of outgrower production. *World Development* 27 (2): 381–401.

Khazan, O. 2015. The selling of the avocado. *The Atlantic*. https://www.theatlantic.com/health/archive/2015/01/the-selling-of-the-avocado/385047/ (Accessed May 10, 2017).

Kruskal, J. 2016. Avocado demand fueling deforestation, unrest in Mexico. *International Policy Digest*. https://intpolicydigest.org/2016/09/07/avocado-demand-fueling-deforestation-unrest-mexico/ (Accessed May 10, 2017).

Kumara, H.N., M. Ananda Kumar, Anantha Krishna Sharma, H.S. Sushma, Mridula Singh, and Mewa Singh. 2004. Diversity and management of wild mammals in tea gardens in the rainforest regions of the Western Ghats, India: A case study from a tea estate in the Anaimalai Hills. *Current Science* 87 (9): 1282–1287.

Lowder, Sarah K., J. Skoet, and T. Raney 2016. The number, size, and distribution of farms, smallholder farms, and family farms worldwide. *World Development* 87, 16–29.

Marin-Burgos, V., J.S. Clancy, and J.C. Lovett 2015. Contesting legitimacy of voluntary sustainability certification schemes: Valuation languages and power asymmetries in the roundtable on sustainable palm oil in Colombia. *Ecological Economics*117: 303–313. doi:10.1016/j.ecolecon.2014.04.011.

Martínez, R. Villalta, E. Soto, G. Murillo, and M. Guzmán. Manejo de la Sigatoka negra en el cultivo del banano. http://www.infoagro.net/programas/Ambiente/pages/adaptacion/casos/Sigatoka.pdf.

Martinelli, L. and S. Filoso. 2008. Expansion of sugarcane ethanol production in Brazil: Environmental and social challenges. *Ecological Applications* 18(4): 885–898.

McCarthur, John W. 2016. What does 'agriculture' mean today? Assessing old questions with new evidence. The Brookings Institution.

Mendez López, M. 2015. Programa Multiregional y Multisectorial de Tecnología e Innovación para la Competitividad de PYMES en Mercados Globalizados. Cooperativa Comon Yaj Noptic S.S.S.

Meyer, J., P. Rein, P. Turner, and K. Mathias. 2011. Good management practices manual for the cane sugar industry. Prepared by PGBI Sugar & Bio-Energy (Pty) Ltd for the International Finance Corporation.

Miller, G. and S. Spoolman. 2012. *Environmental Science*. Cengage Learning. p. 62. (Accessed December 27, 2017).

Moguel, P. and V. Toledo. 1999. Biodiversity conservation in traditional coffee systems of Mexico. *Conservation Biology* 11–21.

Mulderij, R. 2016. Overview global avocado market. *Fresh Plaza*. http://www.freshplaza.com/article/156557/OVERVIEW-GLOBAL-AVOCADO-MARKET (Accessed May 10, 2017).

National Coffee Association. n.d. Coffee around the world. http://www.ncausa.org/ (Accessed April 15, 2017).

Odegard, I., M. Bihleveld, and N. Naber. 2015. Global GHG footprints and water scarcity footprints in agriculture. Delft, CE Delft, August 2015.

Oosterveer, P., B.E. Adjei, S. Vellema, and M. Slingerland. 2014. Global sustainability standards and food security: Exploring unintended effects of voluntary certification in palm oil. *Global Food Security* 3 (3–4): 220–226. doi:10.1016/j.gfs.2014.09.006.

Osuri, Anand, Jagdish Krishnaswamy, Ajith Kumar, and Archana Bali. 2010. Sustaining biodiversity conservation in human-modified landscapes in the Western Ghats: Remnant forests matter. *Biological Conservation*. 143: 2363–2374.

Perez, M. G., and M. Durisin. 2017. Avocado prices are skyrocketing. *Bloomberg*. https://www.bloomberg.com/news/articles/2017-04-28/guacamole-costs-to-jump-as-avocado-shortage-sparks-record-prices (Accessed May 10, 2017).

PurProject Alto Huayabamba 2016. http://www.purprojet.com/project/alto-huayabamba/.

Queensland Government. 2017. https://www.qld.gov.au/environment/agriculture/sustainable-farming/canefarming-impacts (Accessed 22, 2017).

Rajab, Y.A., C. Leuschner, H. Barus, A. Tjoa, and D. Hertel. 2016. Cacao cultivation under diverse shade tree cover allows high carbon storage and sequestration without yield losses. *PLoS One* 11 (2): e0149949. https://www.ncbi.nlm.nih.gov/pmc/articles/PMC4771168/.

Ruf, F.O. 2011. The myth of complex cocoa agroforests: The case of Ghana. *Human Ecology* 39 (3): 373–388. https://www.ncbi.nlm.nih.gov/pmc/articles/PMC3109247/.

Sen, A. 2017. Pathways to deforestation-free food. Briefing Paper. Oxfam International.

Senapati, B.K. 2014. *Restoring Soil Fertility and Enhancing Productivity in Indian Tea Plantations with Earthworms and Organic Fertilizers* (Case Study A1)

Senapati, B. K., P. Lavelle, P. K. Panigrahi, S. Giri, and G. G. Brown. 2002. Restoring soil fertility and enhancing productivity in Indian tea plantations with earthworms and organic fertilizers. *Program, Abstracts and Related Documents of the International Technical Workshop on Biological Management of Soil Ecosystems for Sustainable Agriculture, Série Documentos* 182: 172–190.

Sidhu, Swati, T.R. Shankar Raman, and Divya Mudappa. 2015. Prey abundance and leopard diet in a plantation and rainforest landscape, Anamalai Hills, Western Ghats. *Current Science* 109 (2): 323.

Somarriba, E. and J. Beer. Cocoa based agroforestry production systems. Smithsonian Migratory Bird Center. https://nationalzoo.si.edu/scbi/migratorybirds/research/cacao/somarriba.cfm (Accessed March 17, 2017).

The Development of Agriculture. 2016. *National Geographic*. Archived from the original on 14 April 2016. Retrieved 20 June 2016.

The New York Times. 2016. https://www.nytimes.com/2016/12/01/world/australia/great-barrier-reef coral-bleaching.html?mcubz=1 (Accessed August 22, 2017).

United Nations Educational, Scientific, and Cultural Organization (UNESCO), World Heritage Conservation. Western Ghats. http://whc.unesco.org/en/list/1342 (Accessed May 10, 2017).

United States Department of Agriculture (USDA). 2017. Economic Research Service. https://www.ers.usda.gov/topics/crops/sugar-sweeteners/background/ (Accessed August 22, 2017).

United States Department of Agriculture, Forest Service. Migration and Overwintering. https://www.fs.fed.us/wildflowers/pollinators/Monarch_Butterfly/migration/ (Accessed May 10, 2017).

United States Fish and Wildlife Service. 2017. Assessing the status of the monarch butterfly. https://www.fws.gov/savethemonarch/SSA.html (Accessed May 10, 2017).

USDA NASS. 2012. Census of agriculture, Ag census web maps. www.agcensus.usda.gov/Publications/2012/Online_Resources/Ag_Census_Web_Maps/Overview/. (Accessed August 15, 2017).

Vijay, V., S.L. Pimm, C.N. Jenkins, and S.J. Smith. 2016. The impacts of oil palm on recent deforestation and biodiversity loss. *PLOS One* 11 (7): e0159668. doi:10.1371/journal.pone.0159668.

Webber, D., and Achanah Letchumi. Environment and sustainability-the role of the Roundtable on Sustainable Palm Oil. Planter 91. 1073 (2015): 549–553.

Wich, S.A., J. Garcia-Ulloa, , H.S. Kühl, T. Humle, J.S. Lee, and L.P. Koh 2014. Will oil palm's homecoming spell doom for Africa's great apes? *Current Biology* 24 (14): 1659–1663.

World Cocoa Foundation. "Cocoa Glossary." http://www.worldcocoafoundation.org/about-cocoa/cocoa-glossary/ (accessed October 3, 2017).

World Wildlife Fund. 2005. Sugar and the environment: Encouraging better management practices in sugar production. http://wwf.panda.org/?22255/Sugar-and-the-Environment-Encouraging-Better-Management-Practices-in-Sugar-Production-and-Processing (Accessed May 25, 2017).

World Wildlife Fund. 2017. Which everyday products contain palm oil? https://www.worldwild-
life.org/pages/which-everyday-products-contain-palm-oil (Accessed October 3, 2017).
Zielinski, S. 2015. Illegal cocoa farms are driving out primates in ivory coast. Smithsonian.com.
April 1, 2015. http://www.smithsonianmag.com/science-nature/illegal-cocoa-farms-are-
driving-out-primates-ivory-coast-180954823/.
Zimmerer, K.S. and S.J. Vanek 2016. Toward the integrated framework analysis of linkages
among agrobiodiversity, livelihood diversification, ecoological systems and sustainability amid global charge. *Land* 5: 10.

Section II

Creating Biodiversity-Friendly, Sustainable Solutions

10 Biodiversity and Sustainable Agriculture

Catherine Badgley

CONTENTS

10.1 INTRODUCTION

One of the major challenges facing humanity is to produce enough food without degrading the natural world on farms, pastures, urban gardens, and surrounding native ecosystems. The track record thus far is poor. For centuries, agriculture and food procurement have been a leading cause of soil erosion, greenhouse gas emissions, habitat destruction, and biodiversity loss (Gibbs et al. 2009, Maxwell et al. 2016). These impacts have only intensified since the industrialization of agriculture. By the turn of the 21st century, human activities appropriate 24% of net primary production (the plant base of food webs) in terrestrial ecosystems of the world, with agriculture (cropping and grazing lands) accounting for nearly 80% of this effect (Haberl et al. 2007). Crop production, livestock production, and forest clearing for farms and ranches are the dominant activities over nearly 40% of habitable land areas (excluding Greenland and Antarctica), including regions that harbor vast numbers of native species. Thus, there is an urgent need to recognize and support systems of food production that sustain native biodiversity.

In this chapter, four overarching questions are addressed. First what are the various impacts of the food system on biodiversity globally? Second, how is biodiversity relevant to ecological processes in agriculture? Third, which agricultural practices sustain natural processes and native biodiversity? Fourth, can sustainable agriculture grow enough food to feed the world? There is abundant evidence that the ecologically destructive consequences of industrial agriculture, coupled with overharvesting of wild species on land and at sea, could cause a mass extinction of species and ecosystems. This outcome is clearly not desirable nor is it necessary in order to have a viable, sustainable food system.

10.2 IMPACTS OF THE FOOD SYSTEM ON GLOBAL BIODIVERSITY

Food production and harvesting of wild species comprise the largest burden on global biodiversity of any human activity (Badgley 2013, Maxwell et al. 2016). Much of this impact occurs through land clearing and the growth of industrial monocultures over vast areas in temperate and tropical regions. The replacement of native ecosystems with highly simplified agricultural ecosystems (often reliant on synthetic fertilizers and biocides) displaces or eliminates native plants, animals, and habitats. Another kind of impact occurs through the eradication of native predators and designated "pest" animals (for example, gophers in ranchlands of the western United States with concomitant losses in black-footed ferrets, Matthiessen 1959, Badgley 2002). The eradication of predators on behalf of ranchers and farmers is part of the trophic downgrading pattern (loss of top predators) and consequent disruptions occurring across global ecosystems (Estes et al. 2011). A third kind of impact is overharvesting of targeted species for food. Overharvesting affects both geographically restricted species, such as rare forest lemurs in Madagascar, as well as widespread abundant species, such as the passenger pigeon, once the most abundant bird species in North America and hunted to extinction at the turn of the 20th century (Badgley 2013, Maxwell et al. 2016).

A fourth impact of the food system on biodiversity involves biocides—pesticides, herbicides, and fungicides. These chemicals affect a broad range of organisms beyond their intended target species both as poisons and endocrine disruptors, and may persist in biological tissues for many years (Gibbs et al. 2009, Hayes and Hansen 2017). For example, DDT was applied to crops, in military camps, and across neighborhoods for several decades in the mid-20th century to control disease-bearing insects, including mosquitoes. The insect predators and secondary predators, such as birds and fishes, accumulated DDT in their tissues. At high concentrations, DDT interfered with normal reproduction, including egg production in birds, resulting in the decline of birds of prey over several decades (Carson 1962). After the use of DDT was banned in 1972 in the United States, populations of birds of prey, including peregrine falcons and bald eagles, started to recover over the next decade (New York Times 1982). A contemporary example of harmful pesticides involves neonicotinoids, which are a class of widely used systemic pesticides used to control insect damage on crops. Sublethal exposure of honey bees to neonicotinoids in field experiments in France reduced bee foraging success and increased hive mortality (Henry et al. 2012). In the Netherlands, declines in insectivorous farmland bird populations were found to be correlated over space and time with the concentration of a neonicotinoid pesticide in local waterways (Hallmann et al. 2014).

Given the severity and breadth of these impacts, it is imperative to ask whether it is possible to feed the human population in the 21st century and maintain native species and ecosystems in agricultural landscapes. The global food system could push the Earth into another mass extinction. But there are farming systems around the world that utilize and maintain biodiversity. Understanding how biodiversity supports agriculture provides a basis for supporting farming systems that promote biodiversity.

10.3 THE RELEVANCE OF BIODIVERSITY TO AGRICULTURE

The term "biodiversity," or biological diversity, includes several aspects of biological organization that occur in wild nature and in human-dominated ecosystems (Soulé and Wilcox 1980). Three aspects of biodiversity relevant to agriculture are genetic diversity, species diversity, and habitat diversity. In agriculture, it is useful to distinguish between planned biodiversity—the kinds of plants, animals, and other organisms that farmers deliberately cultivate—and associated biodiversity, which includes all of the other species in the ecosystem (Vandermeer 2011). Both components provide substantial benefits to farmers and humanity at large.

10.3.1 GENETIC DIVERSITY

Genetic diversity refers to individual variation in genetic makeup within species and its expression in different environmental contexts. The genetic diversity of crop and livestock species provides the basis for adaptations of local populations to the climate, soils, pests, and agronomic practices of different regions. For example, indigenous cultures in the Andes Mountains domesticated the potato, *Solanum tuberosum*, and selected different traits for different montane soils and elevations, culinary qualities, and storage properties (Reader 2008). Over 400 varieties of potato grown in the Andes today, reflecting their genetic diversity and its expression in different environments. Following the spread of the devastating fungal disease that caused the Irish potato famine in the mid-19th century, breeders attempted to develop a variety of potato that was resistant to blight. This effort finally achieved success when a European breeder crossed his own variety with wild potato plants from Mexico and could take advantage of the genetic makeup of the wild potato for breeding disease resistance to fungal blight (Reader 2008).

One of the hallmarks of agriculture is the selective breeding of specific traits in plants and animals for favorable properties of growth (e.g., drought tolerance, disease resistance), storage, taste (sweet or starchy, fatty or lean), and other attributes. In the wild, genetic diversity is the raw material for natural selection. Farmers and plant breeders continue to manipulate genetic diversity in developing new cultivars or adding new traits to established cultivars.

10.3.2 Species Diversity

In biology, a species is a basic unit of biological organization involving multiple, closely related individuals. For animals and plants, a species consists of one or more populations of individuals that are capable of interbreeding and producing fertile offspring (http://www.biology-online.org/dictionary/Species). In agriculture, *species diversity* refers to the different kinds of cultivated crops and livestock animals, as well as organisms used in biological control of pests or weeds. It also includes all species in the associated ecosystem. Planned species diversity varies widely among agroecosystems. Industrial agriculture has specialized in large areas dedicated to single species—monocultures—of crop plants. The livestock equivalent is the confined animal operation, in which hundreds to thousands of individual animals are raised in high density. These monocultures offer convenience for standardized management by a few workers and are justified by practitioners as representing economies of scale. In contrast, traditional peasant agriculture, most organic agriculture, and diversified farming systems feature multiple species of plants or animals grown in planned combinations (Kremen and Miles 2012, Gliessman 2014).

The associated species diversity includes the microbes, plants, and animals that grow on farms or in the farm landscape. Some of these species may also be managed by farmers—either encouraged or suppressed. The vast majority of associated diversity has neutral to positive effects on the planned species diversity; associated species may provide substantial ecosystem services in the form of stabilizing soil, hosting beneficial predators for biological control, or moderating local microclimates (Vandermeer and Perfecto 2005, Gliessman 2014).

10.3.3 Habitat Diversity

Habitat diversity includes the natural variation in topography, microclimate, soils, and biota found across terrestrial ecosystems and occurs at spatial scales of hectares (100 m × 100 m) to hundreds of square kilometers. Farmers may take advantage of this variation to grow different crops in different microhabitats—for example, raising moisture-loving crops in poorly drained areas and drought-tolerant crops or deeply rooted trees in well drained areas. Planting (or leaving) trees in shelterbelts, in shade stands, or as living fences is another way of managing habitat diversity on farms. For farmers who raise many kinds of plants or animals, habitat diversity is a valuable resource since it facilitates different growing conditions. In industrial agriculture, habitat diversity is often a nuisance since it signifies non-uniform growing conditions across the farm landscape. Precision agriculture is a technological management system in industrial agriculture that uses field and crop-production data to vary inputs according to variation in field conditions (McLoud et al. 2007). Typically, precision agriculture utilizes GPS (global positioning systems) and multiple sensors to adjust rates of seeding and application of fertilizer and biocides in response to microhabitat variation.

All three aspects of biodiversity on farms and ranches present a combination of opportunities and challenges to farmers. Industrial agriculture has taken the approach of restricting most of the planned and associated genetic diversity, species diversity, and habitat diversity on farms. Traditional peasant agriculture, organic agriculture, and modern diversified farming systems (Kremen and Miles 2012) have utilized these aspects of diversity to provide ecological services, such as soil fertility and autonomous pest control (see following section). The more that we learn about ecological interactions between the planned and associated biodiversity on farms, the more we realize how important all aspects of biodiversity are to the long-term health of farms and the landscapes in which they are embedded (Perfecto et al. 2009).

10.4   BIOLOGICAL DIVERSITY AND ECOLOGICAL PROCESSES

Biological diversity in its several dimensions contributes to ecological processes that are essential for healthy agroecosystems. Nearly 100 years of agroecological research—from the time of Sir Albert Howard and Lady Eve Balfour—have built upon indigenous knowledge to develop a series of principles and practices for farming based on a variety of ecological processes (Altieri 1995, Vandermeer 2011, Gliessman 2014). Also, the classic reference books for organic and agroecological gardening emphasize the value of biodiversity in garden and farm design for the agronomic goals described below (Bradley et al. 2009, Jeavons 2012). Described below are the five properties and processes whereby biological diversity contributes to the ecology of agriculture.

10.4.1   SOIL FERTILITY

Soil fertility is critical to agriculture. The structure, texture, chemistry, and microbial content of soils determine their ability to provide plants with sufficient macronutrients, micronutrients, and moisture for optimal growth. As a substrate, soil influences the growth pattern and depth of root systems, which determine their ability to take up nutrients and water (Brady and Weil 2016). A vast diversity of organisms contributes to soil fertility, including several major groups of microbes, many kinds of invertebrates, some vertebrates, and plants. These organisms contribute to nutrient cycling, soil texture and structure, and soil organic matter. The complex feedbacks between the biodiversity in soils and the plant diversity above ground are active areas of research.

Two recent studies document the positive influence of plant diversity on soil fertility. Balvanera et al. (2006) summarized the results of hundreds of published studies about the effects of increased species diversity on ecosystem functions. Their analysis demonstrated positive effects of plant diversity on microbial biomass and decomposer activity, and of plant and belowground mycorrhizal fungal diversity on nutrient storage in the soil. Experiments in the long-term grassland field trials in Jena, Germany, (modeled after European hay meadows) showed that higher plant diversity resulted in more diverse, active microbial communities below ground and consequently in higher rates of carbon storage in soil (Lange et al. 2015). Stored carbon is a source of nutrition for soil microbes, animals, and plant roots, as well as an important mechanism of sequestering carbon from the atmosphere.

Although plants obtain most of their carbon for growth from the atmosphere (CO_2) via photosynthesis, carbon in soil organic matter is important in several ways. Plants absorb some organic compounds from the soil, and the amount of carbon in soil has a positive influence on microbes that participate in nutrient cycling (see 10.4.2 below). Organic matter, including humus—which is resistant to decay, enhances the capacity of soil to retain moisture (Brady and Weil 2016). Soil organic matter supports large root systems and fungal (mycorrhizal) hyphae that bind soil particles together, thereby holding water and resisting erosion.

10.4.2 Nutrient Cycling

The microbial ecosystem in soils provides essential macronutrients to plants. Particularly important are the bacteria that facilitate biological nitrogen fixation and the fungi that mobilize phosphorus, since nitrogen and phosphorus are the most common limiting nutrients for plant growth (Gliessman 2014). Certain bacteria (diazotrophs) are able to transform the abundant nitrogen in the atmosphere into forms of reduced nitrogen that plants can utilize directly, a process known as biological nitrogen fixation. Some nitrogen-fixing bacteria (such as *Rhizobium*) live symbiotically in nodules on the roots of plants in the legume family (peas, *Acacia*, clover), as well as on roots of other agriculturally important plant species. Other nitrogen-fixing bacteria (such as *Azotobacter*) are free-living in soils. Fungi, especially mold fungi such as *Penicillium* and *Fusarium*, are capable of decomposing complex plant compounds, which become available to other organisms. Some fungi are able to mobilize phosphorus from inorganic sources and transform it into a soluble form for uptake by plant roots (Hendrix et al. 1990, Montgomery and Biklé 2015). Plants have a wide array of partnerships with bacteria, fungi, and other microbes, whereby plant exudates are exchanged for nutrients or for suppression of plant pathogens. This belowground diversity responds positively in terms of microbial biomass and activity to above-ground plant diversity.

Agroecosystems that entail greater plant diversity sequester more carbon and thereby support more microbial activity. In field trials of organic versus conventional cropping systems, the organic systems sequestered more carbon in soils (Delate et al. 2015). The organic systems, in comparison with industrial monocultures, had greater plant diversity, either by inclusion of cover crops or by rotations involving more crop species, than the conventional systems. The increased carbon storage under the organically managed soils was found to support greater microbial biomass and activity, increased moisture retention, as well as greater carbon sequestration.

The high short-term yields of industrial cropping systems may be undermining the long-term fertility of soils by compromising microbial activity in the presence of synthetic fertilizers. In structured field comparisons, organic systems have higher plant-available nitrogen over the long term than their conventionally managed counterparts (Teasdale et al. 2007, Delate et al. 2015). A meta-analysis of the nitrogen cycle in a variety of agricultural systems revealed that application of synthetic nitrogen fertilizer on crop fields suppresses biological nitrogen fixation (Mulvaney et al. 2009).

Soil fertility and nutrient cycling depend on high microbial diversity, biomass, and activity. These properties appear to be enhanced by plant diversity above ground. In turn, vigorous microbial ecosystems support the yields, water infiltration capacity, drought resistance, and carbon sequestration that characterize multi-species grain and vegetable systems under agroecological management.

10.4.3 MUTUALISM AND FACILITATION

In ecology, mutualism involves interactions in which two or more species each provide a benefit to the other (Vandermeer 2011). Facilitation, also known as commensalism, occurs when one species provides a service to others without substantial reciprocation or harm (Boucher et al. 2001). Mutualistic and facilitative interactions among species are common in farming systems that follow agroecological principles. Most examples of intercropping, in which multiple species are grown together, are based on mutualism or facilitation.

A classic example of mutualistic interactions involves the "three sisters" of Mesoamerican agriculture. Corn, beans, and squash provide mutual ecological benefits in the field and show higher yields when grown together than in equivalent areas planted in monoculture (Gliessman 2014). Corn provides tall sturdy stalks as climbing support for beans and a strong root system; beans climb the corn stalk and provide fertility via biological nitrogen fixation from their symbiotic association with bacteria; squash plants meander through the corn rows at ground level and suppress some weeds through shading by their large leaves and through negative allelopathy. Allelopathy is the condition in which one kind of organism produces chemical compounds that affect the life history (negatively or positively) of other organisms.

Other mutualistic systems involve cover crops and agroforestry. Cover crops are plantings of single or multiple species in the presence of a primary harvest crop, such as clover (cover crop) intersown with wheat (primary crop). Cover crops have several beneficial roles. By covering otherwise bare ground, they reduce soil erosion and evaporative water loss from the soil surface. They may also improve soil structure and fertility, suppress weed growth, and deter pests through negative allelopathy (Wezel et al. 2014). Leguminous cover crops, including clover, vetch, and peas, increase nitrogen for the main harvest crop, sometimes for more than one growing season.

Agroforestry, the incorporation of trees into field plantings and pastures, offers a range of benefits for the associated crops or livestock animals. Trees provide shade, wind protection, and often fertility or fodder from leaves or seeds. In addition, trees with long roots tap deep sources of water and nutrients and can draw them upward in the soil profile (Gliessman 2014). The same interacting species can exhibit both mutualistic (or facilitative) and competitive interactions, either simultaneously or at different growth stages. The ecologically informed farmer must manage the diversity in the agroecosystem to optimize the advantages across the farm.

10.4.4 COMPETITION

Plants often compete intensively for space, nutrients, water, and light. These interactions are typically strongest among individuals of the same species because their resource requirements are similar. Self-thinning occurs when some individuals monopolize resources and stifle other individuals completely. In farming, competition from weeds poses recurring challenges. Mechanical tilling and herbicide application are strategies to reduce the competitive effects of weeds on the planned plant diversity. Both practices have destructive effects on parts of the agroecosystem (Wezel et al. 2014). Tilling disrupts soil structure and increases the likelihood of erosion and loss of nutrients, including carbon. Herbicides directed at specific weeds affect many non-target organisms, including soil biota, and may linger in soils and on plant tissues after harvest. Farmers following agroecology eschew herbicides but may use some kind of tillage. There is ongoing research to develop mechanical methods of weed control that reduce disruption of the soil surface.

Some of the facilitation strategies mentioned above (see 10.4.3 above) exemplify the addition of species diversity for weed control in agroecosystems. A strategy with underutilized potential is the use of plants that produce compounds that are negatively allelopathic (see 10.4.3 above), either when the plants are alive or during decomposition of crop residues (Wezel et al. 2014). For example, rye, sorghum, and sunflower release root exudates that inhibit weed germination (De Albuquerque et al. 2011). The residues of brassica (mustard family) crops have negative allelopathic effects on some weeds, fungal diseases, and nematodes (Médiène et al. 2011, Ratnadass et al. 2012).

10.4.5 PREDATION

Since the major goal of agriculture is to produce food or fiber for human consumption, it is not surprising that many other consumers are attracted to the same agricultural products. In some cases, the consumers and parasites (all considered "predators" in ecology) are the same species that eat wild relatives of the cultivated plants and animals, thereby extending the food webs that are present among the associated biodiversity. In many cases, the consumers are novel, either because the cultivated species are introduced into ecosystems far from their original geographic distribution or because the consumers themselves have been introduced. The mouse that eats beets, the larva of the corn earworm, and the cabbage-looper caterpillar are designated as pests, whereas the weasel that eats the mouse, the bat that eats the earworm moth, and the bluebird that eats the caterpillar are considered beneficial natural enemies.

The principle of biological control involves understanding and promoting the predator-prey interactions that are appropriate for particular agroecosystems. In order for biological control to work beyond a single boom-and-bust cycle (i.e., massive release of a natural enemy that consumes the pest population and then collapses), it is important to maintain a large enough pest population or enough alternate prey for the enemy-predator population to persist (Vandermeer 2011). The most effective biological control strategies are those that involve a diversity of natural enemies that reside in the native ecosystem, along with agronomic practices, such as crop rotation, that inhibit the annual cycle of pest populations. A diverse set of interacting predators, parasites, parasitoids, mutualists, and diseases—on par with the ecological complexity of natural ecosystems—can provide checks and balances resulting in "autonomous biological control" such that pests never achieve outbreaks even though they persist in the agroecosystem (Vandermeer et al. 2010).

This brief summary of contributions of biological diversity to agroecological processes illustrates three points. First, much of the associated biodiversity in agroecosystems has positive to neutral effects on the growth of cultivated plants and animals and aids in the maintenance of ecological services over decades and longer. Even industrial monocultures benefit from the soil microbes and natural enemies in the agroecosystem. Second, ecological theory in combination with empirical studies and farmer experience provides a foundation in knowledge and practice for agroecology to manage biodiversity so as to maintain soil fertility and to control weeds and pests without synthetic inputs, even though much remains to be learned about the best practices in different settings. Third, just as biodiversity contributes to ecological processes, farms that manage this diversity for agronomic goals have opportunities to conserve native species and habitats on farms and ranches.

10.5 PERSISTENCE AT THE LANDSCAPE SCALE

Ecologists since Aldo Leopold (1991) and Rachel Carson (1962) have emphasized that the farm is an integral part of a larger landscape. The fate of native species depends on the ability of individual organisms to disperse across the landscape from one patch of suitable habitat to another. Thus, the number, distribution, and management of farms and ranches have a strong influence on the persistence or extinction of populations and species at the landscape scale.

By the 21st century, over 50% of the Earth's habitable terrestrial regions have become managed ecosystems, consisting primarily of agricultural landscapes in temperate and tropical regions (Scherr and McNeely 2008). Natural habitats occur as patches of small to large size at varying distances from each other, surrounded mainly by an agricultural "matrix" (Perfecto et al. 2009). Ecological theory specifies that populations in habitat fragments—essentially islands—are prone to extinction. The likelihood of extinction is proportional to the area of the habitat fragment, other factors being equal; the smaller the fragment, the higher the likelihood of extinction. The extinction of a population in a single habitat patch does not spell the extinction of the species, as long as individuals from other patches can recolonize the empty patch. Recolonization can occur when individuals from populated patches are capable of dispersing through the intervening areas to colonize the empty patches of natural habitat. If dispersal through an inhospitable matrix is unsuccessful, then populations will become extinct more rapidly than empty habitats are recolonized. As long as the dispersal rate is greater than the extinction rate in habitat fragments, then a species can persist as a set of populations distributed across the landscape. These principles are the foundation of metapopulation ecology (Hanksi 1999). They highlight the importance of planning farming systems at the landscape scale (Landis 2017).

These principles are borne out by studies of biodiversity in different agricultural systems. Consider, for example, coffee farms. In the tropics, coffee is grown under a wide variety of management styles, ranging from "rustic" and "shade" coffee farms—which closely resemble natural forests—to "sun" coffee farms, in which the natural forest is completely replaced with an industrial monoculture of coffee bushes (Perfecto and Vandermeer 2015). Across this management spectrum, the diversity of birds, ants, and butterflies is high in shade and rustic coffee farms and drops substantially in intensive coffee monocultures (Perfecto et al. 2009). In the highlands of southern Mexico, which are hotspots of biodiversity for birds, mammals, and arthropods, the native forest occurs as fragmentary patches in a matrix of coffee farms. Species that require large areas of mature forest for survival are able to persist by dispersing among forest fragments. Many such species can persist in shade-coffee farms, but not in sun-coffee monocultures. In addition, the high diversity of arthropods, especially ants, in shade-coffee farms provide natural biological control of the major insect pests of coffee, as described above (see 10.4.5).

Two recent studies conclude that agricultural intensification, i.e., the prevalence of industrial agriculture over large areas, reduces the persistence of native species at the scale of their geographic ranges (the landscape scale). Karp et al. (2012) compared the diversity of birds in low-intensity agriculture (small, diversified farms), high-intensity agriculture (large industrial monocultures), and native forest in Costa Rica. They evaluated changes in species number, composition, and abundance across habitats (turnover rates) in order to assess how agricultural-management styles impacted geographic variation in bird faunas across the landscape. Turnover rates in bird faunas were similar for native forest and low-intensity agriculture but were 40% lower in areas of high-intensity agriculture. The overall abundance of birds, the number of species, and their ecological diversity were lower in areas dominated by industrial agriculture. Karp et al. (2012) found that industrial agriculture disrupted spatial variation in natural vegetation structure and diversity and attributed the reduced bird diversity to this change.

The second study involves insects in temperate Europe. Hallmann et al. (2017) documented startling declines in the biomass of flying insects from protected areas across Germany. Over a period of 27 years (late 20th century to the current decade), insect biomass declined by 77% across multiple habitats; the losses were even greater during midsummer, when insect biomass is typically highest during the annual cycle. Changes in neither local climatic conditions, land cover, nor site habitat variables were substantive predictors of the decline in insect biomass. The authors noted that most of the sampling sites were surrounded by agricultural fields and speculated that increase in agricultural intensification, especially the widespread use of pesticides, was an important factor. Essentially, the protected areas have become islands of natural habitat in a matrix of industrial agriculture; the results are consistent with a reduction in dispersal rate across an inhospitable matrix and extinction of isolated populations in habitat fragments.

10.6   EXAMPLES OF BIODIVERSE AGRICULTURE

Farming that supports biodiversity entails design and practices that maintain both planned and associated biodiversity. Small-scale (<1 ha) plantings of diverse crops, intercropping over larger areas (>1 ha), and multi-species hay meadows are examples with regard to planned biodiversity. Farms and ranches that include areas of native habitat can support native biodiversity, including top predators (Imhoff 2003). Ideally, the size and distribution of patches of native habitat are managed at the landscape scale to enable dispersal of individuals among patches.

Three agroecological approaches are especially relevant: (1) natural-systems agriculture (see below, 10.6.2), in which the agroecosystem mimics the structure and processes of the native ecosystem that it replaces (Soule and Piper 1992) (2) ecoagriculture, in which conservation of native species is a purposeful goal of the farming system (Scherr and McNeely 2008) (3) diversified farming systems, in which the farm design includes different components of biodiversity (native and introduced) to maintain essential ecosystem services that support the production of crops or livestock (Kremen et al. 2012). These approaches overlap with the practices of organic, multifunctional, and regenerative agriculture but are not synonymous.

Three examples of biodiverse farming systems illustrate how both the planned and associated biodiversity contribute to the functioning of the agroecosystem. In these examples, the ecological complexities of biodiverse agroecosystems provide ecological services important to farmers and the food system.

10.6.1 Diversified Organic Vegetable and Fruit Production

In the United States, thousands of small (~10 ha) farms have started up in the last two decades with a focus on vegetable and fruit production, mainly to supply local markets (Kleppel 2014). Produce farms that also raise livestock are typically larger to include hay meadows and pasture. Many of these farms follow agroecological practices, as certified organic, as organic-compliant without certification, or as biodynamic. Such farms may raise more than 50 kinds of vegetables and fruits. Agronomic practices typically include crop rotation through the growing season and between growing seasons, intercropping, cover crops and green manures during fallow or non-growing seasons, strategic placement of allelopathic plants and trap crops, as well as protection or cultivation of native habitats for natural enemies—ranging from birds to parasitic wasps. Such farms may include hedgerows, woodlots, natural wetlands, and buffer strips throughout the farm to maintain habitat complexity for both agronomic and aesthetic purposes (Baumgartner 2006). The natural and semi-natural habitats support beneficial predators and pollinators and disrupt the spatial distribution of herbivore pests. Several studies have documented lower rates of crop damage as the area of semi-natural habitat increases (e.g., Östman et al. 2001, Thies et al. 2003, Altieri and Nicholls 2004).

10.6.2 Natural-Systems Agriculture of the Land Institute

Under the leadership of Wes Jackson, The Land Institute in Salina, Kansas, is developing a new approach to grain agriculture modeled after the tallgrass prairie, the native ecosystem of central Kansas (Jackson 1980, Soule and Piper 1992). Grains are a focus because of their large caloric contribution to modern human diets, their utility as forage crops, and the prevalence of grasses in the native ecosystems of many agricultural regions. A major motivation is to develop an alternative paradigm to the industrial monocultures of the Green Revolution with their massive environmental damage on the farm, downstream, and beyond. The new paradigm involves "perennial polycultures," perennial plants grown in mixtures. Perennials have deeper roots than those of most annuals; these long roots tap deep sources of water and nutrients, are more drought-tolerant, and sequester more carbon than annuals do.

With the plant functional diversity of the prairie as a model, the perennial polycultures suited to central Kansas and much of the U.S. grain belt include cool-season (C_3) grasses, warm-season (C_4) grasses, legumes and sunflowers (Jackson 1980). Research focuses on breeding perennial versions of annual grasses; on developing agronomically desirable traits (e.g., larger seeds); and experimenting with different numbers and proportions of species and functional groups for yields, drought tolerance, and natural pest control. The Land Institute has achieved substantial gains toward all of these goals (www.landinstitute.org/research). Research shows that perennial systems have yields comparable to those of grain monocultures, sequester more carbon, and maintain higher numbers of arthropod species, including natural enemies (Glover et al. 2010).

10.6.3 SHADE COFFEE

Coffee is grown under a wide range of management regimes, from monocultures of coffee bushes in full sun to organic shade coffee within managed forests. Long-term studies of the shade-coffee system in Chiapas, Mexico, demonstrate that these systems can support high proportions of the native biodiversity (ants, birds, butterflies, mammals) found in natural forests (Perfecto and Vandermeer 2015), thereby contributing to conservation of species and habitats in some of the most biodiverse regions of the world.

Coffee grows as a shrub in the understory of trees that are planted or part of the natural forest. In the montane regions where coffee is grown, trees stabilize soils and reduce wind speed and evaporation. The forest supports pollinators and predators and parasites of the pests and diseases of coffee. A remarkable system of autonomous pest control keeps the major pests—the coffee berry borer and the green coffee scale insect—and the coffee rust disease below economically damaging levels. A series of ecological interactions involving arboreal ants and the spatial clustering of their nests, a parasitoid fly, beetles, fungi, the scale insect, and the coffee berry borer, keeps the coffee pests at low levels over most of the system (Vandermeer et al. 2008, 2010). Management involves maintaining trees for the arboreal ants to nest in and avoiding applications of pesticides that would depress insect populations that are part of the natural biological-control system.

10.7 CAN WE FEED THE WORLD WITH BIODIVERSE AGRICULTURE?

Can biodiverse agriculture based on agroecological principles feed the world? This question is often implicitly meant as "can agriculture based on agroecology produce as much food as the industrial system does?" The more appropriate question is: "Can agriculture based on agroecology produce sufficient food for the human population?" Since these are different questions, they have different answers.

Several studies have compared yields for different major food categories from organic practices versus industrial practices; the difference between the yields of the two production systems is called the yield gap (and can range from negative to zero to positive). Organic agriculture is one of the farming approaches that largely follow agroecological principles. Badgley et al. (2007) compiled yield comparisons from 91 studies. For data from developed countries, the yield gap varied from −18% to positive (i.e., organic yields were greater) among food categories. For developing countries, where the comparison was between organic methods and traditional peasant agriculture, modern organic methods yielded 80% more, on average. Assuming the lower yield gaps determined for developed countries, organic agriculture could still provide enough calories and nutrients to feed the entire human population. This study also investigated rates of biological nitrogen fixation as a potential substitute for synthetic fertilizer. The authors estimated that biological nitrogen fixation could generate enough nitrogen to replace all of the synthetic fertilizer currently in use, based on measured rates of biological nitrogen fixation in temperate and tropical agroecosystems, extrapolated to agricultural land where synthetic fertilizers are currently in use. Other estimates suggest that biological nitrogen fixation, recycled nitrogen from crop residues, and animal manures could come close to replacing the nitrogen from synthetic fertilizer (Smil 2002, Seufert and Ramankutty 2017).

More recent meta-analyses comparing yields between organic and industrial methods have documented average yield gaps of −19% to −25% for organically grown food (Seufert et al. 2012, Ponisio et al. 2015, Kniss et al. 2016), varying in magnitude depending on the cropping system and food category. For example, the yield gap between organic polyculture systems and industrial monoculture is smaller than the gap between organic monoculture and industrial monoculture (Ponisio et al. 2015). Cereal crops showed high yield gaps (~20%) in two of the meta-analyses, which may reflect the decades of intensive breeding programs for high-yielding varieties developed for industrial management practices, without comparable investments in varieties grown under agroecological management.

A recent survey of six long-term field trials (over 18–35 years) of organic versus industrial methods in the United States provides insights about yields, soil fertility, performance under drought conditions, and greenhouse gas emissions (Delate et al. 2015). Five of the six trials focused on cereals, soybeans, and alfalfa; one trial included cereals, two vegetable crops, and an oil crop. Yields across the six systems varied widely, depending on weather conditions and management of fertility and weeds. For some systems and years, there was no yield gap; in other years, organic yields were substantially (36%) to moderately (8%) lower. Over time, organic yields improved with changes in management. Notably, in drought years, the organic plots yielded more than the industrial plots (Lotter et al. 2003). In all six trials, measures of soil health and carbon sequestration were greater in the organic systems than in the industrial systems.

Thus, for the first question about organic versus industrial yields, organic yields are often lower than industrial yields for the same crops in the same context, but the yield gaps can decline over time with improved management. For the second question of whether organic agriculture could produce sufficient food to feed the world, even if yields are 20% lower across the board, organic agriculture could, in principle, produce sufficient food. Currently, the global food system provides 2,884 calories (kcal)/person/day for consumption; for most high-income countries, the amount is greater than 3,600 kcal/person/day (Roser and Ritchie 2017).

Reducing these amounts by 20% still provides sufficient calories to meet the average recommended daily caloric intake of 2,000 kcal/person (Smil 2004).

Other aspects of the current global food system place these analyses of yield gaps in perspective. First, estimates of food loss and waste are one-third globally (FAO 2011). For the United States, the estimate is that 40% of food produced is lost across stages of harvest, processing, sale, and final use (Hall et al. 2009). This amount of waste represents 1,400 kcal per person per day, or 124 kg per person per year, 300 million barrels of oil per year (for fertilizer production, harvesting, and transportation), and the associated greenhouse gas emissions (Buzby and Hyman 2012).

Second, over 40% of the global grain supply is diverted to livestock feed, biofuels, and processing of high fructose corn syrup (FAO 2002). The proportion is much higher for the grain supply of the United States (Gurian-Sherman 2008; USDA National Agricultural Statistics Service 2016a). This reallocation of potentially nutritious food away from direct human consumption is a questionable use of agricultural resources.

A third consideration is that many diets are unsustainable in terms of resource use, environmental impacts, and health outcomes. In high-income countries, food availability exceeds 3,000 kcal per person per day, when the actual food requirement is about 2,000 kcal (Smil 2004, FAO 2017). Artificially cheap foods that are high in sugar, salt, or fat promote unhealthy eating patterns (Carolan 2011). Animal products, which are artificially cheap in the United States through overproduction and subsides for grain, forage, and water, have much greater greenhouse gas emissions per calorie than plant foods (Tilman and Clark 2014; FAO 2017).

A final consideration is the sustainability of farming systems over decades and longer, in terms of maintenance of soil fertility and responses to climate change. Although projected climate changes vary substantially for different regions of the world (FAO 2017), persistent themes include increasing growing-season temperature and evapotranspiration, along with forecasts of severe droughts over large regions of croplands that are currently productive (Cook et al. 2015). Agroecological farming practices increase soil carbon and organic matter, which enhance water infiltration and the moisture-holding capacity of topsoils. These properties enable agroecological systems to perform better than industrial systems under drought conditions (Rodale Institute 2011).

These points illustrate that agroecological practices have the potential to feed the world, even if yields are lower in agroecological systems than in industrial systems. Reducing food waste by reducing the number of livestock consumed altogether and allowing those animals to graze naturally would allow a substantial amount of grain to be redirected toward human consumption. Additionally, the cropland could be repurposed for increased production of other foods, such as legumes, nuts, vegetables, and fruits. Furthermore, farming systems based on agroecological principles, which promote biodiversity from the field to farm to landscape, have greater inherent sustainability and provide more ecosystem services than industrial systems do.

10.8 CONCLUSION

Biodiversity—from microbes to pollinators to predators—serves agriculture in myriad ways. Yet food production and food harvesting from the wild are the major causes of elevated extinction rates around the world. This trend ultimately affects agricultural productivity since the decline of wild populations and species includes pollinators and natural enemies of pests. Thus, the imperative to promote and expand biodiverse farms and ranches is great. Planning the size and configuration of farms and natural habitats at the landscape scale is critical for maintaining species and ecosystem services over the long term.

Both traditional forms of peasant agriculture (such as shade coffee) and recent innovations (such as perennial-grain polycultures) feature species and habitat diversity and ecological processes as fundamental to the design and operation of farms. Transforming agriculture to become sustainable and regenerative must involve diversified farming systems and conservation of biodiversity as the norm. Scaling up the many successful examples of biodiverse farming is an urgent goal for both humanity and nature.

VIGNETTE 10.1   Understanding Veganic Agriculture

Mona Seymour

INTRODUCTION

Veganic agriculture refers to organic farming without inputs from farmed animals. In going "beyond organic," veganic growing not only avoids synthetic fertilizers, pesticides, fungicides, and GMOs, but also farmed animal wastes and remains such as manure, blood meal, feather meal, fish meal, and bone meal that are typically used to enhance soil fertility in organic agriculture (Veganic Agriculture Network 2014). A veganic system enhances soil fertility through the use of inputs including plant-based composts and mulches, green manures (plants that are grown and returned to the soil for fertility purposes), chipped branch wood, seaweed fertilizers, and mineral amendments. Veganic agriculture incorporates agroecological and regenerative techniques such as planting to attract beneficial insects and creating barriers to eliminate pests rather than using synthetic products (Hall and Tolhurst 2007, Veganic Agriculture Network 2012, 2014, 2016).

Historically, agriculture without synthetic and farmed animal inputs has been practiced around the world in societies without access to these resources. For instance, some horticultural societies did not keep domesticated animals and thus had no ready source of manure (Mt. Pleasant 2011, Richerson et al. 1996). The "three sisters" system of planting beans, corn, and squash together that was practiced by indigenous peoples of northeastern North America is an example of an indigenous cropping system free of chemical and farmed animal inputs. As mentioned previously, corn stalks provide support for climbing beans, which fix nitrogen in the soil to the benefit of the corn. Squash leaves suppress weeds and keep the ground cool and moist as decomposing plant residues provide nutrients essential to growth (Mt. Pleasant 2009). Interestingly, veganic growing encompasses many approaches and can be implemented at multiple scales.

As opposition rises both to conventional chemical-based agriculture and to intensive animal agriculture, veganic agriculture is garnering increased attention around the world although it remains a fringe activity. There are thought to be fewer than 50 commercial veganic farms in the United States, about a quarter of which are certified organic, (Seymour 2017) in comparison to 12,818 certified organic farms (USDA National Agricultural Statistics Service 2016b). However, research trials point to the viability of veganic systems. For instance, U.S. trials have demonstrated veganic corn and soybean yields to be similar to those of comparator animal organic and conventional systems—and sometimes outperform one or both of those systems in drought years (Lotter et al. 2003, Pimentel et al. 2005). Trials in the United Kingdom (U.K.) have shown yields of a veganic system generally comparable to or exceeding average organic yields in the U.K. (Watson et al. 2000; Welsh et al. 2002).

ENVIRONMENTAL HEALTH BENEFITS

Veganic growing shares the environmental benefits conferred by organic agriculture. For instance, consistent with organic principles, veganic systems avoid synthetic pesticides. They use green manures and create habitat for wildlife. Crop rotation and low or zero tillage principles are employed. These practices support on-farm plant and wildlife biodiversity while conserving water and minimizing soil loss. Further, fossil fuel inputs are minimized while soil organic matter content is enriched—all while improving the soil's carbon dioxide sequestration potential (Bengtsson et al. 2005; Gomiero et al. 2011; Hole et al. 2005; Mondelaers et al. 2009).

Veganic farmers avoid animal waste and other by-products to avoid introducing likely contaminants into the environment. Manure obtained from conventional farms may contain veterinary pharmaceuticals (such as antibiotics and hormones that have been fed to the animals for reasons including infectious disease suppression and growth acceleration) as well as naturally occurring hormones. These compounds will enter soils and waterways and adversely impact terrestrial and aquatic ecosystems (Kemper 2008; Sarmah et al. 2006). For instance, estrogens from manure-treated soils can be transported into water bodies where they have the potential to negatively affect the reproductive biology of aquatic species (Kjær et al. 2007). Use of animal manures can also lead to soil salinization, soil phosphorous loading, and nitrate pollution of groundwater (Cherr et al. 2006; Dahan et al. 2014).

Veganic growing has the potential to diminish agriculture's contribution to global warming. Organic green manure-based systems may in some cases require less fossil energy inputs than organic systems that incorporate animal manure, reducing the amount of carbon dioxide released into the atmosphere (Pimentel et al. 2005; Clark and Tilman 2017). Animal agriculture is responsible for substantial greenhouse gas emissions and global warming, as well as air and water pollution and biodiversity loss (Food and Agriculture Organization of the United Nations 2006). Veganic agriculture avoids such environmentally damaging externalities through refraining from the purchase and use of farmed animal waste products.

The broad vision of some veganic farmers is a plant-based food system. Such a shift would constitute a less wasteful mode of food production, as it is more efficient for humans to consume the grain directly as indicated in

Chapter 3 (Cassidy et al. 2013, Goodland 1997, Pimentel 1984, West et al. 2014). Furthermore, the land used to raise livestock and the land used to grow feed for livestock could be redirected toward growing plant food for people. As an example, a rough calculation of the amount of land required to feed the population of Britain using vegan organic cultivation (one approach to veganics) and producing a vegan diet shows a reduction in agricultural land needs from 18.5 to 7.3 million hectares (Fairlie 2010). The millions of hectares of land removed from cultivation could be restored as native habitat, promoting biodiversity while mitigating climate change. These benefits would accrue at a smaller scale and magnitude if the shift to veganic cultivation and veganism were not universal.

BENEFITS TO HUMAN HEALTH

Like organic systems, veganic systems avoid the health risks to farm workers, agricultural community residents, and consumers who are exposed to chemical pesticides and pesticide residues associated with conventional agriculture. These include increased risks of certain cancers, neurological damage, reproductive effects, developmental disorders, immune system suppression, and acute poisoning (Alavanja et al. 2004, Lozowicka 2015, Lu et al. 2000, Muñoz-Quezada et al. 2016, Pimentel 2005).

Veganic growers avoid additional sources of contaminants in rejecting fertility inputs from farmed animals. Manure can harbor pathogens such as *Salmonella*, *Escherichia coli*, and *Campylobacter*. Application of contaminated manure to farm fields is one way contaminated crops may reach consumers (Heaton and Jones 2008, Mukherjee et al. 2004, Nicholson et al. 2005). The use of animal wastes and remains can also lead to soil and crop contamination by antibiotics and other drugs (Kumar et al. 2005). For instance, feather meal produced from broiler chickens, which are commonly fed arsenical drugs, has been shown to contain levels of inorganic arsenic. When used as organic fertilizer, this feather meal may contribute to arsenic exposure in farmers and gardeners through inhalation and dermal contact, and in consumers through the ingestion of crops that have accumulated arsenic from fertilized soil (Nachman et al. 2012).

OTHER VALUES OF VEGANIC GROWING

Farmers and gardeners may implement a veganic approach to realize additional values may include the following:

- Veganic methods eliminates concern for animal exploitation. This is a key value for many veganic growers.
- Veganic agriculture offers additional economic benefits. Animal-based fertility can be difficult to source in regions that are inhospitable to animal agriculture. Local sourcing or on-farm preparation of resources that are readily available such as green manures and composts eliminates the need for growers to purchase and import synthetic inputs and fertility from distant animal-based farms or slaughterhouses. Farmers without the capital to

invest in livestock for their holding can take a veganic approach to enhance soil fertility.

* Like organic agriculture, veganic growing has the potential to be practiced as a closed-loop system, with all inputs derived from the holding. This appeals to farmers and gardeners who value self-sufficiency, efficiency (for instance, the direct return of nutrients to the soil in the form of grass rather than manure), resource conservation, and low-impact lifestyles. However, factors including site, scale, growing method, and desired yield dictate whether some veganic fertility sources must be imported.

CONCLUSION

In summary, veganic agriculture is a promising approach to agriculture that is sustainable and regenerative (Hagemann and Potthast 2015, Taylor and Morone 2005). As the need for regenerative agriculture becomes increasingly urgent, expanded research will help to discern the potential of veganic methods to bolster our approach to organic and regenerative agriculture as well as biodiversity.

SELECTED VEGANIC AGRICULTURE RESOURCES

The following websites are recommended as resources for further information on veganic approaches, including instructional articles, key books, and videos:

Stockfree Organic Services http://stockfreeorganic.net/

Vegan Organic Network http://veganorganic.net/

Veganic Agriculture Network http://www.goveganic.net/

Vegan Permaculture www.veganicpermaculture.com

Veganic.World http://veganic.world/

REFERENCES

Alavanja, M. C. R., J. A. Hoppin, and F. Kamel. Health effects of chronic pesticide exposure: cancer and neurotoxicity. *Annu Rev Public Health* 25: 155–197.

Altieri, M. A. 1995. *Agroecology: The Science of Sustainable Agriculture*, 2nd edition. Boulder, CO: Westview Press.

Altieri, M. A. and C. I. Nicholls. 2004. *Biodiversity and Pest Management in Agroecosystems*. New York, NY: Food Product Press.

Badgley, C. 2002. Can agriculture and biodiversity coexist? In: *Fatal Harvest: The Tragedy of Industrial Agriculture*, edited by A. Kimbrell, 279–284. Washington, DC: Island Press.

Badgley, C. 2013. Modern biodiversity crisis. In: *Grzimek's Animal Life Encyclopedia, Extinction* (2 vols), edited by N. MacLeod, 617–634. Detroit, MI: Gale/Cengage Learning.

Badgley, C., J. Moghtader, E. Quintero, E. Zakem, M. J. Chappell, K. Avilés-Vázquez, A. Samulon, and I. Perfecto. 2007. Organic agriculture and the global food supply. *Renewable Agriculture and Food Systems* 22: 86–108.

Balvanera, P., A. B. Pfisterer, N. Buchmann, Jing-Shen He, T. Nakashizuka, D. Raffaelli, and B. Schmid. 2006. Quantifying the evidence for biodiversity effects on ecosystem functioning and services. *Ecology Letters* 9: 1146–1156.

Baumgartner, J. A. 2006. Making organic wild. In: *Farming and the Fate of Wild Nature*, edited by D. Imhoff and J. A. Baumgartner, 103–113. Healdsburg, CA: Watershed Media.

Bengtsson, J., J. Ahnström, and A. Weibull. 2005. The effects of organic agriculture on biodiversity and abundance: a meta-analysis. *J Appl Ecol* 42: 261–269.

Boucher, D. H., S. James, and K. H. Keeler. 2001. The ecology of mutualism. *Annual Review of Ecology and Systematics* 13: 315–347.

Bradley, F. M., B. W. Ellis, and E. Phillips, eds. 2009. *Rodale's Ultimate Encyclopedia of Organic Gardening*. New York, NY: Rodale Press.

Brady, N. C. and R. R. Weil. 2016. *The Nature and Properties of Soils*, 15th edition. Harlow, UK: Pearson Education Limited.

Buzby, J. C. and J. Hyman. 2012. Total and per capita value of food loss in the United States. *Food Policy* 37: 561–570.

Carolan, M. 2011. *The Real Cost of Cheap Food*. London: Earthscan.

Carson, R. 1962. *Silent Spring*. Boston, MA: Houghton Mifflin.

Cassidy, E. S., P. C. West, J. S. Gerber, and J. A. Foley. 2013. Redefining agricultural yields: from tonnes to people nourished per hectare. *Environ Res Lett* 8: 1–8.

Cherr, C. M., J. M. S. Scholberg, and R. McSorley. 2006. Green manure approaches to crop production: a synthesis. *Agron J* 98: 302–319.

Clark, M and Tilman, D. 2017. Comparative analysis of environmental impacts of agricultural production systems, agricultural input efficiency, and food choice. *Environ. Res. Lett.* 12: 064016–11. https://doi.org/10.1088/1748-9326/aa6cd5

Cook, B. I., T. R. Ault, and J. E. Smerdon. 2015. Unprecedented 21st century drought risk in the American Southwest and Central Plains. *Science Advances* 1: e1400082.

Dahan, O., A. Babad, N. Lazarovitch, E. E. Russak, and D. Kurtzman. 2014. Nitrate leaching from intensive organic farms to groundwater. *Hydrol Earth Syst Sci* 18: 333–341.

De Albuquerque, M. B., R. C. Santos, L. M. Lima, P. A. Melo Filho, R. J. M. C. Nogueira, C. A. G. Da Câmara, and A. R. Ramos. 2011. Allelopathy, an alternative tool to improve cropping systems: A review. *Agronomy and Sustainable Development* 31: 379–395.

Delate, K., C. Cambardella, C. Chase, and R. Turnbull. 2015. A review of long-term organic comparison trials in the U.S. *Sustainable Agriculture Research* 4: 5–14.

Estes, J. A., J. Terborgh, J. S. Brashares, M. E. Power, J. Berger, W. J. Bond, S. R. Carpenter, et al. 2011. Trophic downgrading of Planet Earth. *Science* 333: 301–306.

Fairlie, S. 2010. *Meat: A Benign Extravagance*. White River Junction: Chelsea Green.

FAO (Food and Agriculture Organization). 2002. *World Agriculture: Towards 2015/2030*. Rome, Italy: FAO.

FAO (Food and Agriculture Organization). 2006. *Livestock's Long Shadow: Environmental Issues and Options*. Rome: FAO.

FAO (Food and Agriculture Organization). 2011. *Global Food Losses and Food Waste—Extent, Causes and Prevention*. Rome, Italy: FAO.

FAO (Food and Agriculture Organization). 2017. *The Future of Food and Agriculture—Trends and Challenges*. Rome, Italy: FAO.

Gibbs, K. E., R. L. Mackey, and D. J. Currie. 2009. Human land use, agriculture, pesticides and losses of imperiled species. *Diversity and Distributions* 14: 242–253.

Gliessman, S. R. 2014. *Agroecology: The Ecology of Sustainable Food Systems*, 3rd edition. Boca Raton, FL: CRC Press.

Glover, J. D., J. P. Reganold, L. W. Bell, J. Borevitz, E. C. Brummer, E. S. Buckler, C. M. Cox, et al. 2010. Increased food and ecosystem security via perennial grains. *Science* 328: 1638–1639.

Gomiero, T., D. Pimentel, and M. G. Paoletti. 2011. Environmental impact of different agricultural management practices: conventional vs. organic agriculture. *Crit Rev Plant Sci* 30 (1–2): 95–124.

Goodland, R. 1997. Environmental sustainability in agriculture: diet matters. *Ecol Econ* 23: 189–200.

Gurian-Sherman, D. 2008. *CAFOs Uncovered: The Untold Costs of Confined Animal Feeding Operations*. Cambridge, MA: Union of Concerned Scientists.

Haberl, H., K. Heinz Erb, F. Krausmann, V. Gaube, A. Bondeau, C. Plutzar, S. Gingrich, et al. 2007. Quantifying and mapping the human appropriation of net primary production in earth's terrestrial ecosystems. *Proceedings of the U.S. National Academy of Sciences* 104: 12942–12947.

Hagemann, N., and T. Potthast. 2015. Necessary new approaches towards sustainable agriculture – innovations for organic agriculture. In *Know Your Food: Food Ethics and Innovation*, ed. D. E. Dumitras, I. M. Jitea, and S. Aerts, 107–113. Wageningen: Wageningen Academic Publishers.

Hall, K. D., J. Guo, M. Dore, and C. C. Chow. 2009. The progressive increase of food waste in America and its environmental impact. *PLoS ONE* 4 (11): e7940.

Hall, J., and I. Tolhurst. 2007. *Growing Green: Animal-Free Organic Techniques*. White River Junction: Chelsea Green.

Hallmann, C. A., R. P. B Foppen, C. A. M. van Turnhout, H. de Kroon, and E. Jongejans. 2014. Declines in insectivorous birds are associated with high neonicotinoid concentrations. *Nature* 511: 341–343.

Hallmann, C. A, M. Sorg, E. Jongegans, H. Siepel, N. Hofland, H. Schwan, W. Stenmans, et al. 2017. More than 75 percent decline over 27 years in total flying insect biomass in protected areas. *PLoS ONE* 12 (10): e0185809.

Hanski, I. 1999. *Metapopulation Ecology*. Oxford: Oxford University Press.

Hayes, T. B. and M. Hansen. 2017. From silent spring to silent night: Agrochemicals and the Anthropocene. *Elementa Science of the Anthropocene* 5: 57.

Heaton, J. C., and K. Jones. 2005. Microbial contamination of fruit and vegetables and the behavior of enteropathogens in the phyllosphere: a review. *J Appl Microbio* 104: 613–626.

Hendrix, P. F., D. A. Crosskey, Jr., J. M. Blair, and D. C. Coleman. 1990. Soil biota as components of sustainable agroecosystems. In: *Sustainable Agricultural Systems*, edited by C. A. Edwards, R. Lal, P. Madden, R. H. Miller and G. House, 637–654. Boca Raton, FL: CRC Press.

Henry, M., M. Beguin, F. Requier, O. Rollin, J. F. Odoux, P. Aupinel, J. Aptel, et al. 2012. A common pesticide decreases foraging success and survival in honey bees. *Science* 336: 348–350.

Imhoff, D. 2003. *Farming with the Wild: Enhancing Biodiversity on Farms and Ranches*. San Francisco, CA: Sierra Club Books.

Jackson, W. 1980. *New Roots For Agriculture*. Lincoln, NE: University of Nebraska Press.

Jeavons, J. 2012. *How to Grow More Vegetables*, 8th edition. New York, NY: Ten Speed Press.

Karp, D. S., A. J. Rominger, J. Zook, J. Ranganathan, P. R. Ehrlich, and G. C. Daily. 2012. Intensive agriculture erodes ß-diversity at large scales. *Ecology Letters* 15: 963–970.

Kemper, N. 2008. Veterinary antibiotics in the aquatic and terrestrial environment. *Ecol Indic* 8: 1–13.

Kjær, J., P. Olsen, K. Bach, et al. 2007. Leaching of estrogenic hormones from manure-treated structured soils. *Environ Sci Technol* 41: 3911–3917.

Kleppel, G. 2014. *The Emergent Agriculture: Farming, Sustainability and the Return of the Local Economy*. Gabriola Island, BC: New Society Publishers.

Kniss, A. R., S. D. Savage, and R. Jabbour. 2016. Commercial crop yields reveal strengths and weaknesses for organic agriculture in the United States. *PLoS ONE* 11 (8): e0161673.

Kremen, C., A. Iles, and C. Bacon. 2012. Diversified farming systems: An agroecological, systems-based alternative to modern industrial agriculture. *Ecology and Society* 17 (4): 44.

Kremen, C. and A. Miles. 2012. Ecosystem services in biologically diversified versus conventional farming systems: benefits, externalities, and trade-offs. *Ecology and Society* 17 (4): 40.

Kumar, K., S. C. Gupta, S. K. Baidoo, Y. Chander, and C. J. Rosen. 2005. Antibiotic uptake by plants from soil fertilized with animal manure. *J Environ Qual* 34: 2082–2085.

Landis, D. A. 2017. Designing agricultural landscapes for biodiversity-based ecosystem services. *Basic and Applied Ecology* 18: 1–12.

Lange, M., N. Eisenhauer, C. A. Sierra, H. Bessler, C. Engels, R. I. Griffiths, P. G. Mellado-Vázquez et al. 2015. Plant diversity increases soil microbial activity and soil carbon storage. *Nature Communications* 7707. DOI:10.1038/ncomms7707.

Leopold, A. 1991. The farmer as a conservationist. In *The River of the Mother of God and Other Essays by Aldo Leopold*, edited by S. L. Flader and J. B. Callicott, 121–129. Madison, WI: University of Wisconsin Press.

Lotter, D. W., R. Seidel, and W. Liebhardt. 2003. The performance of organic and conventional cropping systems in an extreme climate year. *American Journal of Alternative Agriculture* 18: 146–154.

Lozowocka, B. 2015. Health risk for children and adults consuming apples with pesticide residue. *Sci Total Environ* 502: 184–198.

Lu, C. S., R. A. Fenske, N. J. Simcox, and D. Kalman. 2000. Pesticide exposure of children in an agricultural community: evidence of household proximity to farmland and take home exposure pathways. *Environ Res* 84: 290–302.

Matthiessen, P. 1959. *Wildlife in America*. New York, NY: Viking Press.

Maxwell, S. L., R. A. Fuller, T. M. Brooks, and J. E. M. Watson. 2016. The ravages of guns, nets and bulldozers. *Nature* 536: 143–145.

McLoud, P. R., R. Gronwald, and H. Kuykendall. 2007. Precision agriculture: NRCS support for emerging technologies. Agronomy Technical Note 1, Natural Resources Conservation Service, U.S. Department of Agriculture, Greensboro, NC.

Médiène, S., M. Valantin-Morison, U.-P. Sarthou, S. De Tourdonnet, M. Gosme, M. Bertrand, J. Roger-Estrade, et al. 2011. Agroecosystem management and biotic interactions: A review. *Agronomy for Sustainable Development* 31: 491–514.

Montgomery, D. R. and A. Biklé. 2015. *The Hidden Half of Nature: The Microbial Roots of Life and Health*. New York, NY: W.W. Norton.

Mt. Pleasant, J. 2011. The paradox of plows and productivity: an agronomic comparison of cereal grain production under Iroquois hoe culture and European plow culture in the seventeenth and eighteenth centuries. *Agr Hist* 85 (4): 460–492.

Mt. Pleasant, J. 2009. The science behind the three sisters mound system: an agronomic assessment of an indigenous agricultural system in the northeast. In *Histories of Maize: Multidisciplinary Approaches to the Prehistory, Linguistics, Biogeography, Domestication, and Evolution of Maize*, ed. J. E. Staller, R. H. Tykot, and B. F. Benz, 529–537. Walnut Creek: Left Coast Press.

Mukherjee, A., D. Speh, E. Dyck, and F. Diez-Gonzalez. 2004. Preharvest evaluation of coliforms, *Escherichia coli, Salmonella*, and *Escherichia coli* O157:H7 in organic and conventional produce grown by Minnesota farmers. *J Food Prot* 67 (5): 894–900.

Muñoz-Quezada, M. T., B. A. Lucero, V. P. Iglesias, et al. 2016. Chronic exposure to organophosphate (OP) pesticides and neuropsychological functioning in farm workers: a review. *Int J Occup Environ Health* 22 (1): 68–79.

Mulvaney, R. L., S. A. Khan, and T. R. Ellsworth. 2009. Synthetic nitrogen fertilizers deplete soil nitrogen: A global dilemma for sustainable cereal production. *Journal of Environmental Quality* 38: 2295–2314

Nachman, K. E., G. Raber, K. A. Francesconi, A. Navas-Acien, D. C. Love. 2012. Arsenic species in poultry feather meal. *Sci Total Environ* 417-418: 183–188.

New York Times. 1982. Bird populations rise after DDT ban. *New York Times*, March 11, 1982.

Nicholson, F. A., S. J. Groves, and B. J. Chambers. 2005. Pathogen survival during livestock manure storage and following land application. *Biores Tech* 96: 135–143.

Östman, O., B. Ekbom, and J. Bengtsson. 2001. Landscape heterogeneity and farming practice influence biological control. *Basic and Applied Ecology* 2: 365–371.

Perfecto, I. and J. Vandermeer. 2015. *Coffee Agroecology*. Abingdon, OX: Routledge.

Perfecto, I., J. Vandermeer, and A. Wright. 2009. *Nature's Matrix: Linking Agriculture, Conservation, and Food Sovereignty*. London: Earthscan.

Pimentel, D. 2005. Environmental and economic costs of the application of pesticides primarily in the United States. *Environ Dev Sustain* 7: 229–252.

Pimentel, D. 1984. Energy flow in the food system. In *Food and Energy Resources*, ed. D. Pimentel, and C. W. Hall, 1–24. Orlando: Academic Press, Inc.

Ponisio, L. C., L. K. M'Gonigle, K. C. Mace, J. Palomino, P. deValpine, and C. Kremen. 2015. Diversification practices reduce organic to conventional yield gap. *Proceedings of the Royal Society B* 292: 1799.

Ratnadass, A., P. Fernandes, J. Avelino, and R. Habib. 2012. Plant species diversity for sustainable management of crop pests and diseases in agroecosystems: A review. *Agronomy for Sustainable Development* 32: 273–303.

Reader, J. 2008. *The Propitious Esculent: The Potato in World History*. New York, NY: Random House.

Richerson, P. J., M. Borgerhoff Mulder, and B. J. Vila. 1996. *Principles of Human Ecology*. Needham Heights: Simon & Schuster.

Rodale Institute. 2011. The farming systems trial: Celebrating thirty years. Report, Rodale Institute. https://rodaleinstitute.org/our-work/farming-systems-trial/farming-systems-trial-30-year-report/ (Accessed October 22, 2011).

Roser, M. and H. Ritchie. 2017. Food per person. Published online at OurWorldinData.org. https://ourworldindata.org/food-per-person/ (Accessed November 9, 2017).

Sarmah, A. K., M. T. Meyer, and A. B. A. Boxall. 2006. A global perspective on the use, sales, exposure pathways, occurrence, fate and effects of veterinary antibiotics (VAs) in the environment. *Chemosphere* 65: 725–759.

Scherr, S. J. and J. A. McNeely. 2008. Biodiversity conservation and agricultural sustainability: Towards a new paradigm of 'ecoagriculture' landscapes. *Philosophical Transactions of the Royal Society B* 363: 477–494.

Seufert, V. and N. Ramankutty. 2017. Many shades of gray—the context-dependent performance of organic agriculture. *Science Advances* 3: e1602638.

Seufert, V., N. Ramankutty, and J. A. Foley. 2012. Comparing the yields of organic and conventional agriculture. *Nature* 485: 229–232.

Seymour, M. 2017. Unpublished findings.

Smil, V. 2002. Nitrogen and food production: Proteins for human diets. *Ambio* 31: 126–131.

Smil, V. 2004. Improving efficiency and reducing waste in our food system. *Environmental Sciences* 1: 17–26.

Soule, J. D. and J. K. Piper. 1992. *Farming in Nature's Image*. Washington, DC: Island Press.

Soulé, M. E. and B. A. Wilcox. 1980. *Conservation Biology: An Evolutionary-ecological Perspective*. Sunderland, MA: Sinauer Associates.

Taylor, R. and P. Morone. 2005. Diversity in food systems: the case of stockfree organic. Paper presented at Complexity, Science & Society Conference, Liverpool.

Teasdale, J. R., C. B. Coffman, and R. W. Mangum. 2007. Potential long-term benefits of no-tillage and organic cropping systems for grain production and soil improvement. *Agronomy Journal* 99: 1297–1305.

Thies, C., I. Steffan-Dewenter, and T. Tscharntke. 2003. Effects of landscape context on herbivory and parasitism at different spatial scales. *Oikos* 101: 18–25.

Tilman, D. and M. Clark. 2014. Global diets link environmental sustainability and human health. *Nature* 515: 518–522.

Union of Concerned Scientists. 2013. The healthy farmland diet. Published online by the
    Union of Concerned Scientists at https://www.ucsusa.org/sites/default/files/legacy/
    assets/documents/food_and_agriculture/healthy-farmland-diet.pdf (accessed February
    15, 2017).
USDA National Agricultural Statistics Service. 2016a. Crop production 2015 summary.
    Washington, DC.
USDA National Agricultural Statistics Service. 2016b. Certified organic survey: 2015 sum-
    mary.   http://usda.mannlib.cornell.edu/usda/current/OrganicProduction/Organic
    Production-09-15-2016.pdf.
Vandermeer, J. 2011. *The Ecology of Agroecosystems.* Sudbury, MA: Jones and Bartlett
    Publishers.
Vandermeer, J. and I. Perfecto. 2005. *Breakfast of Biodiversity: The Political Ecology of
    Rainforest Destruction*, 2nd edition. Oakland, CA: Food First Books.
Vandermeer, J., I. Perfecto, and S. Philpott. 2008. Clusters of ant colonies and robust criticality
    in a tropical agroecosystem. *Nature* 451: 457–459.
Vandermeer, J., I. Perfecto, and S. Philpott. 2010. Pest control in organic coffee production:
    Uncovering an autonomous ecosystem service. *BioScience* 60: 527–537.
Veganic Agriculture Network. 2012. Veganic fertility: growing plants from plants. http://
    www.goveganic.net/article205.html?lang=en.
Veganic Agriculture Network. 2014. Introduction to veganics. http://www.goveganic.net/
    article19.html.
Veganic Agriculture Network. 2016. Green manures. http://www.goveganic.net/spip.
    php?article125.
Watson, C. A., D. Younie, E. A. Stockdale, and W. F. Cormack. 2000. Yields and nutrient bal-
    ances in stocked and stockless organic rotations in the UK. *Asp Appl Biol* 62: 261–268.
Welsh, J. P., L. Philipps, and W. F. Cormack. 2002. The long-term agronomic performance
    of organic stockless rotations. In *UK Organic Research 2002: Proceedings of the COR
    Conference*, ed. J. Powell et al., 47–50. Aberystwyth, Wales.
West, P. C., J. S. Gerber, P. M. Engstrom, et al. 2014. Leverage points for improving global
    food security and the environment. *Science* 345 (6194): 325–328.
Wezel, W., M. Casagrande, F. Celette, J.-F. Vian, A. Ferrer, and J. Peigné. 2014. Agroecological
    practices for sustainable agriculture: A review. *Agronomy for Sustainable Development*
    34: 1–20.

11 The Importance of Saving Seeds

Bill McDorman and Stephen Thomas

CONTENTS

11.1 INTRODUCTION: RESTORING DIVERSITY WITH SEEDS

Modern science has given us the unprecedented power to dissect and understand the natural world. It also has shown us nature's interconnectedness. While we often think of our food system as a carefully managed, scientific operation, it is important to realize that it is intimately connected to the Earth system that supports us all. As in all natural systems, the resilience and sustainability of our food system depends upon its *diversity*.

As the human population continues to grow and the climate continues to change, new and unexpected pest and disease vectors are emerging to threaten our fragile food system. At the same time, the health of our soil and supplies of fresh water are diminishing. This combination of factors presents serious risks for the stability of our industrial agriculture model. The need for a broad diversity of crop varieties to adapt to these new conditions and challenges has never been greater.

Restoring our seed diversity is the key to replenishing diversity in our food system. More diverse crop varieties help create resilient farms and gardens that can weather the pressures of climate change and environmental stresses. This chapter provides essential information about seeds—from the global history of how the industrialization of our food system undermined our vital seed diversity—to the time-honored practices of seed saving that can help us rebuild it. In other words, we will explore how seeds offer us a tested, credible, and hopeful response to the crises we face in our food system.

11.2   THE SEEDS OF MODERN FOOD CROPS

Modern agriculture has come to be defined by the "hybrid" seeds that emerged with the Green Revolution after World War II and the genetically modified organisms (also known as GMOs—organisms whose genetic material have been altered using genetic engineering techniques) that are developed today. These newfangled creations did not appear from out of nowhere. The first modern plant breeders of the late 19th and early 20th centuries began to create new varieties out of existing lines of seeds that had been grown and stewarded by seed savers for generations. These "landrace" varieties, as they are known today—commonly used varieties like Turkey Red wheat or Reid's Yellow Dent corn—were the result of the thousands of years of careful seed saving. Almost all of our modern food crops were developed from wild plants as far back as 10,000 years ago. The original plants are sometimes so different that they are difficult to recognize as the ancestors of today's familiar grains, fruits, and vegetables. For example, modern wheat originally came from *einkorn*, a wild grass ("Ancient Grains: Einkorn" 2016); corn (also known as *maize*) arose from *teosinte*, a tropical grass (Carroll 2010); and modern chile peppers evolved from the *chiltepin* plant, a perennial bush found in northern Mexico ("Crop Wild Relatives" 2013).

It is important to remember that the vast majority of the initial work done to create landraces from wild plants took place before the science of genetics began in the early 20th century. Bill Tracy, an agronomist at the University of Wisconsin-Madison, eloquently describes the process of creating landraces during the long and distant span of years that gave rise to modern agriculture:

> Early in crop domestication, changes likely occurred in populations without conscious direction, but people quickly recognized that they could select for desirable characteristics. For roughly the next 9,850 years there were literally millions of breeders around the globe. Simply by saving seed each farmer selected for adaptation to the local environment. Selection for local cultural and culinary needs required more conscious effort. Artificial selection along with mutation and introgression from wild relatives resulted in the enormous diversity of adaptation, morphology, and physiology we see in crop species today. While the first 9,850 years of breeding might not have been efficient in modern terms, it was highly effective
>
> **Tracy 2016**

The process described here is actually not that complicated in practice. Seeds are simply saved and replanted based on their desirable characteristics. People saved seeds for a host of possible reasons. Perhaps the parent plants survived a frost or heat wave, indicating a special hardiness. Seeds were also saved from crops based on their flavor (i.e., less bitter or more sweet), ease of harvest (i.e., they don't "shatter"), or because they had some other important cultural or religious or religious value.

Seed Term Glossary

Selection – The process of saving the seeds from plants that exhibit desirable characteristics and traits. To identify desirable characteristics, breeders plant the same variety in different environmental conditions, or plant different varieties in the same environmental conditions.

Landrace – A domesticated, locally adapted, traditional variety developed over time, through adaptation to its natural and cultural environment.

Open-pollinated – Stable varieties resulting from the uncontrolled pollination between the same or genetically similar parents. Not hybrid.

Hybrid – Varieties resulting from controlled pollination between distinct (inbred) parents. F1, the notation used for most hybrids, is the uniform, 1st generation offspring (filial) after pollination. F2 hybrids, seed saved from F1s, lack the consistency of F1s but usually retain desirable traits that can be stabilized with further selection.

GMO – (Genetically modified organism) Any organism whose genetic material has been altered using genetic engineering techniques.

FIGURE 11.1   "Basic Seed Saving", McDorman, (1994)

Through seed saving, farmers are able to take the best characteristics of each harvest and carry them into the next season—and the next, and so on. Seeds are like self-replicating hard drives, allowing farmers to store newfound improvements and pass them onto future generations. Only now are we beginning to recognize or more accurately *remember* this as the powerful breeding technique it really is. Plant scientists call it "selection." Before the discoveries of genetic science opened up a brave new world of crop modification, this elegantly simple process transformed and refined a menagerie of wild edible plants into the colorful, diverse, and familiar foods of our modern diet (Figure 11.1).

11.3   BIODIVERSITY LOST

In a relatively short span of time, industrial models of crop production converged with breakthroughs in genetic science to bring about dramatic changes in agriculture and plant breeding. Tracy (2016) goes on to summarize this radical transformation:

> Over the last 150 years the landscape of plant breeding has changed nearly completely. The changes can be represented by a number of trends: from all farmer breeders to nearly all professional breeders, millions of breeders to a few thousand, highly local adaptation to broad adaptation, breeding in every environment in which the crop is grown to breeding for only highly profitable areas, breeding every crop to only the few highly profitable to seed companies, decisions on breeding targets and goals [made] by many people to very few people.

The changes represent a monumental shift in humanity's relationship to growing food and stewarding seeds, which culminated in the Green Revolution. Following World War II, chemical companies involved in weapon manufacturing converted their production to create pesticides and fertilizers for agriculture (Philpott 2013). When used alongside hybrid seeds, this gave rise to the first "monocropping" growing

operations—vast fields of genetically homogenous crops reliant on industrial chemicals to thrive and resist pests. Laboratory scientists in white coats replaced peasant
farmers as the force behind seed breeding, appropriating the seed varieties created
over countless generations and shaping them to fit the new industrial paradigm.

The Green Revolution dramatically reduced the diversity available to farmers and,
thus, to the food system as a whole. Today, there are only a tiny fraction of plant
breeders compared to the multitudes of seed savers in our ancestral past. Their work
is typically focused on developing a small number of crops with uniform genes suited
for industrial agriculture—characteristics that make them highly profitable for large
seed companies. This is true even in our nation's land-grant universities. These public institutions were historically involved in producing diverse seed varieties adapted
to their local bioregions and made available for public use. But after the passage of
the Bayh-Dole Act in 1980, our land-grant colleges began protecting the intellectual
property rights of the university before releasing new varieties to the public (Tracy
2016). The resulting partnerships and licensing agreements with big businesses created what amounts to a takeover of research at our publicly funded land-grant institutions. Agribusiness companies fund the majority of research in agricultural science
departments (Philpott 2012). As a result, university seed breeders now focus on creating profitable, patented varieties for industrial use that benefit corporations and ensure
continued corporate funding for the colleges.

The success of the Green Revolution (and the massive shift toward genetic uniformity in agricultural systems around the world) has created a precarious situation
for global food security. With our crop diversity dwindling, there are growing fears
that we lack the resilience in our food system to overcome new pests and diseases,
as well as the mounting pressures of climate change and environmental degradation.
Agriculture's modern history is filled with stories of entire industries being saved by
traits of disease or pest resistance found in a single forgotten or little-used variety.
This wealth of crop genetic diversity that modern breeders turn to in hopes of saving
a threatened hybridized crop was, of course, created by traditional seed savers with
different aims in mind.

Instead of planting genetically uniform varieties bred to produce the greatest yield
(despite their vulnerability), traditional farmers stewarded a broad diversity of crops,
with the ragtag assortment of genetic variability acting as a safeguard to protect
their harvests from extreme, unpredictable conditions and new, unexpected pests.
Drought-tolerant varieties would better survive a long dry spell. Fungus-resistant
varieties might make it through an unusually wet season. Unlike their modern
equivalents who put profits above sustainability, our seed-saving ancestors seemed
to inherently understand that, in the long run, creating and preserving diversity is the
essence of good farming.

11.4   MEASURING LOST DIVERSITY

Over the past 40 years, the United Nations, national governments, corporations,
and regional non-government organizations (NGOs) have all pushed to preserve
our remaining crop diversity and estimate just how much has been lost. While the
increase in genetic uniformity is obvious, measuring or quantifying the actual loss of

crop diversity is extremely difficult. Two reports are often cited by popular articles examining the impacts of industrial agriculture on crop diversity. The first was published in 1983 by the Plant Genetic Resources Project of the Rural Advancement Fund (RAFI). This study compared a 1903 USDA inventory of seeds found in commercial seed catalogs with those present at the time in the United States' largest seed bank, the National Seed Storage Laboratory (NSSL) in Fort Collins, Colorado. The report concluded that 94% of the varieties commercially available in 1903 could not be found in the NSSL seed bank—a statistic suggesting that only 430 out of 7262 varieties remained available (Fowler and Mooney 1990).

The other oft-quoted report, as summarized here by University of Georgia researchers Paul Heald and Susannah Chapman, was published in 1999 by the United Nations Food and Agriculture Organization (FAO) and describes the loss of diversity worldwide:

> Since the 1900s, some 75 percent of plant genetic diversity has been lost as farmers worldwide have left their multiple local varieties and landraces for genetically uniform, high-yielding varieties.
>
> **FAO 2009**

Both of these statistics have been challenged for their accuracy and have become somewhat controversial. Colin Khoury, a scientist at the International Center for Tropical Agriculture, notes that doing studies like these is difficult because "there aren't many good ways to count the diversity that existed before it disappeared" (2017). Khoury spent two years searching for many of the plant varieties that were suggested to be "lost" in the original RAFI report. He was able to find a sample of every variety he searched for, sowing doubts about the actual percentage of varieties that have disappeared (Khoury et al. 2014).

Another report by Heald and Chapman (2009) revisited the RAFI study and found that, although only 6% of the original varieties could be found in 1983, other varieties of these same vegetable crops were commercially available:

> In 1903, buyers of seeds had the choice of 7262 varieties of the 48 vegetable crops studied. In 2004, buyers had the choice of 7100 varieties of the same set of vegetables, only 2 percent fewer than one hundred years earlier. By this measure, consumers of seeds have seen almost no loss of overall varietal diversity. (2009)

Although much publicity surrounding the RAFI and FAO reports used the words "disappeared" or "extinct" when describing the presumably lost seed varieties, the Khoury and Heald studies found the opposite to be true. Missing varieties were being found. One explanation for the rediscovery of this diversity is the growth of a grassroots movement beginning in the early 1980s to find and share rare heirloom seeds, as well as to start new, small, bioregional seed companies. To be clear, the diversity represented by thousands of forgotten varieties has not completely disappeared. Still, this good news does not solve the problems posed by the overwhelming uniformity of the crops growing on modern industrial farms. As the FAO report observes, "More than 90 percent of crop varieties have disappeared from farmers' fields" (Heald and Chapman 2009).

While the scientists of the world may still have access to much of the diversity (or are able to find it after a concerted search), farmers are no longer using it. This is problematic for several reasons. For one, seeds have a shelf life. If left unused, locked away in seed banks or stashed in shoeboxes in a gardener's cellar, they will eventually die. Just as importantly, seeds that aren't actively growing are no longer adapting. The creative process that happens as a result of farmers selecting new seeds for new conditions stops in its tracks. As the naturalist and author Gary Paul Nabhan (1989) puts it in his classic book *Enduring Seeds*, "When plants are removed from frequent contact with field conditions, their evolution is put on hold." Finally, we must ask the question: "What good is this seed diversity to protect our food system if it isn't being grown and used?" The vast monocultures of genetically identical crops that dominate industrial agriculture are incredibly susceptible to pests and environmental pressures. Without diversified crop varieties being grown together, a farmer's entire harvest—and the food system that depends on it—is precariously vulnerable to failure and collapse.

11.5   BIODIVERSITY SAVED: EX-SITU OR IN-SITU CONSERVATION?

In the late 1970s, the world began to respond seriously to the loss of diversity in our food system. One of the first orders of business was to gather the seeds of remaining varieties before they too disappeared and store them safely in seed banks outside their natural habitats, a practice known as *ex-situ* (or "off-site") conservation. These seed storage facilities are known as "gene banks," a term emphasizing the genetic information held in the seeds rather than the seeds themselves. Today more than 1,700 gene bank facilities exist around the world. Central to this network of gene banks is the Consultative Group for International Agricultural Research (CGIAR) started in 1971 by the World Bank, the Rockefeller Foundation, the FAO, and other UN organizations. CGIAR is primarily composed of 15 research centers around the world including the Center for Wheat and Maize (CIMMYT), the International Rice Research Institute (IRRI) and Biodiversity International. In 2006, the Global Crop Diversity Trust, an international non-profit, was formed by the FAO and CGIAR to focus specifically on ex-situ conservation. The Crop Trust currently provides $2.4 million annually to support 20 international collections of 17 major food crops in nine CGIAR gene banks. The famous "doomsday" Svalbard Seed Vault in Norway, a Global Crop Diversity Trust project, now provides safety backup for 930,000 accessions from the world's gene banks (Figure 11.2).

As effective and important as the now decades-old effort to save the disappearing diversity caused by industrial agriculture has been, serious questions remain about how best to keep the seeds in ex-situ collections viable. Continually growing out and replenishing the seed samples stored in gene banks (known as "accessions") is a costly endeavor, prompting explorations into ways to lengthen their lifespan. Huge efforts by gene banks have focused on storing seeds at colder and colder temperatures to make them live longer. Massive databases have been created among gene banks to avoid the duplication of growing out shared varieties and make the system more efficient. These stopgap efforts cost considerably less than actually re-growing seeds to keep them from dying.

Ex-situ and In-situ Conservation

Seed conservationists employ the terms *ex situ* and *in situ* to describe different approaches to preserving seed diversity. Ex-situ (or "off-site") conservation involves conserving seeds outside of their natural environment. This typically takes place in gene banks (also called "seed banks" or "seed vaults"), which are storage facilities built to safely house seed varieties for long-term viability.

In-situ (or "in-place") conservation means conserving seeds within their natural habitats, such as in a farmer's field or a garden bed. This is the type of seed conservation practiced by seed savers of the past who grew, saved, and replanted seed varieties each season, thereby keeping them alive (and continuously adapting) through active use. In-situ conservation is also called "on-farm" conservation.

FIGURE 11.2 "Conservation of Plant Genetic Resources for Food and Agriculture" FAO (Food and Agriculture Organization of the United Nations)

According to the Global Crop Diversity Trust website, "It requires, on average, only $625 to conserve an accession in [a gene bank] collection for everyone, forever." This means the cost of ex-situ conservation of the world's 7.4 million accessions could eventually reach more than $4.6 billion. Journalist Jennifer Duggan summarized the financial predicament faced by the world's gene banks in an online piece for *Time*:

> Woefully underfunded, many [gene-banks] lack the resources to properly store or protect the seeds they hold. The Crop Trust is now raising money for an endowment fund to ensure that the world's 1,700 gene-bank facilities are able to continue acting as guarantors of global biodiversity ... a lack of resources is probably the biggest threat facing the world's gene banks. (n.d.)

The Global Crop Diversity Trust is currently soliciting the world's governments, corporations, wealthy individuals, and social media users to raise $850 million (a figure recently expanded from $150 million) to preserve the world's seeds in ex-situ facilities ("The Endowment Fund" 2017). This is far less than the $4.6 billion in projected costs needed to take care of the accessions already held by the gene banks.

In addition to funding constraints, gene banks face threats from war and weather:

> The gene bank in Aleppo was not the first to be threatened by war. Gene banks in Afghanistan and Iraq have been destroyed, along with them genetic material that wasn't backed up in Svalbard. But it is not just armed conflict that threatens these valuable resources. Some have been hit by natural disasters, like the Philippine national gene bank, which was damaged by flooding from a typhoon and later a fire.
>
> **Duggan, 2017**

Because of these and other reasons, many around the world now seriously question the limits of ex-situ conservation to preserve the diversity needed for a sustainable future.

11.6 IN-SITU CONSERVATION

Farmers around the world—especially small, urban, and indigenous farmers—are awakening to the critical importance of, and opportunities involved in, saving and producing their own seeds again. The unregulated, spontaneous sharing of seed is (and always has been) the foundation of in-situ conservation; this is the wellspring of diversity that made modern agriculture possible. The appearance of community and tribal seed banks, seed libraries, and organized seed exchanges in one form or another represent a new level of sophistication in the modern, planet-wide, grassroots movement to conserve and create more seed diversity.

Many examples of this rising movement can be found worldwide. In Canada, "Seedy Saturday" seed exchanges have grown in a few short years to include more than 100 community events each year ("Everything You Want to Know About Seedy Saturdays" Seeds of Diversity Canada 2018). Navdanya, a network of researchers, seed keepers, and organic producers in India, count among their efforts 122 community seed banks, 5,000 crop varieties stewarded, and training opportunities serving more than 500,000 farmers. The Peliti Seed Festival in Greece now hosts the world's largest seed exchange each April and stewards more seed varieties than the Greek National Seed Bank.

Since 2010, more than 500 seed lending libraries have been created worldwide, with at least 400 in the United States alone (Seed Libraries, 2018). A seed library is an institution that lends or shares seed. It is distinguished from a seed bank in that the main purpose is not to store or hold seeds against possible destruction but to disseminate them to the public, a model which preserves plant varieties through propagation and sharing of seed. Seed libraries in the United States can now be found in many public libraries. Perhaps the most impressive example is the Pima County Library Seed Library in Tucson, Arizona. Seeds can be checked out from nine different branches in the countywide library system using a computer-based interlibrary loan network, which allows anyone in the 22-library system to "check out" seeds for free. More than 28,000 packets of seed were checked out by library users in 2017.

11.7 PUSH BACK

The growth of the modern seed diversity movement and its focus on in-situ conservation has not been without controversy and conflict. Seed libraries and seed exchanges have been criticized and opposed, even facing threats of closure by state regulators. Seed control officials in Pennsylvania, for instance, cracked down on a local community seed library in attempt to regulate it as a commercial seed distributor (Smith 2014). The library, they insisted, must register as a seed dealer, abide by state seed laws, and implement controls to assure commercial standards for seed uniformity and purity (McFetridge 2014). At the very least, officials wanted the seeds in the seed library to be properly labeled and meet minimum germination standards like all commercially available seeds—a labor-intensive and costly requirement that would be impossible for the small community project to follow (McCartney and Baird 2014).

Some seed-saving advocates felt that this opposition was a sinister attempt to shut down local food resilience efforts. Upon investigation, however, it seems more likely that the conflict arose because of a fundamental misunderstanding of the seed diversity movement by government seed officials. By its nature, grassroots seed saving functions as a decentralized, uncontrolled means of creating crop diversity and producing seeds. This age-old, do-it-yourself practice has gone overlooked by most seed control officials, university plant breeders, and even commercial seed growers. The conventional seed industry and its regulators operate from a radically different paradigm. Uniformity, profitability, and genetic stability are the benchmarks of seed "quality" for industrial agriculture. State and federal seed regulations are written according to these market-driven concepts, which need not apply to home gardeners and small, subsistence farmers interested in diversity and sharing. Home gardeners and small growers, especially when trained in seed saving practices, can afford to be more tolerant of genetic variability in their seeds—and more importantly, can take advantage of any "surprises" through intentional selection. This is, of course, the way that seed savers created the world's crop diversity in the first place.

Conventional seed officials who characterize grassroots seed saving and seed sharing as somehow inferior, misleading, or even threatening to industrial seed systems are missing this very important point. On the other hand, seed diversity advocates often demonize multinational seed corporations and overlook the critical importance of quality and uniformity in the industrial seed supply for farmers who are locked into the current food system and depend upon their crops for a living. In this time of transition and accelerating change, both approaches have value and need to be acknowledged for the role they play in our shifting and complex food system.

In response to the Pennsylvania seed library incident, a committee of dedicated seed librarians and seed diversity activists met for almost a year with representatives of the American Association of Seed Control Officials with the hope of coming to an understanding. In August of 2016 they reached an agreement for an amendment to the Recommended Uniform State Seed Law (RUSSL). The amendment allows seed libraries to continue operating in the commons without penalty. This means no fees, no germination testing, and no expiration dates are required. It recommends that seed libraries be exempt from the laws of seed businesses as regulated by state agricultural departments. As the name implies, the RUSSL amendment is not codified legislation but a recommendation. It must be approved legislatively state by state in order to have the force of law. Importantly, this agreement marks a huge step forward by governing bodies and the seed industry at large in recognizing the significance and promise of the grassroots seed diversity movement.

11.8 REALISTIC GLOBAL CAPACITY

How realistic is it to imagine that disparate grassroots organizations can produce and conserve the seed diversity needed for humanity's future? This question often arises in serious discussions about overhauling the industrial seed and food systems paradigm. Within the context of the modern food system as it now exists, the standard answer is "no." Individual and community seed saving efforts are often seen as "quaint" or "interesting," but dismissed as inadequate to feed a population of seven billion people and growing. To meet the demands of global hunger, the conventional argument goes, the world will need industrial agriculture, biotechnology, and gene banks.

As discussed above, there are hard limits to the capacity of gene banks to properly conserve the world's wealth of seed diversity. Much evidence also argues against the use of industrial farming and biotechnology for long-term food security and resilience. More to the point, the claim that small-scale, traditional farming practices can't possibly "feed the world" ignores evidence to the contrary. There is immense global capacity to reintroduce agricultural diversity and increase sustainable food production via grassroots seed saving. According to a 2013 FAO report, 70% of the world's food is actually still produced on small farms (Wolfenson, 2013). Subsistence and indigenous farmers around the world and in the United States still have access to the traditional seed-saving practices of their parents and grandparents. Seed savers on small farms are better able to create new crop varieties adapted to changing climates and unique cultural needs. In many places they are beginning to serve as a model for the deindustrialization of all food production. Not only does this increase seed diversity, but it is also achieving environmental, economic, and human health benefits (Ruelas 2014).

11.9 POLICY HURDLES

The seed industry worldwide has seen tremendous consolidation in the past few decades with only a handful of companies now controlling the majority of seed sales worldwide. Government policies around the world, and especially in the United States, largely support the interests of these companies over those advocating a return to the kind of dispersed traditional plant breeding so effective for creating diversity. For instance, current USDA funding for plant breeding research in the United States tilts as much as 70 to 1 in favor of biotechnology and GMOs.

Major court cases in recent decades have allowed a nearly unrestrained application of intellectual property rights to seeds. Until the passage of the Plant Variety Protection Act (PVP) of 1970, owning (e.g., patenting) the seeds of seed-producing plants was prohibited. Although PVP restricted seed saving for the first time in human history, the original legislation made exceptions for farmers saving their own seeds and plant breeders needing to save seeds to continually create new varieties. These exceptions effectively ended in 1980 as the result of a U.S. Supreme Court ruling, *Diamond v. Chakarbarty*. In the decision, Chief Justice Warren Burger stated that patents could extend to "anything under the sun made by man" ("*Diamond v. Chakrabarty*" 1980). From this landmark decision, utility patents granted for seed-producing plants now restricted any and all seed saving.

A 2001 challenge to this ruling failed ("*J.E.M. Ag Supply, Inc. v. Pioneer Hi-Bred International, Inc.*" 2001), and seed saving for utility-patented crops was effectively outlawed. Now, in the 21st century, more and more utility-patented varieties are showing up in seed catalogs targeted toward gardeners and small farmers. Popular utility-patented varieties include non-hybrid, open-pollinated, and even certified organic seeds, a circumstance that puts seed savers in legal jeopardy.

11.10 THE PATH FORWARD

As daunting as these hurdles may seem, the seed diversity movement is growing worldwide with a renewed passion and urgency. Seeds represent the greatest opportunity we have for sustainability. This is because seeds have the miraculous power to self-replicate. They contain the software and hardware necessary to evolve in real-time based on information from the environment. With a curious gardener or farmer behind this process, seeds can morph and adapt season after season to meet our changing needs, tastes, and climates. This incredible potential for *adaptability* is unparalleled in any form of our modern, human-made technology.

11.11 EDUCATION

Creating a network of seed savers across the United States to preserve seed diversity is entirely possible. To be sure, this interconnected web of seed stewards once existed. Until the turn of the last century, most every gardener and farmer in the developed world was a still a seed saver. Thomas Jefferson famously practiced and promoted seed saving. When he signed the Morrill Act in 1862, Abraham Lincoln reinforced federal support for seed saving by creating the land-grant college system so important to early seed testing and production in each state ("Abraham Lincoln—His Lasting Gift to Farmers" 2017).

While the number of farmers has steadily decreased over the past century, gardening has grown to become one of the most popular outdoor hobbies in America. The 2016 edition of the *National Gardening Study* found that 76% of all U.S. households participated in lawn and garden activities that year (Butterfield 2016). Vegetable gardening has been particularly on the rise since the 2008 recession, according to the study. Millennials comprised the largest new demographic of food gardeners with more than six million young people taking up the spade in 2016. Among the top reasons stated by millennials for their new hobby are the desire to access healthy food and to live more sustainably (Butterfield 2016).

When these idealistic young gardeners and market farmers discover that the seeds at the source of their homegrown food come from industrial fields thousands of miles away, a light bulb goes off. Suddenly, the crucial importance of seed saving for true sustainability becomes obvious. This is the awakening that is driving the burgeoning local seed movement. Education is a powerful force in this growing awareness—whether this be through seed libraries, hands-on seed-saving workshops, local mentors, books, documentary films, or any of the emerging forms of knowledge sharing for seed wisdom.

11.12 STARTING POINT

Where does one begin to learn to save seeds? Many myths exist that seed saving is too complicated and esoteric for the average time-stressed gardener or overworked farmer to tackle. Rules to avoid unwanted cross-pollination or the need to learn necessary minimum population numbers to avoid inbred depression can dissuade at any potential new seed saver. Fortunately, the process is relatively easy, especially in the beginning stages. Self-pollinating plants like tomatoes and peas are a great place to start. Lovingly referred to as "selfers," these clever crops have hermaphroditic flowers that can pollinate themselves, typically before they open. This is a boon for seed savers, preventing unwanted pollen from a neighboring garden or field from crossing in. Selfers also need very small numbers of plants to carry enough genetics to ensure a stable variety, making it easy for a small gardener to create a robust new variety.

By starting with the right plants, beginning seed savers can experience success without much extra work or planning. In addition, even if undesirable "sexual encounters" occur through cross-pollination, the resulting offspring can still be eaten. By the same token, genetic accidents sometimes create remarkable new varieties. The "pumpzini"—a combination of a pumpkin and zucchini—is one of example of these delicious, haphazard experiments. This is the beauty of small-scale, intimate seed saving. Planned or unplanned, diversity is created.

11.13 LOCAL ECOSYSTEMS AND RESILIENCE

The larger a farm operation, the more profitable it can be. However, the smaller a farm is, the greater its potential for ecological health and resilience. Our agriculture system has become super-sized around the principle of profit, and at the expense of environmental and human health. Profits result from greater yields in industrial farming systems. Within our current era of degraded environments and disappearing species all pressured by climate change, the value of an interconnected web of small, ecologically regenerative farming systems becomes clear. Across the planet, communities, and non-profit entities are localizing food production, shrinking supply lines, and finding ways to interface more sensitively with their regional environments. Resilience and profit are seeking a new balance. Central to this revised equation is the need for enough new seed diversity to sustain the system. The most efficient and durable way to produce and preserve this diversity is through a broad, interwoven web of local seed savers growing and adapting varieties where they live. This isn't a biased speculation; it is a biological truth. In other words, the creation of crop diversity must be a grassroots activity. To quote the ecologist Paul Hawken, "You can't run elegant systems from command central" (1993).

11.14 BUILDING COMMUNITY

Seeds offer an unprecedented opportunity to both grow our local economies and bring our communities together. Every region, town, and neighborhood has the opportunity to understand its own role and forge a path forward. Many communities are beginning to see this as not only a necessary responsibility, but also a source of incredible opportunity for prosperity, resiliency, and positive progress. Growing local food from local seeds offers a distinctive, valuable niche in food markets. Communities can promote their unique culinary palette based on their own climate and culture. Seeds and local selection provide an unparalleled tool to make this happen. In addition to the food, fiber, and medicinal value of local crops, the seeds themselves can provide economic benefits as products to be shipped and shared with other regions.

The importance of unique, place-based plant varieties and value-added foods for the health, identity, and economic prosperity of local communities has long been recognized. The United Nations Education, Scientific, and Cultural Organization (UNESCO)'s Creative Cities list recognizes international capitals of gastronomy like Tucson, Arizona, alongside cities in Mexico, Thailand, and the Mediterranean that boast rich traditions of regional cuisines (Nalewicki, 2016). The European Union employs a range of labels such as "protected designation of origin" (PDO) and "traditional specialty guaranteed" (TSG) to serve as seals of quality protecting the cultural heritage of locally produced crops and artisanal food products ("Agricultural Quality Policy" 2017). Radicchio, a colorful winter salad green hailing from Italy, has several registered variety names corresponding to their towns of origin. For example, the historic *Variegato di Castelfranco* radicchio is from CastełO, a town in the northern Italian region of Veneto, and *Rosso di Treviso* is from the province of Treviso. Both distinctive regional varieties carry the PDO logo as a stamp of authenticity.

Many countries have similar registration programs of their own. Prominent examples include the appellation *d'origine contrôlée* (AOC) in France, the *denominação de origem controlada* (DOC) in Portugal, and the *denominación de origen* (DO) system used in Spain ("Geographical Indications and Traditional Specialties in the European Union" 2017). In the United States, the USDA's Marketing Orders program protects hundreds of U.S.-developed crop varieties and products ("Marketing Orders and Agreements" 2017). For example, only onions grown within the Walla Walla valley spanning the border regions of Washington and Oregon can be legally sold as "Walla Walla sweet onions."

These lists were created as marketing tools to benefit both consumers and producers: Buyers of food anywhere in the world can be assured they're receiving the most authentic product, and the regions that originally created these delicacies have their intellectual property and economic rights protected. In order to participate, a community or region must steward something distinctive. By finding, saving, and growing a unique crop variety, a community steps up to help preserve seed diversity while also enjoying economic, cultural, and culinary rewards.

To help communities find important foods and varieties to steward, in 1996 the organization Slow Food International created the Ark of Taste, a living catalog of delicious and distinctive foods facing extinction around the world. More than 3500 products from over 150 countries have been added to the list, including more than 200 from the United States ("Ark of Taste in the USA" 2018). It was created as a tool for farmers, ranchers, fishers, chefs, grocers, educators, and consumers to seek out and celebrate a region's diverse biological, cultural, and culinary heritage before it disappears.

11.15   SEEDS FOR ENVIRONMENTAL CARE AND RESPONSIBILITY

As members of a complex society facing an uncertain future, we must continue to search for effective tools to help us solve the converging crises of environmental degradation and resource depletion on a finite planet. Gus Speth, a U.S. advisor on climate change, offers an important insight into this challenge:

> I used to think that top environmental problems were biodiversity loss, ecosystem collapse, and climate change. I thought that thirty years of good science could address these problems, I was wrong. The top environmental problems are selfishness, greed and apathy, and to deal with these we need a cultural and spiritual transformation. And we scientists don't know how to do that.
>
> **2015**

Saving seed diversity is scientifically and biologically necessary for resilience, stability, and weathering the storms ahead from climate change and dwindling resources.

Seeds themselves offer a simple tool that is available to everyone, everywhere. These humble, tiny objects have the power to spark the vital cultural and spiritual transformation that Speth speaks of.

Seeds are one of the most widely available tools we have offering real, tangible hope. They are truly universal, found in nearly all cultures throughout the world. Like rare jewels, they shimmer with beauty. They disperse themselves ingeniously and are remarkably easy to transport, store, and share. They can multiply exponentially. Each seed carries a story. These stories connect us to our history as a people to our sense of place, to our families, and to our communities. Planting seeds we have saved connects us directly to the larger environmental cycles we are a part of, and that we need to better understand. They are our patient teachers in a crucial time of learning and remembering.

11.16 CONCLUSION

Around the world, seeds are being embraced as the solution to solve the problems of our modern world. Many are beginning to recognize that our only hope of saving our current food system and making it more resilient and sustainable is by reuniting with the power, wisdom, and potential of seeds. Our indigenous ancestors knew this. They worshipped seeds. The Hopi Indians still see them as their children. They honor them as the ultimate gift of the Creator, and protect them under a sacred responsibility that defines their very identity as a people. On a profound level, perhaps seeds are returning to us in this pivotal time to provide the spiritual salvation we need—the courage, wisdom, and guidance to steward our planet, and ourselves.

BILL MCDORMAN'S PRINCIPLES OF SEED DIVERSITY

1. No one should suffer from hunger, food insecurity or malnutrition.
2. The survival of the food system depends upon its seed diversity.
3. Every crop seed is a gift resulting from thousands of years of human care and should not be privatized.
4. With seeds we inherit a responsibility to care for and pass on seed diversity to future generations.
5. More seed diversity is created when more gardeners and farmers save seeds.
6. Seed education is fundamental to the creation of more seed savers and thus more seed diversity.
7. Complicated rules to assure uniformity need not be applied to small-scale seed saving for diversity.
8. Each region has a responsibility to provide safety back-up for its seed diversity.
9. Seed stories teach us how to care for our seeds and ourselves, they must also be preserved.
10. Saving your own seeds is important. Joining forces with other seed savers is transformative.

VIGNETTE 11.1   Rehydrate the Earth with Swales

Lydia Neilsen

HOW WATER, EARTH, AND FORESTS INTERACT

Forests (and to some extent all vegetation) have an enormous influence on the functioning of the Earth's water cycle and the stability of our planet's climate. Healthy and diverse perennial-dominated ecosystems create the ideal conditions for water to soak into the Earth's surface, recharging groundwater, and maintaining natural waterways. They then draw that water back up through their bodies and re-release it, stabilizing the composition and distribution of water vapor in the atmosphere. The impact of these processes on our global climate is enormous, yet they have been negatively altered by human activity over the last 100 years, resulting in many of our current climate and weather challenges (Bartholomew 2003). Fortunately, this damage can be repaired. Restoration practices informed by a deeper comprehension of these relationships can enable individuals and communities to replicate forests' ecosystem services on a variety of scales. Thus, we can "rehydrate the Earth" both individually and collectively (Mollison 1988, Hemenway 2009).

Forests protect, stabilize, and cool soil. Cool shaded soil readily absorbs warm rain, whereas hot exposed soil repels it (Bartholomew 2003). Organic matter from trees and their inhabitants feeds the soil biota and creates *humus*, a thick spongy carbon-rich material, which covers the forest floor. Humus provides stable long-term nutrients for plants and soil biota and absorbs large quantities of water from rain or condensation.

Once the humus layer is saturated, water sinks slowly downward through the topsoil into the mineral subsoil. Water travels through pores made by soil microorganisms and along the channels of roots, whose sugary exudates also feed the microorganisms. Water (1) can be drawn by roots into the bodies of plants, or (2) remain held in the interstitial spaces as groundwater (slowly feeding natural waterways and vegetation), and (3) can be stored even more deeply as an aquifer. Water is filtered and purified by its journey both through the mineral earth and the living bodies of microorganisms, releasing and absorbing nutrients on its way (Bartholomew 2003).

Water that is taken up by trees is eventually released as vapor through the leaves in a process is called *transpiration*. Transpiration combined with evaporation is called *evapo-transpiration*, which comprises all atmospheric vapor. Clouds formed over oceans are primarily evaporated vapor, while clouds formed over forests are high in transpired vapor. (Bartolomew 2003). The transformation of vapor into rain depends on air temperature and vapor density, yet it also requires the presence of a particle around which to condense. These particles can be mineral, chemical, or biological, and are called *cloud seeds* or *condensation nuclei*. Evapo-transpired vapor from forests is rich in organic cloud seeds, which have been shown to induce rain more readily than non-organic particulates from oceanic vapor (Pearce, 2011).

In addition to promoting the infiltration of rain and the formation of rain atmospherically, forests "comb" water out of the air by condensing vapor on cold leaf surfaces. This water, which is not measured as precipitation, can add up to five times more water to the Earth than rain alone. Like rain, this water supplies subterranean storages, springs and streams, and is taken up and re-released via transpiration. This additional water vapor feeds additional clouds, creating more rain and distributing it further inland (Schwartz 2016).

Furthermore, moisture-laden airstreams cool and condense as they are pulled inland and drawn upward over forests or mountains. Clouds increase as forests add warm transpired vapor and organic cloud seeds. Compressed airstreams dragging over the forest canopy stratify like waves until upper layers overtake and eddy underneath lower layers in a wind pattern known as Ekman spirals, which form at regular intervals perpendicular to the wind and produce bands of rain. This additional rain infiltrates and is transpired, subsequently moving vapor and rain inland (Mollison 1988).

When trees or other full-cover perennial ecosystems are removed, not only is the influence of forests on airstreams eliminated and the source of transpiration vapor and cloud seeds removed, but the Earth's surface is completely exposed. Unprotected soil experiences extreme temperature fluctuations and is beaten by the full impact of the rain, washing away organic matter. Roots and soil life disappear, and with them the tunnels and pores that water and air moved through. The surface can become as impermeable as concrete. When water cannot soak in, the groundwater table drops, natural waterways dry up, and spontaneous regeneration becomes impossible (Bartholomew 2003).

RESTORATION WITH DESIGN

Fortunately, the pattern of surface impermeability can be reversed with conscious intervention. Though high infiltration and deep-rooted plants for transpiration are necessary, complete forest cover is not required, as the climatic effects can be produced by correctly placed bands of trees on a variety of scales (Mollison 1988). Urban and suburban dwellers can mimic the ecosystem services of the forest by restoring the infiltration capacity of the ground and re-vegetating in an appropriate pattern, fostering the plants and soil organisms that create cool, protected earth and porous soil structure for water infiltration—as well as producing organic matter and cycling nutrients to maintain a healthy ecosystem. With informed landscape design that is productive, easy to maintain, diverse, and beautiful, the formation of Ekman spirals is reestablished. Hence, rain patterns are distributed further inland, and the rehydration of the Earth commences (Mollison 1988).

In urban and de-vegetated areas, the conditions required for water infiltration are now largely absent and intervention is required. Compacted earth must be contoured to allow it to hold water, and organic matter must be introduced. Moisture and food trigger the development of diverse soil biota, which can then support larger plants. Trees shade and cool the earth and supply additional organic matter and habitat and food for biodiversity. This jump-starts the rehydration process, restores the cycle, and enables the entire ecosystem to accelerate on its own (Hemenway 2009).

A simple contouring technique to promote the infiltration of water is digging a *swale*. A swale is a ditch with a flat level bottom which is dug perpendicular to the downward flow of surface water. The soil taken from the ditch is used to create a mound or *berm* immediately downhill, increasing the capacity of the swale, and creating an undulating form or contour. The swale and berm interrupt runoff and enable infiltration, sometimes filling up like a long skinny pool while water waits to soak in through compacted soil. Ideally, swales are filled behind the berm with woodchips or other organic debris creating the appearance of a flat terrace. This mulch cools and protects the infiltration surface and provides a seam of carbonaceous food for soil organisms, which proliferate in the moist organic matter. As water is caught in the swale, sediment, pollutants, and additional organic matter are filtered out by the mulch, and are consumed and broken down by the diverse soil biota as shown in Figures V11.1 and V11.2. Humus formation begins (Hemenway 2009).

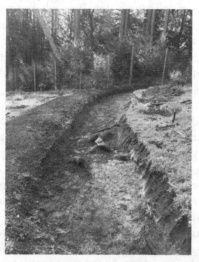

FIGURE V11.1 Digging the swale. (Courtesy of Ms. Lydia Neilsen, Rehydrate the Earth, Santa Cruz, California.)

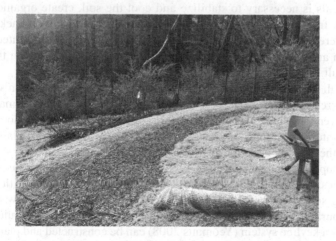

FIGURE V11.2 Swale filled with wood mulch. (Courtesy of Ms. Lydia Neilsen, Rehydrate the Earth, Santa Cruz, California.)

Over the course of the rainy season, large quantities of water infiltrate in each swale, creating a *lens*, or zone of saturated soil underground. This saturated area slowly sinks and creeps downhill, increasing in size and capacity for several years as the soil biota, plant roots, and soil porosity develop. Over time the lens will provide sufficient water to sustain the deep-rooted perennials and trees planted on the berm and a considerable distance downhill. In some situations, swales near the top of a slope have restored springs and wells at the bottom. (Hemenway 2009). The trees require several years of growth to provide shade and protection, so it is critical to cover and protect berms initially by planting cover crops and smaller perennials.

After a few years, an ecosystem develops where trees shade and cool the ground, feed and support a diverse soil biota, and provide physical and chemical mechanisms for water to enter, be retained by, and filtered through the soil. As the trees access this deep water, they draw it up and release it through transpiration back into the air as vapor. This transpired vapor joins the airstreams which rise and cool, become clouds, condense, and fall again as rain (Mollison 1988).

Depending on the degree of slope, amount of runoff, intensity of rain events, area to be worked, and existing features such as trees and buildings, swales can be installed singly or in an overlapping series across a large area. They can be short and shallow or long and deep. To gauge what is needed for a given situation, consider the permeability of the earth, the amount of rain in a given interval, and the stability of the slope. Less permeable soil will require larger swales to hold the water while it soaks in. Larger rain events require larger swales to hold the high volume. Less stable slopes, however, require smaller swales to avoid oversaturating and causing slumps or slides. In these cases an off-contour ditch might be recommended to shunt water to another area more appropriate for high infiltration. In all cases however, the establishment on the berm of deep-rooted perennials (especially trees) and fast-growing full-coverage annuals is necessary to stabilize and cool the soil, create organic matter, and draw from the lens of infiltrated water in order to transpire it back into the atmosphere and continue vapor cycling. If excessive water is infiltrated but not drawn in and transpired by plants, boggy conditions downhill from the swale may result.

Though swale systems can be implemented on a micro to medium scale, the effect increases with size and scope. While no effort is too small to make a difference, very small systems, through infiltrating water in the swales locally, will supply water vapor not to themselves but downwind of their installation. This benefits the ecosystem even if there is not an onsite benefit.

A group of friends with shovels in a backyard can dig one swale and plant a few trees, catch enough water to sustain the trees, and set up a little oasis of cool rich soil teeming with life, feeding whatever happens to grow downhill and encouraging rain downwind. With multiple acres, a system of multiple long swales or a keyline system (Yeomans 2008) can be constructed and planted with trees initiating Ekman spirals and bands of rain, potentially impacting an entire bioregion.

CONCLUSION

Individual swales and swale systems alike increase the complexity of the surface topography and the diversity of food sources and microclimates above and below ground. They, in turn, support a greater diversity of plants, insects, and larger animals—positively impacting biodiversity as a whole. This productive, underutilized, and self-enhancing strategy is a powerful way for individuals and communities to restore biodiversity, stability, and resilience in local ecosystems and beyond.

REFERENCES

Abraham Lincoln—His lasting gift to farmers. *AgWeb* April 14, 2017. https://www.agweb.com/blog/straight-from-dc-agricultural-perspectives/abraham-lincoln-his-lasting-gift-to-farmers.

Agricultural product quality policy. *European Commission*. https://ec.europa.eu/agriculture/quality_en (Accessed January 12, 2018).

Ancient grains: Einkorn. *PennState College of Agricultural Sciences*. http://plantscience.psu.edu/research/projects/grains/heritage-grains/einkorn (Accessed January 12, 2018).

Ark of taste in the USA. *Slow Food USA*. https://www.slowfoodusa.org/ark-of-taste-in-the-usa (Accessed January 12, 2018).

Bartholomew, A. 2003. *Hidden Nature: The Startling Insights of Viktor Schauberger*. Floris Books.

Butterfield, Bruce. 2016. *National Gardening Survey, 2016 Edition*. Burlington, VA: National Garden Market Research Company.

Carroll, Sean B. May 24, 2010. Tracking the ancestry of Corn Back 9,000 years. *The New York Times*. http://www.nytimes.com/2010/05/25/science/25creature.html

Crop wild relatives. *USDA Forest Service*. https://www.fs.fed.us/wildflowers/ethnobotany/wildrelatives.shtml (Accessed January 12, 2018).

Diamond v. Chakrabarty. n.d. *Justia*. https://supreme.justia.com/cases/federal/us/447/303/casc.html (Accessed January 12, 2018).

Duggan, Jennifer. Inside the 'Doomsday' Vault. *Time*. http://time.com/doomsday-vault (Accessed January 12, 2018).

Everything you want to know about seedy saturdays. n.d. *Seeds of Diversity*. http://www.seeds.ca/Seedy-Saturday"EU (Accessed January 12, 2018).

FAO. 1999. "Women: users, preservers and managers of agrobiodiversity" (available at www.fao.org/FOCUS/E/Women/Biodiv-e.htm). What is Happening to Agrobiodiversity. http://www.fao.org/docrep/007/y5609e/y5609e02.htm.

Fowler, Cary and Pat Mooney. 1990. *Shattering: Food, Politics, and the Loss of Genetic Diversity*. Tucson: University of Arizona Press.

Geographical indications and traditional specialties in the European Union. *Wikipedia.org*. https://en.wikipedia.org/wiki/Geographical_indications_and_traditional_specialities_in_the_European_Union (Accessed January 12, 2018).

Hawken, Paul. 1993. *The Ecology of Commerce*. New York: HarperCollins.

Heald, Paul, and Susannah Chapman. August 27, 2009. Crop diversity report card for the twentieth century: diversity bust or diversity boom? Unpublished paper, http://dx.doi.org/10.2139/ssrn.1462917.

Hemenway, T. 2009. *Gaia's Garden: A Guide to Homescale Permaculture*. White River Junction: Chelsea Green.

Hole, D. G., A. J. Perkins, J. D. Wilson, I. H. Alexander, P. V. Grice, and A. D. Evans. 2005. Does organic farming benefit biodiversity? *Biol Conserv* 122:113–30.

J. E. M. Ag Supply, Inc., v. Pioneer Hi-Bred International, Inc. 2001. *Justia*. https://supreme.justia.com/cases/federal/us/534/124/ (Accessed January 12, 2018).

Khoury, Colin. 2017. How diverse is the global diet? *CIAT Blog*. http://blog.ciat.cgiar.org/how-diverse-is-the-global-diet (Accessed May 15, 2017).

Khoury, C., A. D. Bjorkman, H. Dempewolf, J. Ramirez-Villegas, L. Guarino, A. Jarvis, L. H. Rieseberg, and P. C. Struik. 2014. Increasing homogeneity in global food supplies and the implications for food security. *PNAS* 111 (11):4001–6. doi:10.1073/pnas.1313490111

Marketing orders and agreements for fruits, vegetables & specialty crops. n.d.*United States Department of Agriculture*. https://www.ams.usda.gov/rules-regulations/moa/fv (Accessed January 12, 2018).

McCartney, Kelly and Sarah Baird. August 7, 2014. Pennsylvania seed library investigated by department of agriculture. *Shareable*. https://www.shareable.net/blog/pennsylvania-seed-library-investigated-by-department-of-agriculture

McFetridge, Scott. December 28, 2014. Seed libraries struggle with state laws limiting exchanges. *The Washington Times*. https://www.washingtontimes.com/news/2014/dec/28/seed-libraries-struggle-with-state-laws-limiting-e

Mollison, B. 1988. *Permaculture: A designer's manual*. Tagari Publications.

Nabhan, Gary Paul. 1989. *Enduring Seeds*. San Francisco: North Point Press, p. 97.

Nalewicki, Jennifer. January 13, 2016. What makes Tucson deserving of the title of the United States' First Capital of Gastronomy. *Smithsonian.com*https://www.smithsonianmag.com/travel/introducing-americas-first-capital-gastronomy-180957793/

Paul J. Heald. 2009. Crop Diversity Report Card for the Twentieth Century: Diversity Bust or Diversity Boom? University of Illinois College of Law, Susannah Chapman, University of Georgia Department of Anthropology.

Pearce, F. 2011. The long strange journey of earth's travelling microbes. Yale Environment 360, Yale School of Forestry and Environmental Studies.http://e360.yale.edu/features/the_long_strange_journey_of_earths_traveling_microbes.

Philpott, Tom. May 9, 2012. How your college is selling out to big Ag. *Mother Jones*.http://www.motherjones.com/food/2012/05/how-agribusiness-dominates-public-ag-research.

Philpott, Tom. April 19, 2013. A brief history of our deadly addiction to Nitrogen fertilizer. *Mother Jones*, http://www.motherjones.com/food/2013/04/history-nitrogen-fertilizer-ammonium-nitrate

Pimentel, D., P. Hepperly, J. Hanson, D. Douds, and R. Seidel. 2005. Environmental, energetic, and economic comparisons of organic and conventional farming systems. *BioScience* 55 (7):573–82.

Richerson, P. J., M. Borgerhoff Mulder, and B. J. Vila. 1996. *Principles of Human Ecology*. Needham Heights: Simon & Schuster.

Ruelas, Richard. August 22, 2014. Hayden flour mills grows tradition and heritage grain. *AZCentral.com*. https://www.azcentral.com/story/life/az-narratives/2014/08/22/hayden-flour-mill/14121683

Schwartz, J. D. 2016. *Water in Plain Sight: Hope for a Thirsty World*. New York, NY: St. Martin's Press.

Sister libraries. n.d.*Seed Libraries*. http://seedlibraries.weebly.com (Accessed on January 12, 2018).

Smith, Heather. August 8, 2014. The little seed library that could... get busted by a state Ag department. *Grist*. https://grist.org/food/the-little-seed-library-that-could-get-busted-by-the-state-agriculture-department

Speth, James G. 2015. *Angels by the River: A Memoir*. White River Junction: Chelsea Green.

The endowment fund. *Global Crop Diversity Trust*. https://www.croptrust.org/our-mission/crop-diversity-endowment-fund/ (Accessed January 12, 2018).

Tracy, Bill. 2016. Intellectual property rights and public plant breeding. *Conference Proceedings*, Raleigh, NC. http://host.cals.wisc.edu/agronomy/wp-content/uploads/sites/16/2016/05/Proceedings-IPR-Final.pdf.

Wolfenson, Karla D. M. 2013. Coping with the food and agriculture challenge: Smallholders' agenda. Conference Report, Rome. http://www.fao.org/docrep/018/ar363e/ar363e.pdf.

Yeomans, P. A. 2008. *Water for Every Farm: Yeomans Keyline Plan*. Queensland, Australia: Keyline Designs.

12 Urban and Regional Planning for Biodiversity and Food Systems

Kimberley Hodgson and Tara Moreau

CONTENTS

12.1 INTRODUCTION

The loss of biodiversity defines one of the most critical sustainability issues of our time. While humans have altered ecosystems and impacted biodiversity for thousands of years through hunting, gathering, agriculture, and human settlement, the past few centuries have experienced an unprecedented loss of species. Rapid population growth and the sprawling nature of agriculture and urban development are driving this loss (de Oliveira et al. 2014). In particular, the intensification and expansion of agriculture worldwide has significantly impacted biodiversity through ecosystem degradation.

Scientists describe a sixth mass extinction of species that is underway and immediate action is needed to preserve, enhance, and regenerate biodiversity and ecosystem services (Ceballos et al. 2015). Sustainable development, the antithesis of current urbanization and development patterns, aims to reduce the impact of development on natural systems while ultimately optimizing quality of life for people. Urban and regional planning is considered to be an important tool for achieving sustainable development, thereby preserving, enhancing, and regenerating biodiversity (UN-Habitat 2009).

In North America, local and regional planners have typically planned for a range of issues, but food has not always been one of them. Food systems planning has advanced as a specialization within the planning profession, due in part to a combination of factors including: Sprawling urban development and its impact on the rapid loss of farmland in metropolitan areas; rising poverty rates and associated food insecurity; loss of open space and biodiversity within urban areas; unsustainable food production, processing, and distribution; and waste management practices and their impact on air, water, and soil health.

As a result, planning has emerged as an important tool for strengthening and enhancing community food systems. In cities across the United States and Canada, local and regional governments are bringing forward innovative plans and policies to provide a roadmap for achieving sustainable development and sustainable food systems.

This chapter describes how planning for sustainable development *and* sustainable food systems can positively contribute directly and indirectly to biodiversity conservation and planetary health. Urgent action to replicate and scale up successful plans and policies is needed. In this chapter, planning tools and processes, including community-wide plans and various policies, programs, projects, and public finance decisions used to implement them, are identified. Agriculture production and food systems plans and policies from North America are explored as key tools for biodiversity conservation and regeneration.

12.2   BIODIVERSITY, SUSTAINABLE DEVELOPMENT, AND PLANNING

The term biodiversity describes the total of all living species on Earth such as plants, animals, fungi, viruses, bacteria and more. It is vital to the health of our planet and all forms of life. The biodiversity of genes, species, and ecosystems is the foundation of our natural environment, which is connected by the Earth's physical and biological systems. With over 3.5 million taxa and 1.7 million species inventoried, biodiversity is a complex resource to manage (Catalogue of Life Partnership 2017).

Human's use of ecosystem services (benefits that people obtain from nature) and production of goods has dramatically altered the landscape and reduced biodiversity on Earth leading to the mass extinction and extirpation (local extinction) of animals, plants, microorganisms, genes, and all their interconnected relationships (Ceballos et al. 2015). The most crucial drivers to biodiversity and ecosystem service loss include habitat degradation through land-use change, climate change, overexploitation, agriculture production, invasive species, pollution, and urbanization (Assessment 2005; Royal Botanic Gardens Kew 2016). While cities take up 2% of the Earth's land surface, their inhabitants consume 75% of the Earth's resources (de Oliveira et al. 2014). Cities and urbanizations are responsible for habitat destruction and the introduction of alien species, but also contribute to air and water pollution and climate change (de Oliveira et al. 2014).

In addition to urbanization, how we feed ourselves has significantly impacted biodiversity. Agriculture is the cornerstone of food security and human civilization; however, its expansion over the past 10,000 years has changed the face of Earth's terrestrial and aquatic surfaces. Agriculture involves the growing of crops and rais-ing of animals for food, feed, fibers, oils, ornamentals, and industrial purposes. In the 1900s, the Green Revolution and the subsequent industrialization of agriculture was credited with increasing crop yields, global food supply, and human population. However, the focus on intensification displaced interest in sustainable agriculture practices that support and enhance on- and off-farm biodiversity (practices such as crop rotation, intercropping, cover cropping, etc.). The advancement of plant and animal breeding, distribution of hybridized seeds, irrigation expansion, increased mechanization and distribution of new technologies (e.g. agro-chemicals such as fer-tilizers and pesticides), clearing of forests for croplands, and the use of waterways for aquaculture have contributed to a rise in greenhouse gas emissions (GHGs) and the dramatic loss of sensitive ecosystems.

In the face of these challenges, local and regional governments across the globe are developing and implementing a range of strategies that mitigate the impact of human populations on biodiversity. Urban and regional planning is the profession dedicated to building and shaping the places in which we live—human settlements including cities, towns, and neighborhoods. Local and regional government planners determine how the built environment can be shaped and formed to create a healthy, livable place that can offer social, cultural, and economic opportunities for current and future populations (UN-Habitat 2009; American Planning Association [APA] 2000). The built (or human) environment includes the design, location, and network of gray infrastructure (such as buildings, public plazas, roads, and utilities, and other paved areas) across a city, town or neighborhood (APA 2000; UN-Habitat 2009; APA 2016). People experience the built environment as part of their daily life—in the places where they live, work, and recreate (APA 2016).

Local and regional planning also influences the protection and restoration of the natural environment used by cities for both recreation and biodiversity purposes; water systems used for water supply, waste disposal, and recreational purposes; agri-culture, forestry, soil, climate and air systems that provide healthy air (UN-Habitat 2009). The natural environment is the Earth's interrelated systems of air, water, soil, and vegetation used by human settlements (APA 2016). Human health and well-being depends on the natural environment to provide a range of services, such as healthy air, water and food, fiber, energy, waste dispersion, hazard protection, and a reliable climate (UN-Habitat 2009; 2APA 2016). The natural environment is located both within urban and non-urban areas. In urban areas, it includes green space or green infrastructure, which is the interconnected network of natural areas and open spaces across an urban area. Examples include local and regional parks, lawns, private and community gardens, green roofs, landscaping, urban forests, beaches, streams and rivers, etc.

Urban and regional planning in North America occurs at local and regional levels of government, but is influenced and guided by policies, plans and actions of state, provincial, federal and international governments. In their roles, planners must con-sider and balance many competing needs of human society, as well as the compet-ing policies and actions enacted by multiple levels of government to address those needs. Planners typically address issues related to land use, transportation, air and water quality, housing affordability, economic and community development, parks and open space, and emerging issues such as climate change, green infrastructure and biodiversity, public health, social equity, and food systems.

Local governments—typically cities, towns and counties—prepare many types of plans to address a variety of social, economic and environmental opportunities and problems. *Comprehensive plans* are community-wide plans that establish a roadmap for the long-range future of an entire community and highlight the dependencies and interrelationships between planning topics, such as housing, transportation, land use, and economic development. *Strategic plans* often highlight new or emerging issues, such as climate change or health equity, and identify a suite of policy options for addressing the issue(s). And *neighborhood or area plans* provide detailed guidance on how to deal with specific issues at the neighborhood level or within a specific geographic area.

Common to the development of most plans is the process for creating them. The *planning process* typically begins with an assessment of social, economic, and/or environmental conditions within a community. This assessment of current conditions helps to provide an "understanding of the strengths, gaps, and obstacles" of a community. This is followed by a community visioning and goal-setting process to identify the needs and goals of a community. Planners develop a set of actions, or a plan, to help the community achieve its vision and goals. Actions often include a range of local government policies, programs, projects, and public finance decisions. Often called a *blueprint for action*, a plan provides a community with a roadmap for implementing various local government decisions and actions that are needed to achieve desired community goals.

Historically, urban and regional planning has disregarded the impact of the human systems on natural systems, including the loss and degradation of biodiversity within and outside of cities. With rising concern for climate change, exponential population growth, sprawling urbanization, resource consumption, poverty and growing income inequality, food security, health inequities, and other issues facing cities across the globe, the planning profession has had to evolve.

One area of planning that has gained considerable traction in the past decade is planning for sustainable development. In the 1990s, the United Nations (UN) Commission on Human Settlements coined the term *sustainable development* as a "new concept of economic growth, which provides for fairness and opportunity for all people in the world without destroying the world's natural resources and without further compromising the carrying capacity of the globe" (UN-Habitat 2009). The goal of sustainable development is to reduce human impact on natural systems, while simultaneously optimizing quality of life for people (UN-Habitat 2009). In 2015, the UN General Assembly approved the 2030 Sustainable Development Goals (UN 2016). The 2030 Sustainable Development Goals address a number of global issues aimed broadly as a blueprint for planet and people. This framework of 17 goals and targets is consistent with other international biodiversity commitments such as the Strategic Plan for Biodiversity with its 20 Aichi Biodiversity Targets (Convention on Biological Diversity 2016).

While cities are responsible for biodiversity loss, they are also part of the solution. Urban biodiversity supports an urban area's resiliency and capacity to endure changing conditions when confronted with climate change. Urban ecosystems and the biodiversity within them can reduce the negative impacts of extreme weather events and improve food and water security. Urban green spaces can provide a number of ecosystem services that help mitigate the impact on biodiversity loss. These services include air pollution regulation, microclimate regulation (when plants and soil alter temperature, moisture, and air flow), noise reduction (through absorption of sound), rainwater drainage, sewage treatment, in addition to recreational/cultural services, well-being, and mental health (de Oliveira et al. 2014).

Over the past two decades, organizations such as the UN and the International Council for Local Environmental Initiatives (ICLEI), Local Governments for Sustainability, and more recently, the APA, have pushed for a new framework for cities—one that acknowledges the relationship between cities and the bioregions or "life-places" in which they reside (Newman and Jennings 2008). A bioregion is "a unique region definable by natural (rather than political) boundaries within a geographic, climatic, hydrological, and ecological character capable of supporting unique human and nonhuman living conditions" (Newman and Jennings 2008).

As a result, there has been a shift in how local governments view their impact on both human and natural systems, specifically related to climate change, water and air pollution, natural resource consumption, population growth, and sprawling urban development. This is evidenced by the growing number of local and regional government sustainability plans and climate action plans, as well as comprehensive plans that integrate sustainability and sustainable development as a key principle.

For example, in 2007, the Mayor of New York City adopted an overarching 20-year sustainability plan called PlaNYC: A Greener, Greater New York. The plan addressed sustainability issues related to land (housing, open space, and brownfields), water (quality and network), transportation (congestion and repair), energy, air quality, and climate change. The plan included goals and actions related to greening the cityscape; requiring greening of parking lots; providing incentives for green roofs; protecting wetlands; reforesting parkland; increasing tree plantings on lots; and capturing the benefits of existing open space and transportation plans. Since its adoption, the City adopted an updated sustainability plan (2012) in response to Hurricane Sandy. This updated plan, called PlaNYC: A Stronger, More Resilient New York, provided recommendations on how the city could adapt to the projected impacts of climate change, such as rising sea levels and extreme weather events. And, in 2015, the City adopted One New York: The Plan for a Strong and Just City, which builds on the city's existing efforts related to growth, sustainability, and resilience. This plan focuses on principles of growth, equity, sustainability and resiliency, and outlines a number of goals and actions related to GHGs, air quality, zero waste, water management, parks and natural resources, and coastal defense.

New York City is one of many cities across the globe that has recognized and embraced its role in reducing the impact of the built environment on the natural environment (UN-Habitat 2009). Planning for biodiversity can help to develop, conserve, and manage a network of new and existing green/natural spaces, which is thought to be one of the "most effective instruments by which to preserve and enhance urban biodiversity" (de Oliveira et al. 2014).

In 2016, the APA officially adopted The Sustainability Policy Framework for the profession of urban and regional planning in the United States (APA 2016). The APA was created in 1978 and serves over 3,500 members from 100+ countries by helping planners create better communities. The APA Sustainability Policy Framework states that principles of sustainability, or sustainable development, are "essential characteristics of good planning" and "infiltrate all facets of planning." Sustainability is "overarching and is best considered as an umbrella to many, if not almost all, planning topics." The Framework defines sustainability as "improving the quality of people's lives while living within the capacities of supporting natural and human systems." While not explicitly addressing biodiversity and ecosystem services loss, the APA Sustainability Framework offers recommended actions that directly or indirectly impact the preservation, enhancement, or regeneration of natural systems, specifically ecosystems within and outside urban boundaries (APA 2016).

There are a range of direct and indirect strategies local and regional governments can take to preserve, enhance, and regenerate biodiversity and ecosystems within and outside urban boundaries (Newman and Jennings 2008a; Godschalk and Rouse 2015; UN-Habitat 2009; de Oliveira et al. 2011; de Oliveira et al. 2014). Examples include mitigating land-use change (or preventing the conversion of natural environment to the built environment), adopting climate change mitigation and adaptation actions, increasing urban density, preventing sprawling urban development, and reducing air and water pollution. Little attention, however, has been paid to the role of food systems planning as a subset of urban planning in preserving, enhancing and regenerating ecosystems and biodiversity.

12.3   FOOD SYSTEMS PLANNING

In North America, local and regional planners have typically planned for a range of issues, but food has not always been one of them. However, in recent years this field of food systems planning has advanced. The APA's Food Systems Planning Interest Group defines food systems planning as a dynamic profession that works to improve the well-being of people and their communities by building more sustainable, equitable, self-reliant, and resilient community and regional food systems for present and future generations. The food system is the complex set of activities, processes, and relationships related to: (1) food production (2) processing (3) distribution (4) marketing (5) retailing (6) acquisition (7) preparation (consumption) and (8) waste management (APAAPA's Food Systems Planning Interest Group 2017).

The process of food systems planning includes several key steps (Table 12.1). Food systems planning emphasizes, strengthens, and makes visible the interdependent and inseparable relationships between individual sectors and offers solutions to food systems issues by seeing and leveraging their connections to other health, social, economic, and environmental issues. Essential and integral to the work of food systems planners is the active and meaningful engagement of the community (both governmental and non-governmental stakeholders) in food systems planning and policy-making processes and decisions. Planners, both within and outside of government, are leading these efforts in alliance with community groups such as food policy councils (citizen advisory groups made up of stakeholders across the food system that provide guidance and advice to municipal and county government staff and elected officials on food systems issues), non-government organizations,

TABLE 12.1

An Overview of the Food Systems Planning Process

Step 1: Community engagement	The active, meaningful identification and engagement of stakeholders including governmental, community groups (non-governmental stakeholders, including a diverse range of cultures, and marginalized groups) and allied professionals (food policy councils or similar entities; public health, economic development, etc.) in food systems planning and policy-making processes and decisions
Step 2: Plan development and implementation	The preparation, development, implementation and evaluation of food system related elements/components of community-level plans (this could include neighborhood, area, municipal, county, multi-jurisdictional, regional, and state/provincial plans with a local/regional impact, or stand-alone plans)
Existing conditions	The identification, tracking and analysis of food system challenges and opportunities (including social, health, economic, and environmental factors) within a community
Goal setting	The development of community food systems-related goals and objectives
Policy identification	The identification of potential local, regional, and state/provincial policies (regulations, programs, projects, or public finance decisions that have a local or regional impact) that can help a community strengthen its food system, provide solutions to community food system challenges, and achieve community goals and objectives
Implementation and evaluation	The implementation of identified local, regional, and state/provincial policies and the evaluation of their impact on community food systems goals and objectives. This includes adapting to changing needs
Step 3: Integration	The integration of food systems planning with land use, transportation, economic development, parks and recreation, housing and other areas of urban and regional planning practice

Source: Adapted from American Planning Association's Food Systems Planning Interest Group. (n.d.). Retrieved July 28, 2017, from https://apafig.wordpress.com/about/

and other community-based organizations (APA's Food Systems Planning Interest Group 2017) (Table 12.1).

Today, local and regional governments across North America—large and small—are actively integrating sustainable food systems actions and initiatives in their comprehensive plans, developing stand-alone food systems plans, and crafting a range of policies, programs and projects to implement these plans. For local and regional governments, planning for a healthy, just and sustainable food system can help achieve a wide range of social, economic and environmental goals.

There are many direct and indirect strategies urban and regional planners can take to strengthen community food systems. While the planner's main tool for doing so is the plan—whether it is a comprehensive, strategic, functional or an area plan—additional actions and policy changes needed to implement a plan are also important. Plan implementation typically involves a range of governmental and non-governmental actors, with the planner acting as the coordinator and facilitator of change and involving a range of policies, projects, programs, and public investment decisions.

Many resources provide a comprehensive overview of planning strategies (Raja et al. 2008; Hodgson et al. 2011; Dillemuth and Hodgson 2016b 2015, 2016a; Freedgood and Fydenkevez 2017; Growing Food Connections 2017). While there is a range of strategies local and regional governments can take to support community food systems, there is an opportunity for these governments to enact plans, policies, and programs that support sustainable food systems that enhance biodiversity and minimize ecosystem loss.

12.4 PLANNING FOR SUSTAINABLE AGRICULTURE AND FOOD PRODUCTION

All stages of the food system play an important role in protecting, enhancing, and regenerating biodiversity and ecosystems. However, because of agriculture's direct impacts on biodiversity (mainly conversion of land through agriculture, livestock farming, agricultural inputs, etc.), this section focuses on local and regional government planning and policy efforts to support a diversity of sustainable agriculture typologies and practices (Royal Botanic Gardens Kew 2016).

Today's agricultural systems rely heavily on synthetic fertilizers, pesticides, and fossil fuels, which contribute directly to climate change through GHGs. As the climate is changing in expected and unexpected ways, the agriculture sector must participate in both mitigation and adaptation strategies. As delineated in Chapter 3, current agricultural practices contribute to climate change through GHGs associated with nitrous oxide (from fertilizers containing ammonium and nitrate), methane (from animal waste, enteric fermentation, and plant debris), and carbon dioxide emissions (from land-use change, fossil fuels, biomass burning) (Moreau et al. 2012). By working with the natural capacity of soil, plants, animals, and ecosystems, sustainable agriculture aims to maintain high levels of biodiversity while using natural ecological functions to enhance productivity and resilience. Sustainable agriculture takes on different forms based on specific farm practices and principals as discussed in Chapter 10.

12.4.1 SUSTAINABLE AGRICULTURE

Urban and regional planning has a direct impact on agriculture (from rural to urban), specifically the protection of agricultural land; the availability of growing space and land; access to land and land tenure; location and placement of agriculture activities and infrastructure; and training opportunities for new farmers. Planning also influences access to natural resources, namely soil, compost and water, and the ecological health of those resources. There is an opportunity for local and regional governments to enact plans and policies that support not just any type of agriculture, but sustainable agriculture that enhances biodiversity within and surrounding urban areas.

The 1996 *Sustainability Plan for San Francisco*, one of the first comprehensive sustainability plans in North America, identified food and agriculture as "critical components of a sustainability plan even for a dense, highly urbanized city" and called out the need for cities to "consider the production, marketing, and distribution of food, as well as the recycling of food wastes, within their boundaries and bioregions." The plan highlighted the city's influence on regional agriculture and the need to support locally grown, organic food to reduce impacts on regional water quality and wildlife preservation, as well as public health. Furthermore, the plan laid out specific goals and policy actions to encourage sustainable agriculture (City of San Francisco 1997).

The 2008 *King County (Washington) Comprehensive Plan* update called out the need to reduce the impact of the food system on climate change (King County 2008). The 2016 *King County Comprehensive Plan* update goes one step further by presenting new policies that encourage the use of Agricultural Best Management Practices and sustainable farming activities to help protect the environment. The plan outlines several goals to preserve farming within the county that meet county environmental standards, particularly for water and fisheries resources, and provides an overview of agricultural protection policies and incentives. These include "the provision of technical assistance to aid property owners in land management, outreach to owners of properties vulnerable to development, creating opportunities for property owners to sell their development rights, and seeking funding for public acquisition of rural properties that had an existing resource-based use." The plan also includes the goal of developing incentives to encourage agricultural activities in prime farmland areas such as "tax credits, expedited permit review, reduced permit fees, permit exemptions for activities complying with best management practices, assistance with agricultural waste management or similar programs" (King County 2016).

According to a recent publication by the UN, urban agriculture is often "overlooked with regards to its contribution to urban biodiversity, as cities tend to focus on green space and/or areas with natural habitats" (de Oliveira et al. 2014). Urban agriculture however can enhance urban biodiversity by providing habitat for other species and enhance agricultural biodiversity (de Oliveira et al. 2014). Urban agriculture, when replacing impervious surfaces such as parking lots and rooftops, can contribute to stormwater management, increased plant foliage or greening, and reductions in urban heat island effects (Hodgson et al. 2011). Replacing grass lawns and grass areas of parks can reduce the use of fertilizers, herbicides and pesticides as well as the need for mowing and other lawn-maintenance activities. Urban agriculture can also contribute to the productive reuse and environmental management of contaminated land in former industrial areas of a city. All of these benefits contribute to urban biodiversity and species preservation. In addition to these benefits, urban agriculture can also: help connect people to nature; foster food literacy and increase environmental stewardship; support healthy eating behaviors such as increasing the consumption of whole, fresh produce; improve social capital; and raise property values (Hodgson et al. 2011). As a result, local and regional government plans and policies that support urban agriculture, or the production of food within urban boundaries, are important strategies for enhancing urban biodiversity *and* contributing to social and public health goals.

In March 2009, the City of Baltimore adopted *The Baltimore Sustainability Plan* as an official part of the city's comprehensive plan. The plan lays out a broad, inclusive, and community-responsive sustainability agenda for the city and its residents. The plan establishes 29 priority goals surrounding seven themes and a set of recommended strategies for each. The seven themes include cleanliness, pollution prevention, resource conservation, greening, transportation, education and awareness, and green economy. Due to the food system's impact on public health, quality of life, environmental stewardship, and GHGs, the plan included the priority goal of establishing Baltimore a leader in sustainable, local food systems, and lists several food system objectives and actions for achieving that goal. One of the food system objectives states the need to "increase the percentage of land under cultivation for agricultural purposes" and identifies four policy actions to achieve this goal:

- Modify zoning regulations to accommodate urban agricultural production and sales.
- Increase the number of city farms and gardens in parks, on vacant lots, school grounds, and other appropriate and available areas.
- Promote community gardening for food production through programs such as the existing Master Gardener Urban Agriculture Program.
- Develop incentives and support for urban farm enterprises (Baltimore Office of Sustainability 2009).

There are a range of other local government policies that can support sustainable agriculture and biodiversity. These include pollinator programs, alternative water collection and reuse policies, storm water runoff regulations, animal control ordinances, public land use policies, and land disposition policies (Hodgson et al. 2011; Wooten and Ackerman 2011). In 2009, Vancouver's Parks Board along with a number of non-governmental organizations established the *Pollinator Project* for the purpose of making Vancouver's parks and gardens more supportive of pollinator habitat. Vancouver's Pollinator Project has resulted in efforts to enhance habitat in urban parks and green spaces across the city, by increasing vegetation diversity, using native plants, increasing connectivity (linking ecosystems) and providing overwintering habitats (City of Vancouver 2015).

In order to facilitate access to water for urban agriculture and to minimize water loss through evaporation, some municipalities have adopted water access policies. Some municipalities have established "policies requiring the incorporation of soil amendments and organic materials into soil and the use of mulch or other material to cover the ground surrounding plants can help reduce water loss by 10–20%" (Hodgson et al. 2011). In 2011, the city and county of San Francisco adopted the *Water Efficient Irrigation Ordinance* for the purpose of protecting water resources and plant and animal habitats; promoting low water use and climate appropriate plantings; reducing runoff and maximizing water retention in soil and plantings; and lessening the impact of rising water costs on renters and homeowners alike (San Francisco Public Utilities Commission Water Conservation Section 2011). Urban agriculture projects of 1,000 square feet and over are required to provide documentation on how they abide by water efficiency requirements, such as re-circulating water features, mulching, automatic irrigation controllers, restrictions on plant species, and plant groupings by water needs (San Francisco Department of the Environment 2017).

12.4.2 ORGANIC AGRICULTURE

Organic agriculture and the products derived from this method of food production are guided by Codex Alimentarius, the international practices and guidelines used to facilitate harmonization and the design of national standards to support international trade (Codex Alimentarius 2007). Organic agriculture bans the use of synthetic fertilizers, pesticides, and genetically engineered organisms. The primary goal of this type of agriculture is to optimize health and productivity of communities of soil life, plants, animals, and people (Codex Alimentarius 2007). Organic farming was found to increase biodiversity species richness by 30% in a meta-analysis comparing biodiversity under organic versus conventional agriculture systems in developing countries (Tuck et al. 2014). The specific sustainable agriculture practices employed in organic systems are based on principles aimed at:

- maintaining or increasing fertility and biological activity of the soil through the cultivation of legumes, green manures, deep-rooted plants, incorporation of soil organic matter, and crop rotation programs;
- managing pests, diseases, and weeds using methods such as diversified ecosystems, natural enemies, mulching, mowing, grazing animals, mechanical controls (traps, barriers, light, sound), crop rotation and mechanical cultivation;
- using untreated seeds or vegetative plant material;
- using buffer zones that act as biological corridors linking habitats and ecosystems;
- managing livestock production to use natural breeding methods, reduce disease and stress in animals, reduce veterinary drugs (including antibiotics), and maintain animal health and welfare.

Certified organic foods maintain the integrity of the organic product throughout the food supply chain during process, storage, transportation, and sale. For example, processing methods use techniques to limit refining, and the use of additives and processing aids. Ionizing radiation is not permitted in organic systems as a pest control, food preservation, or sanitation method.

Local governments, such as in Marin County, California, and Woodbury County, Iowa, are encouraging organic agricultural practices through various plans and incentives. The award winning 2007 comprehensive plan of Marin County, California (titled *Marin Countywide Plan*), included principles of ecological, social, and economic sustainability as the plan's framework. The plan established indicators and targets for protecting and preserving agricultural land, including acres of land farmed organically, and agricultural resources, including soil, water, and forage (Marin County Community Development 2007). To incentivize the production of organic agriculture, in 2006, Woodbury County, Iowa, passed the Local Food Purchase Policy, requiring county departments that serve food (e.g., the county jail, work release center, and juvenile detention facilities) to purchase local organic food (Woodbury County 2005).

While many state governments in the United States prohibit cities and counties from regulating the use of pesticides (Wooten and Ackerman 2011), some municipalities are encouraging urban farmers to minimize or forgo pesticide use by requiring *farm management plans* as part of the zoning process. The City of Madison, Wisconsin, requires urban commercial farms to prepare an urban farm management plan. These management plans require applicants to describe how they will minimize or avoid negative impacts on neighboring land and natural systems (Wooten and Ackerman 2011). In Canada, municipalities are allowed to prohibit the use of pesticides and fertilizers in urban agriculture. Vancouver, Victoria, and Toronto, in addition to others, prohibit pesticide and fertilizer use in community gardens and urban farms.

Many municipalities have revamped their land use regulations to permit a variety of types and intensities of urban agriculture and some have gone a step farther to encourage and (in some cases) mandate more sustainable production practices. In 2010, Seattle updated the Seattle Land Use Code to "help create a more sustainable and secure local food system by increasing opportunities to grow and sell food in all zones" (Seattle Department of Construction and Inspections 2010). The zoning code update recognizes five different urban agriculture uses—animal husbandry, aquaculture, community gardens, horticulture and urban farms—and specifies additional restrictions in each respective zone. These changes establish definitions for each type of urban agriculture use, detail where each urban agriculture use is permitted or conditionally permitted, and established conditions, or additional requirements, for more intensive urban agriculture uses. In addition to these zoning regulations, the City of Seattle provides guidance on soil testing and environment-friendly gardening, including soil building, composting, water conservation, plant care, and alternatives to pesticide use (Seattle Department of Construction and Inspections 2010).

12.5 BEYOND AGRICULTURE: PLANNING FOR SUSTAINABLE FOOD SYSTEMS

In addition to developing and implementing a range of plans and policies to support sustainable agriculture, there are also a variety of strategies needed to ensure its viability. These include food processing, distribution, marketing, procurement, access, and waste policies. These strategies often require the involvement of other local government departments that are necessary to ensure the viability and success of sustainable agriculture.

12.5.1 Food Aggregation, Processing and Distribution

Food aggregation or "bringing produce together from multiple sources to create a larger and more consistent supply to meet consumer demand" (Dillemuth and Hodgson 2016a), food processing, and food distribution are essential to ensuring that sustainable agriculture and food-related businesses can meet consumer demand for local, sustainably produced products (Dillemuth and Hodgson 2016a). There are many ways in which local governments can support food aggregation, processing, and distribution infrastructure including by providing technical assistance and public financing for food infrastructure projects, and updating and revising land use plans and policies to support food infrastructure needs.

In the update of its Master Plan, Montpelier, Vermont, integrated extensive goals and action items to support its food system. With regards to infrastructure, the plan includes actions to support and enhance processing and distribution facilities for local foods and amend processing regulations so they support local agriculture (Montpelier Planning Commission, enVision Montpelier Stakeholders, and Department of Planning and Community Development 2010). Marin County, California's general plan identifies goals and policies to encourage processing and distribution of locally produced foods (Marin County Community Development 2007). Boulder County, Colorado's *Environmental Sustainability Plan* includes goals and actions related to investment in local food infrastructure and the need to work with local growers to identify infrastructure needs (Dillemuth and Hodgson 2016a).

Howard County, Maryland, updated its zoning ordinance to define "food hub" as "a centrally located facility that facilitates the collection, storage, processing, distribution, and/or marketing of locally produced food products," and permits it as an accessory use to farming in rural zoning districts (Municipal Code Corporation 2015). Sonoma County, California, adopted a zoning ordinance to "allow small-scale food processing facilities in agricultural and rural districts with administrative approval of a simple, low-cost zoning permit" (Dillemuth and Hodgson 2016a; Board of Supervisors of the County of Sonoma California 2014).

12.5.2 FOOD ACCESS PROCUREMENT AND CONSUMPTION

While local governments have little control over what foods people consume, they have influence over promoting, increasing demand for, and improving access to healthy foods, thereby indirectly influencing consumption habits. Local governments can simultaneously increase demand for local foods, strengthen markets for local foods, and improve the availability of healthy foods within a community by adopting local food procurement policies. These often include guidance on the type of food being purchased, provided, or made available by public agencies, such as government departments, schools, parks, and recreation facilities (Dillemuth and Hodgson 2015). Additionally, local governments can establish buy-local campaigns and adopt proclamations to increase awareness about sustainable and traditional indigenous diets.

In 2010, the City of Cleveland adopted an ordinance that provided incentives to businesses that are sustainable and locally-based or purchase 20% of their food locally (Dillemuth and Hodgson 2015). To increase demand for local foods, Cabarrus County, North Carolina, established a buy-local campaign (Hodgson 2015). The Douglas County (Kansas) Commission adopted a proclamation to highlight the importance of indigenous food and the relationships between humans, plants, and animals (Douglas County Commission 2012). In an effort to ensure that local foods are accessible to low-income residents, many local governments in the United States are incentivizing the sale of healthy, local foods at farmer's markets and through Community-Supported Agriculture (CSA) programs. These incentives not only aim to improve the purchasing power of low-income residents and their health, but also support local farmers. Both Seattle and Lawrence-Douglas County, Kansas, established incentive programs

(Fresh Bucks and Market Match, respectively) that double the value of SNAP (Supplemental Nutrition Assistance Program, or food stamps) benefits at area farmer's markets for low-income consumers. The City of Baltimore established an employee farm share program as part of city employees' wellness program (Dillemuth and Hodgson 2016b).

12.5.3 FOOD WASTE

Many local governments are beginning to recognize food waste as a significant issue. Over the past several years, many local governments in North America including Portland, San Francisco, Toronto, and Vancouver have established municipal food-composting programs to divert food waste from the landfill and transform it into healthy soil. Other local governments such as Philadelphia are exploring food recovery and food gleaning programs to collect excess food from area restaurants and farms, respectively, so that it can be distributed to area food banks and the like (Hodgson 2012).

12.6 CITY SPOTLIGHT: VANCOUVER, BRITISH COLUMBIA

While individual plans and policies related to sustainability, climate change, biodiversity, and food systems are important tools for biodiversity conservation, urban and regional planning plays an important role in (1) identifying connections between these issue areas (2) aligning plan goals and policy actions across issue areas to mutually support each other in achieving sustainability and biodiversity goals and (3) ensuring consistency across local, regional, state/provincial, federal—and even international policies.

The City of Vancouver (COV), British Columbia, Canada, is making tremendous progress at meeting sustainable development, biodiversity, *and* food systems planning goals through a number of connected plans and policies. The COV municipal government is leading a coordinated approach to develop a series of plans that address various sustainability topics to collectively support the long-term goal of improving social, ecological, and economic sustainability for the city.

Sustainability as a topic is not new to Vancouverites. The city has a history of being a North American global leader in sustainability. In the early 1990s, Vancouver was one of the first cities in the world to recognize the city's role in mitigating climate change and developed GHG inventories for both community and corporate emissions. Today, the COV has one of the smallest per capita carbon footprints in North America as the result of plans and policies aimed at landfill gas recovery and energy utilization, managed growth of emissions from light-duty vehicles (or passenger cars), and stabilizing emissions from buildings. In 2012, the COV adopted the Climate Change Adaptation Strategy designed to prepare the city for climate change impacts such as increased temperatures, increased intensity of heavy rain events, sea level rise, and appropriate infrastructure (COV 2012a).

In 2012, the COV adopted a comprehensive and innovative community sustainability plan, called the Vancouver Greenest City 2020 Action Plan (GCAP). This plan provides a sustainability framework for the entire city, providing guidance on ten environmental, economic, and social sustainability topics. The plan also makes visible the connections between climate change, the green economy, clean air and water, transportation, buildings, natural systems, and local food (COV 2012b). The vision of the plan is to "create opportunities today, while building a strong local economy, vibrant and inclusive neighborhoods, and...[meeting] the needs of generations to come" (COV 2012b). While the plan does not explicitly delve into the role of sustainable development in protecting and enhancing biodiversity, it does support greenhouse gas reductions in the transportation and building development sectors, decreases in water and air pollutants, and improving green infrastructure and access to green spaces such as parks, community gardens, and greenways. The plan explicitly highlights the role of local food systems in reducing ecological footprints (COV 2012b).

As a result of the GCAP, the Vancouver City Council adopted the Vancouver Food Strategy in January 2013 (COV 2013). This plan provides a coordinated roadmap for food policy in the city and builds upon decades of non-governmental and governmental work towards a just and sustainable food system. The plan provides a single umbrella for previously disparate and fragmented food policies, and helps align food system goals with broader sustainability, housing, transportation, and health goals. The plan includes five goal areas and 70 actions for achieving those goals. In July 2013, the Vancouver Board of Parks and Recreation (VBPR) adopted the Local Food Action Plan, which provides guidance and direction to VBPR staff around the role of land, facilities, and capacity building to support a just and sustainable food system (Jasper et al. 2013). Both plans were a direct result of the sustainability framework established by the Vancouver GCAP.

In 2014, the city adopted the Vancouver Healthy City Strategy, a "long-term, integrated plan for healthier people, healthier places, and a healthier planet." Together with the Vancouver CGAP and the Vancouver Economic Action Plan, the Vancouver Healthy City Strategy provides a sustainability framework for all future government decisions and actions, representing the ecological, economic, and social aspects of sustainability, respectively. These three plans are well aligned and are mutually reinforcing. In follow-up to the Greenest City Action Plan, the COV approved the Renewable City Strategy in 2015 (COV 2015). This plan outlines the target to derive 100% of the energy used in Vancouver from renewable sources before 2050. Energy generation and the consequences of using fossil fuels impacts both biodiversity and food production.

Awareness and celebration of First Nation traditional foods is an important aspect of the food movement in Vancouver. Vancouver lies on the Burrard Inlet, part of the Pacific Ocean, and homelands to three First Nations including the Musqueam, Squamish, and Tsleil-Waututh peoples. Fisheries and seafood plays an important and essential role in First Nations culture and food security. In 2016, the Tseleil-Waututh peoples developed a Burrard Inlet Action Plan to improve the health and integrity of the saltwater inlet (Lilley et al. 2016a). This action plan developed from the Tsleil-Waututh peoples' perspective outlines six priority areas that advance water health and biodiversity with a specific goal to recover shellfish beds, an important food source that was lost due to pollution (Lilley et al. 2016b).

In 2016, the Vancouver Board of Parks and Recreation adopted the Vancouver Biodiversity Strategy. This comprehensive biodiversity plan aims to "increase the size and quality of Vancouver's natural areas including: forests, wetlands, streams, shorelines, and meadows" and "expand vital habitat for pollinators, birds, urban salmon, and herring, [and] wildlife" (Vancouver Board of Parks and Recreation 2016). This plan recognizes the role backyard gardens, community gardens, parks, and green roofs (including rooftop farms) play in sustaining biodiversity and providing natural habitats (see Table 12.2. Excerpt from the Vancouver Biodiversity Strategy Summary).

While Vancouver is a global leader in sustainable development, biodiversity conservation and sustainable food systems, there is room for improvement to reduce fragmentation and ensure alignment between plans and policies. A number of policies, programs, projects, and public investment decisions are underway to implement these plans, some of which were mentioned earlier in this chapter, others are listed in Table 12.3.

The COV is in the process of developing a resilience strategy (as one city of the 100 Resilient Cities), a zero waste 2040 strategy, and a poverty reduction strategy. It is also working to update its Climate Change Adaptation Strategy as well as the Food Strategy. However, the COV lacks a clear, coordinated vision for how all these individual plans are connected and can collectively impact the environmental, economic and social sustainability of the city, including topics such as climate change and biodiversity.

As cities such as Vancouver continue to explore ways to support sustainable development, biodiversity, and food systems, it will be important to align plans so they are supportive and consistent with not only local policies, but regional, state/provincial, federal, and even international sustainability, biodiversity, and climate change policies.

TABLE 12.2

Excerpt from the Vancouver Biodiversity Strategy Summary

Goal

Increase the amount and ecological quality of Vancouver's' natural areas to support biodiversity and enhance access to nature

Objectives

1. Restore habitats and species
2. Support biodiversity within parks, streets, and other City-owned lands
3. Protect and enhance biodiversity during development
4. Celebrate biodiversity through education and stewardship
5. Monitor biodiversity to track change and measure success

Source: Vancouver Board of Parks and Recreation. (2016). *Biodiversity Strategy*. Vancouver. Retrieved from http://parkboardmeetings.vancouver.ca/reports/REPORT-BiodiversityStrategy2016-FINAL.pdf

---

TABLE 12.3

Highlights of the City of Vancouver's Food Plans and Policies

Date	Food Policy
July 8, 2003	City Council Just & Sustainable Food System Motion
December 9, 2003	Vancouver Food Action Plan (adopted)
March 11, 2004	Vancouver Food Action Plan (expenditures approved)
July 14, 2004	Vancouver Food Policy Council
Dec 2004–Oct 2005	Vancouver Food System Assessment
September 19, 2005	Community Gardens Policy
February 27, 2006	Hobby Beekeeping Guidelines
May 30, 2006	2,010 Garden Plots by 2010 Initiative
January 2007	Vancouver Food Charter
2008	Urban Agriculture Steering Committee
January 20, 2009	Urban Agriculture Design Guidelines for the Private Realm
June 10, 2010	Keeping of Chickens Guidelines
2010	Food scraps collection program
2009–2010	Greenest City Grants in support of urban agriculture
2011	Grant to support urban farming forum
2009–2012	Grants to support Neighborhood Food Networks
2012	Greenest City Action Plan
January 2013	Vancouver Food Strategy
May 16, 2013	Rezoning Policy for Sustainable Large Developments Amendment
July 2013	Vancouver Park Board Local Food Action Plan
April 2014	Pollinator Project

12.7 CONCLUSION

Agriculture and food systems are key drivers of biodiversity loss and extinction. Solutions that are coordinated and connected to local and global efforts can be advanced and accelerated through urban and regional planning for sustainable development, food systems, and biodiversity conservation.

The conservation and protection of biodiversity requires immediate and urgent action by stakeholders at all levels. While urban and regional planners have not always explicitly addressed biodiversity, the planning profession provides an essential framework for leveraging solutions and directions to enact change. However, the future is uncertain and as our climate changes in both expected and unexpected ways. Our human settlements and the food systems upon which they depend will need to be planned and managed in a proactive and adaptive manner in order to respond to changes on our planet.

ACKNOWLEDGEMENT

The development of this chapter was supported in part by Growing Food Connections, a five-year project made possible with a grant from the USDA/NIFA AFRI Food Systems Program, NIFA Award #2012-68004-19894.

REFERENCES

American Planning Association. 2000. Policy guide on planning for sustainability. *American Planning Association*. https://www.planning.org/policy/guides/adopted/sustainability.htm.

American Planning Association. 2016. Sustainability policy framework. https://planning-org-uploaded-media.s3.amazonaws.com/document/Sustainability-Policy-Framework.pdf.

American Planning Association's Food Systems Planning Interest Group. 2017. About – American planning association's food systems planning interest group. https://apafig.wordpress.com/about/ (Accessed July 28).

Assessment, Millennium Ecosystem. 2005. *Ecosystems and Human Well-Being: Our Human Planet: Summary for Decision Makers*. 1st edition. Washington, DC: Island Press.

Baltimore Office of Sustainability. 2009. The Baltimore sustainability plan. Baltimore. http://www.baltimoresustainability.org/wp-content/uploads/2015/12/Baltimore-Sustainability-Plan.pdf.

Board of Supervisors of the County of Sonoma California. 2014. *Ordinance No. 6081. Zoning Ordinance*. http://www.sonoma-county.org/prmd/docs/small_scale_ag/ord13-0004_6081_small_ag_processing_adopted_ordinance.pdf.

Catalogue of Life Partnership. 2017. Catalogue of life. January. doi:10.15468/RFFZ4X.

Ceballos, Gerardo, Paul R. Ehrlich, Anthony D. Barnosky, Andrés García, Robert M. Pringle, and Todd M. Palmer. 2015. Accelerated modern human–induced species losses: Entering the sixth mass extinction. *Science Advances* 1 (5) e1400253.

City of San Francisco. 1997. The sustainability plan for the City of San Francisco. San Francisco. http://www.sustainable.org/creating-community/community-visioning/717-the-sustainability-plan-for-the-city-of-san-francisco.

City of Vancouver. 2012a. Climate change adaptation strategy. http://vancouver.ca/files/cov/Vancouver-Climate-Change-Adaptation-Strategy-2012-11-07.pdf.

City of Vancouver. 2012b. Vancouver greenest city 2020 action plan. Vancouver. http://vancouver.ca/files/cov/Greenest-city-action-plan.pdf.

City of Vancouver. 2013. Vancouver food strategy. *Heterocycles*. 87. doi:10.3987/Contents-12-85-7.

City of Vancouver. 2015. Pollinator project. http://vancouver.ca/parks-recreation-culture/pollinator-project.aspx.

Convention on Biological Diversity. 2016. Biodiversity and the 2030 agenda for sustainable development. https://www.cbd.int/development/doc/biodiversity-2030-agenda-technical-note-en.pdf.

de Oliveira, Puppim J. A., O. Balaban, C. N H Doll, R. Moreno-Peñaranda, A. Gasparatos, D. Iossifova, and A. Suwa. 2011. Cities and biodiversity: Perspectives and governance challenges for implementing the Convention on Biological Diversity (CBD) at the city level. *Biological Conservation*. doi:10.1016/j.biocon.2010.12.007.

de Oliveira, Puppim, J. A. Shih, Wan-yu, Raquel Moreno-Peñaranda, and Adele Phillips. 2014. Integrating biodiversity with local and city planning: The experience of the studios in the development of local biodiversity strategies and action plans – LBSAPs. http://collections.unu.edu/eserv/UNU:2568/integrating-biodiversity-with-local-and-city-planning.pdf.

Dillemuth, Ann, and Kimberley Hodgson. 2015. Local, healthy food procurement policies: Driving demand for, and improving the availability of local, healthy foods. Buffalo, NY. http://growingfoodconnections.org/wp-content/uploads/sites/3/2015/11/FINAL_GFCFoodProcurementPoliciesBrief-1.pdf.

Dillemuth, Ann, and Kimberley Hodgson. 2016a. Food aggregation, processing, and distribution: The local government's role in supporting food system infrastructure for fruits and vegetables. Buffalo, NY. http://growingfoodconnections.org/wp-content/uploads/sites/3/2015/11/GFCFoodInfrastructurePlanningPolicyBrief_2016Sep22-3.pdf.

Dillemuth, Ann, and Kimberley Hodgson. 2016b. Incentivizing the sale of healthy and local food the local government's role in promoting access to and purchase of good food. Buffalo, NY. http://growingfoodconnections.org/wp-content/uploads/sites/3/2015/11/GFCHealthyFoodIncentivesPlanningPolicyBrief_2016Feb-1.pdf.

Douglas County Commission. 2012. Indigenous food day. http://www.douglas-county.com/mycounty/news/news_release_details.aspx?record_id=818.

Freedgood, Julia, and Jessica Fydenkevez. 2017. Growing local: A community guide to planning for agriculture and food systems. Washington DC. http://growingfoodconnections.org/wp-content/uploads/sites/3/2013/06/AFT_GFC_Community-Guide_lo_res_04-2017.pdf.

Godschalk, David R., and David C. Rouse. 2015. *Sustaining Places: Best Practices for Comprehensive Plans.* Chicago IL: American Planning Association.

Growing Food Connections. 2017. Local government food policy database. http://growing-foodconnections.org/tools-resources/policy-database/.

Hodgson, Kimberley. 2012. Planning for food access and community-based food systems: A national scan and evaluation of local comprehensive and sustainability plans. *American Planning Association.* Washington, DC. https://planning-org-uploaded-media.s3.amazonaws.com/legacy_resources/research/foodaccess/pdf/foodaccessreport.pdf.

Hodgson, Kimberley. 2015. Advancing local food policy in Cabarrus County, North Carolina : Successes and challenges in a changing political climate. In: *Exploring Stories of Innovation,* 3. http://growingfoodconnections.org/wp-content/uploads/sites/3/2015/04/Cabarrus-COI-Web-Feature_20150715.pdf.

Hodgson, Kimberley, Marcia Caton Campbell, and Martin Bailkey. 2011. *Urban Agriculture: Growing Healthy, Sustainable Places.* Washington, DC: American Planning Association.

Jasper, Aaron, Niki Sharma, Lindsay Cole, Jason Hsieh, Trish Kelly, Ian Marcuse, Wendy Mendes, et al. 2013. The local food action plan of the Vancouver Park Board. Vancouver. http://vancouver.ca/files/cov/Local-food-action-plan.pdf.

King County. 2008. 2008 King County comprehensive plan. King County, Washington. http://www.kingcounty.gov/depts/permitting-environmental-review/codes/growth/CompPlan/archive/2008_2010update.aspx.

King County. 2008. 2016. 2016 King County comprehensive plan. King County, Washington. http://www.kingcounty.gov/council/CompPlan/2016compplan.aspx.

Lilley, Patrick, Peter DeKoning, John Konovsky, and Bridget Doyle. 2016a. Burrard Inlet action plan: A Tsleil-Waututh perspective. Tseil-Waututh Nation. http://www.twnation.ca/en/Band and Community/~/media/John Konovsky/TWN Burrard Inlet Action Plan Summary.ashx.

Marin County Community Development. 2007. Marin Countywide plan. Marin County, CA. http://www.smwlaw.com/files/Marin_CountyWide_Plan.pdf.

Montpelier Planning Commission, enVision Montpelier Stakeholders, and Department of Planning and Community Development. 2010. Master plan Montpelier, VT. Montpelier. http://www.montpelier-vt.org/DocumentCenter/Home/View/1227.

Moreau, Tara, Jennie Moore, and Kent Mullinix. 2012. Mitigating agricultural greenhouse gas emissions: A review of scientific information for food system planning. *Journal of Agriculture, Food Systems, and Community Development* (3)(March): 237–246. doi:10.5304/jafscd.2012.022.007.

Municipal Code Corporation. 2015. *Howard County, MD Supplementary Zoning District Regulations: Municipal Code Corporation.* https://library.municode.com/md/howard_county/codes/zoning?nodeId=HOWARD_CO_ZONING_REGULATIONS_S128.0SUZODIRE.

Newman, Peter, and Isabella Jennings. 2008. *Cities as Sustainable Ecosystems: Principles and Practices: Cities.* Island Press. doi:10.1111/j.1467-9906.2010.00504.x.

Raja, Samina, Branden Born, and Jessica Kozlowski Russell. 2008. A planners guide to
    community and regional food planning: Transforming food environments, facilitating
    healthy eating. Chicago, IL: *American Planning Association.*
RBG Kew. 2016. The State of the World's Plants Report - 2016. Royal Botanic Gardens, Kew.
San Francisco Department of the Environment. 2017. Water conservation requirements.
    https://sfenvironment.org/article/urban-agriculture-permits/water-conservation-
    requirements (Accessed July 28).
San Francisco Public Utilities Commission Water Conservation Section. 2011. Complying
    with San Francisco's water efficient irrigation requirements. San Francisco. http://
    www.sfwater.org/Modules/ShowDocument.aspx?documentID=731.
Seattle Department of Construction and Inspections. 2010. *Urban Agriculture..* Seattle:
    Seattle Permits. http://www.seattle.gov/DPD/Publications/CAM/cam244.pdf.
Tuck, Sean L., Camilla Winqvist, Flávia Mota, Johan Ahnström, Lindsay A. Turnbull, and
    Janne Bengtsson. 2014. Land-use intensity and the effects of organic farming on bio-
    diversity: A hierarchical meta-analysis. *Journal of Applied Ecology*, February, n/a-n/a.
    doi:10.1111/1365-2664.12219.
UN-Habitat. 2009. *Planning Sustainable Cities: Global Report on Human Settlements,*
    edited by UN-Habitat. London: Earthscan. doi:10.1007/s13398-014-0173-7.2.
United Nations. 2016. United Nations sustainable development goals. http://www.un.org/
    sustainabledevelopment/sustainable-development-goals/.
Vancouver, City of. 2015. City of Vancouver: Renewable city strategy. http://vancouver.ca/
    files/cov/renewable-city-strategy-booklet-2015.pdf.
Vancouver Board of Parks and Recreation. 2016. Biodiversity strategy. Vancouver. http://park-
    boardmeetings.vancouver.ca/reports/REPORT-BiodiversityStrategy2016-FINAL.pdf.
Woodbury County. 2005. Organics conversion policy resolution. http://growingfoodconnec-
    tions.org/gfc-policy/organics-conversion-policy-resolution/.
Wooten, Heather, and Amy Ackerman. 2011. Seeding the city: Land use policies to promote
    urban   agriculture.   http://www.changelabsolutions.org/sites/default/files/Urban_Ag_
    SeedingTheCity_FINAL_(CLS_20120530)_20111021_0.pdf.
World Health Organization (WHO) 2007. Codex Alimentarius. *Organically Produced Foods,
    3rd Edition.* Rome, Italy Food and Agriculture Organization of the United Nations
    (FAO).

13 Taking It Outside
The Value Added By Experiential Learning On Food Systems

Alison H. Harmon

CONTENTS

13.1 INTRODUCTION TO EXPERIENTIAL LEARNING

To address today's food system challenges, we need engaged citizens capable of critical thinking and able to learn from experience (Heinrich et al. 2015). Experiential education is an effective pedagogy for developing learners who can understand and address complex, multifaceted problems that span environmental, social, and economic realms (Spence and McDonald 2015; Heinrich et al. 2015). Relevant to sustaining food systems and solving food-related problems, experiential learning has been shown to improve practical competence, civic engagement, an appreciation of diverse ideas and people, and professional networking (Coker and Porter 2015).

In contrast to didactic learning, the experiential learner plays an active role and increases knowledge and awareness by reflecting on the act of "doing". The early proponents of experiential education, including Dewey (1938) and later Kolb (1984), posited that students would learn to form their own opinions from their experiences, which accumulate to create a unique individual while expanding perspective. Kolb's Experiential Learning Theory (2005) includes four stages: (1) concrete experience (2) reflective observation (3) abstract conceptualization and (4) active experimentation (1984). These stages are important components of experiential learning activities. Reflection is described as the rational analytic process by which learners extract knowledge from their experience (Howden 2012; Jordi 2011). It is important to complete the learning by allowing participants time and freedom to process and reflect on their learning, apply it, and then use it further as Kolb (1984) suggests.

In higher education, one clear goal is to prepare graduates for the challenges of the contemporary workplace. Experiential learning often simulates workplace learning, and develops skills needed for being competitive applicants and for starting a career with previous real-world exposure and readiness to make a contribution (Clements 2013). Some examples of experiential education in higher education include internships and practicum courses, study abroad experiences, service learning, hands-on research, and curricular and extra-curricular leadership experiences (Coker and Porter 2015).

There are numerous examples of active and experiential learning that transpire within the confines of a traditional classroom—but the classroom can also be mobile or outdoors (Howden 2012). Outdoor experiential education involves learning through the body—not merely the head. When we participate in an experience, we remember the skills and ideas that we have come to understand (Howden 2012). Outdoor field experiences are said to transform students (Hamlin 2016). Merizow's Transformative Learning Theory (TLT) (1991) provides a foundation for experiential education that seeks to challenge students' perspectives or existing worldviews. The TLT also states that learning entails reflection and openness to others' perspectives and ideas, providing the opportunity to construct a new or revised interpretation of the meaning of one's experiences in order to guide future action (Merizow 1991). Using wilderness as a backdrop, adventure education is a unique application of experiential education where the learner is in a physical and social environment and must adapt and struggle to solve problems, often with other members of a team. Learning in this case is both intense and memorable, with enduring usefulness (Howden 2012).

13.2   EXPERIENTIAL LEARNING AND FOOD SYSTEMS

The food system uses raw materials to create edible foodstuffs through sectors including production, transformation (processing, packaging, and labeling), distribution (wholesaling, storage, and transportation), access (retailing, institutional foodservice, emergency food programs), and consumption (preparation and health outcomes). A pool of human and natural resources serves as the foundation of food systems that are combined with other factors such as technology, policy, economics, sociocultural trends, research, and education that influence how the system functions. Industrial food system operations create externalities that threaten environmental sustainability. Examples include ecological issues related to water pollution and soil erosion; economic issues associated with low wages for producers and industry consolidation; and social issues like food insecurity or food-related chronic disease. Sustaining food systems entails conserving the raw materials or inputs while regenerating the foundation upon which the system is built (Harmon 2007).

Experiential education can be a method for learners to develop a more thorough and intimate understanding of food system issues and problems while actively engaging in formulating solutions. Newly instituted sustainable agriculture and food systems curricula at universities often include introductory courses and capstone courses that are experiential and interdisciplinary in nature and focused on developing critical thinking and problem-solving skills (Jordan et al. 2014; Malone et al. 2014). Many sustainable agriculture programs in land-grant colleges of agriculture have used transformative and experiential food systems education as a way to make students aware of how we have come to our knowledge and about the values that lead us to our perspectives (Galt 2013). Experiential education offers opportunities for students to see, hear, and do things that are out of their current perspective, incorporating new ways of thinking and understanding. Francis et al. (2011) use experiential learning in sustainable agriculture curricula as an opportunity for students to transfer experiences and information from the research laboratory, the experimental field, or the rural community into the classroom.

Campus sustainable food projects can contribute to transformational change toward an alternative food system in the university microcosm and beyond. Components of campus projects might include procurement goals, academic programs, direct marketing on campus, and other forms of experiential learning. Examples include 'farm-to-college' programs in university dining services, civic agriculture on campus farms, and restoration of foodsheds through stimulating the local agricultural economy. Campus food projects build coalitions beyond the classroom, and provide students with opportunities to network with future partners, collaborators, or employers (Barlett 2011).

Service learning in food and nutrition curricula is a powerful experiential education method for teaching and learning about food systems, while also strengthening the food system in the community surrounding the university or college campus. Wadsworth et al. (2012) describes specific examples of projects designed to engage students in partnerships with local entities such as organizing public forums, creating educational newsletters to accompany food assistance boxes, creating local food and farm maps, and developing advocacy tools to assess how well political candidates would address food insecurity.

Harmon et al. (2017) have used experiential education in a community nutrition course to introduce students to the realities of living on food assistance, and in particular the challenges of affording nutritious diets on a limited income. During the "Food Insecurity Experience" students struggle first hand with hunger for a short period of time. The purpose of the activity is for students to develop some understanding of what it is like to be hungry, to create strategies for maintaining a nutritious diet on a limited food budget, and to gain empathy for individuals who are food insecure. Results indicate that the experience is transformational. In addition to accomplishing the stated purposes of the activity, students demonstrate awareness that will contribute to becoming competent food and nutrition professionals. They better understand what is involved in practicing community nutrition, and express the desire to work on community and social issues to address root causes of hunger-related problems rather than developing generalized programs that address only symptoms (Harmon et al. 2017).

13.3 COMMUNITY SUPPORTED AGRICULTURE (CSA): EXPERIENTIAL FOOD DISTRIBUTION

13.3.1 WHAT IS CSA?

Local food systems generate alternative models of social organization that address the problematic aspects and externalities of the food system (Papaoikonomou and Ginieis 2017). One such alternative model is Community Supported Agriculture (CSA). CSA is a food distribution system that brings eaters in close contact with the producers of their food. The economic exchange provides an opportunity for "experiential eating" that contrasts with a more passive acquisition of a food supply that is globally distributed, counter-seasonal, and often heavily processed and packaged from the grocery store or supermarket.

Members of CSAs pay a fee in advance of the season in return for a weekly share of the seasonal harvest (Henderson 1999). Most CSAs provide fresh produce to their members, but some also provide some combination of eggs, flours, bread, grains and legumes, meat and poultry, or fish (Henderson 1999). In addition to providing food, newsletters, recipes, tours, and other events are often included.

The number of CSAs in the U.S. has grown rapidly since the mid-1980s when they were first introduced to more than 6,000 enterprises (Harmon 2014). Compared to the early CSA membership characteristics, today's CSAs are inclusive of a more mainstream audience (Harmon 2014). This is the result of growing public interest in locally and organically grown produce and more healthful food (Brown and Miller 2008).

13.3.2 CSAs, FOOD SYSTEM HEALTH, AND EXPERIENTIAL LEARNING

At the cost of time, convenience, and an upfront fee, CSAs can make a positive contribution to individual and family health. Individuals and families that subscribe to a CSA consume significantly more fresh produce, which displaces other less healthful foods in the diet (Cohen et al. 2012; Curtis et al. 2013). Positive behavior change and health outcomes have been demonstrated (Allen et al. 2017). Members often develop higher expectations for flavors and textures as a result of membership and begin to prefer fresher produce that is consumed close to production in both time and space (Harmon 2014).

Households subscribing to CSAs tend to cook at home more, and enjoy an increased number of family meals eaten together on a weekly basis (Harmon 2014). Cooking with unfamiliar produce provides an opportunity for experimentation and building food preparation skills. For family budgets, CSAs can be an overall cost savings, as weekly shares often exceed the relative portion of the upfront membership fee. If a family makes good use of the weekly produce share, it may also save trips to the supermarket, reducing opportunities to purchase expensive processed foods (Cullen 1994; Abratt and Goodey 1990).

In addition to being a vehicle for improving individual and family health, CSAs support community and food system level health. For example, members assume some of the financial risk of farming by paying ahead of the season. A unique aspect of CSAs is the mutually beneficial relationship they create among producers and consumers resulting in a local food economy, where food is produced exclusively for local consumption and all food produced by an enterprise is marketed directly to consumers (McFadden 2003). CSA members have the opportunity to re-connect with the local or regional agricultural landscape, and to be part of a community of eaters and growers that share food values and a vision for a true alternative to the industrial food system (Galt 2013; Worden 2004).

CSA provides a means for producers to produce a diverse array of crops on a small scale while earning returns that exceed wholesale prices. By providing fair wages for farmers and reasonable working conditions for farm labor, CSAs contribute to the economic viability of sustainable food production. Additionally, farmland that generates revenue near rural communities and urban areas is more likely to be protected from development (Tegtmeier and Duffy 2005). While consolidation and distant industrial control are characteristics of the modern U.S. food system, CSAs are uniquely under local control (Henderson 1999).

CSAs can minimize externalized food system costs by including natural resource stewardship and conservation in the farm's business plan. CSAs typically use fewer chemicals, cause less soil erosion, employ water conservation practices, and sustain a greater level of biodiversity in the farm ecosystem (Lass et al. 2003; Anderson-Wilk 2007; Tegtmeier and Duffy 2005). Additionally, CSA farmers can give careful attention to maintaining a high level of animal welfare. Food processing and packaging is minimized while transportation energy use may be decreased. These features of CSAs are what attract members, also known as "shareholders" (Buttel 2003).

CSAs clearly provide an experiential education for members, but a CSA operation linked to a university or college campus can also provide comprehensive experiential learning for students interested in sustainable community food systems. Wharton and Harmon (2009) describe CSA as a way for students to engage on campus and in the community to make positive change in local food systems.

13.4   THE STUDENT FARM AS A CENTER OF EXPERIENTIAL LEARNING ON FOOD SYSTEMS

Land-grant universities have become important catalysts for developing innovative sustainable agriculture curricula and a major component of these is a campus farm, often operated by students. In 1992 there were approximately 23 farms on university and college campuses, but that number has grown substantially to approximately 300 today (LaCharite 2016). Many student farms pre-date sustainable agriculture degree programs, but more recently student farms have been integrated into formal academic programs for the benefit of students involved and the economic sustainability of the farm operation (Parr and Trexler 2011).

The campus farm provides a unique opportunity for students enrolled in agricultural degree programs to learn about environmental sustainability and to develop critical thinking, personal initiative, management, research, decision-making and communication skills—and to experience a sense of community, belonging with other students who share the mission of having a successful harvest (LaCharite 2016; Reeve et al. 2014). Campus farms can also serve to attract new students to the study of food and agriculture and contribute experiential preparation for the diversity needs of the food system workforce. Students can link community service to curricular activities, spend more time outdoors, make connections with the sources of their food, and interact socially with students of varied academic backgrounds. This provides students with opportunities for personal growth, as well as social, professional, and practical skills (Sayre and Clark 2011).

Overall, campus farms serve important purposes for higher education institutions by providing a real and visible venue for students to apply their classroom learning. They offer ways to integrate agricultural production with other campus services and environmental sustainability initiatives; improving food security by engaging with the community through workshops; offering emergency food by partnering with local food banks; selling food at local farmers' markets; and increasing access to fresh produce for families with limited resources (Biernbaum et al. 2006; Markhart 2006; Wharton and Hamon 2009).

Consistent with the philosophy of experiential education, Parr and Trexler (2011) note that the campus farm learning experience allows students to resolve the tensions between abstract conceptualization and concrete experience, and between reflective observation and experimentation—while constructing knowledge in the process. Students can use the campus farm experience to obtain immediate feedback as they test their content-based theories and methods, all the while developing personal and professional skills. This type of learning is a necessary complement to formal education in classrooms. It is important to revisit the field experience back in the classroom, and integrate it with formal learning experiences to cyclically reinforce the experiential education. Classroom time helps learners process the experience, share observations and reflections, consider modifying behaviors and approaches, and prepare for the next experience.

When preparing students for the work force, it is likely that educational deficiencies are not due to curricular content, but lie in the inability of students to apply what they have learned. Benefits of experiential learning in the context of the campus farm include: The motivation of students, realism, integration of concepts, teachable moments (multiple real illustrations of concepts that can then be explained or explored), inductive learning (sometimes from trial and error), incorporation of cross-disciplinary concepts, and face-to-face encounters with negotiation and ethics, in addition to group or team problem solving (Koontz et al. 1995).

13.5 THE VALUE ADDED BY A STUDENT FARM EXPERIENCE: A CASE STUDY OF TOWNE'S HARVEST GARDEN AT MONTANA STATE UNIVERSITY

13.5.1 History of Towne's Harvest Garden

Towne's Harvest Garden is a three-acre vegetable garden located on Montana State University's (MSU's) agricultural research station and teaching farm. Montana State

University Friends of Local Foods, a student organization, formed in the fall of 2006, began operating Towne's Harvest Garden as a CSA during the summer of 2007. The project is a collaboration among the MSU College of Education, Health, and Human Development (EHHD) and the College of Agriculture (Ag). Land and greenhouse space is rented from the Ag, which over the years has allocated resources to improve the permanent building infrastructure on the farm to support teaching and research. Faculty oversight of production is provided by the Department of Plant Sciences and Plant Pathology. Bookkeeping and human resources support is provided by the College of EHHD along with the marketing and distribution aspects of the garden. Faculty and students from both colleges are involved in the project, which has become the cornerstone of an interdisciplinary degree program called Sustainable Food & Bioenergy Systems (SFBS). In the ten years since its beginning, Towne's Harvest has become a valuable outdoor classroom for experiential learning, a laboratory for studying small-scale biodiverse food production, and an opportunity for community engagement on many levels.

13.5.2 THE FARM-TO-TABLE LEARNING EXPERIENCE

The SFBS degree program, which is structurally inter-departmental, interdisciplinary, and hands-on, links coursework in agriculture with that of human health and nutrition. The original purpose of the program was to create graduates capable of systems thinking while addressing multifaceted, complex problems. Enrollment in the program has grown rapidly after being launched in 2009. Students who enter the program rarely come from traditional agriculture backgrounds. This highly experiential degree program has attracted students to the study of food and agriculture who otherwise might not have chosen this path. Over 100 graduates have entered careers in every sector of the food system.

Majors in the program are required to spend a summer or semester in a Towne's Harvest practicum course or internship. The course is designed to span the harvest season and involve students in every aspect of small-scale production including planning, seeding, transplanting, irrigation, weed and pest control, composting and soil fertility management, harvesting, washing and preparing for distribution, CSA and farm stand marketing, business management, and public communications. The course is entirely field-based, and includes supervised field and market work, outdoor class meetings and discussions with the instructor, as well as individual reflection and writing assignments.

13.5.3 FIVE-YEAR IMPACT STUDY AT TOWNE'S HARVEST GARDEN

As the course was being developed, students completed a qualitative pre/post survey at the beginning and end of the course. The following summary is based on five aggregated years of survey data with approximately 80 students participating. Ninety percent of the students were of traditional college age, with 10% being post-baccalaureate adults. Nearly all were Caucasian, which mirrors state demographics though the gender distribution was even. With few exceptions, students had not been raised on a family farm or ranch.

When asked how the experience would contribute to their career goals, about half of the students expressed wanting to be small-scale producers prior to the experience, and about 30% maintained that after the course. Students claimed in advance that they wanted to promote healthful food, support communities, operate greenhouses, gain business skills, and learn how to make a living. Students who had decided that small-scale production would not be their career path still grew in their appreciation for the work involved, overall respect for producers, and desire to support the local food system.

When asked to comment on the value of field-based learning, students offered a variety of feedback and insight. They revealed that the course offered a high level of interaction, cooperation, responsibility, and accountability. The work was nearly all hands-on, tactile, and was perceived as enjoyable. The course presented "real-life" situations and problems that needed to be solved every day in practical ways. Students particularly valued learning how to "manage the system" that is a small farm enterprise. Some students struggled with the unstructured nature of the course, the unsystematic scheduling of class activities that sometimes occurred, and how the weather often determined what activities would be completed on any given day.

Though most students in the course were enrolled in the SFBS major, they had chosen from one of four academic options within the degree program (agroecology, sustainable food systems, sustainable crop production and sustainable livestock production). Therefore, students came into the course with different academic backgrounds and different career interests. When asked about the benefits and challenges associated with mixing academic backgrounds, students generally felt positive. They shared like-minded attitudes with their classmates despite differences in skills and backgrounds, and could each share their own unique experiences. Students shared a variety of viewpoints on issues and had differing perspectives. They enjoyed learning and solving problems collaboratively, as each individual could offer unique but useful skills and ideas. Students learned the importance of clearly written and verbal communication when working with individuals from different experience levels. They noticed that occasionally, students from differing academic backgrounds interpreted explanations given by the instructor differently. They also noticed varying work ethics among students.

Students came into the course knowing most about food safety and garden maintenance, and the least about integrated pest management, irrigation, CSA, and farm planning. At the conclusion of the course, they felt they knew comparatively more about post-harvest handling, CSAs, food production, and marketing, but still wanted more content and experience about integrated pest management, composting, and irrigation. Students generally responded that the most important topics they learned about were farm planning, and how to run a successful operation.

Before the course, students were asked which areas of professional development would be most important for them to advance in the course. The most common answers included project planning and implementation, conflict resolution, ethical responsibility, systems thinking, problem solving, and overall professionalism. After the hands-on experience, students responded that they had developed the most skill in customer service, taking initiative, ethical responsibility, leadership, teamwork, networking, and systems thinking.

13.6 SUSTAINED LEARNING TO PROMOTE BIODIVERSITY IN FOOD SYSTEMS

The Towne's Harvest Practicum experiential learning course has been offered continuously for the past eight years. Changes in the course include having a more structured schedule and shortened course length so that students can plan ahead for paid summer employment also engage in other outdoor experiences. Students who cannot complete the experience during the summer have an alternative experience during the spring or fall that is also diverse and hands-on, but focuses on different aspects of seasonal small-scale farm management. More academic content has been added to the course with the involvement of additional faculty, and a weekly meal is prepared by students using farm produce. Teaching and learning at Towne's Harvest has become more integrated with nearby research, including season extension methods, diverse tree fruit production, integration of animals for weed control, crop diversity and rotation for soil fertility, and pollinator gardens adjacent to beehives. Communication with all students involved in Towne's Harvest has improved and better farm infrastructure has created a more consistent class experience in spite of unpredictable weather. In recent years, more students have been involved in paid management and oversight of production and marketing at Towne's Harvest. Several students who have graduated now operate their own successful farms in the vicinity and serve as hosts for field trips and additional internships for SFBS students.

13.7 CONCLUSION

Experiential learning as a teaching methodology holds tremendous opportunity for supporting the sustainable food system movement and for sustaining biodiversity in food systems. Nearly every aspect of the food system, from food production to hunger and social justice issues, can be explored in experiential ways. CSA provides an experiential eating education for individuals and families who become members. When CSAs are operated as college campus farms, their potential to serve the surrounding community grows while food system learning opportunities expand. Those students involved in experiential education on campus farms enjoy transformational learning. This creates skilled future leaders with a deep understanding of food and agricultural systems who can address contemporary food-related problems.

VIGNETTE 13.1 World Challenge

Learner-Driven Teaching for Interdisciplinary, Global Problems

Michael Berger

INTRODUCTION

A novel two-week interdisciplinary "World Challenge" course was created in 2012 to identify issues under the broad topic of food security. While the problem of food security isn't new, this student-centered and student-led interdisciplinary course challenged students to take ownership of this complex issue and create practical local solutions.

Students were challenged with the question: "How can students learn about and engage in complex world problems (such as world hunger or food security) in a sustainable and meaningful way on campus and in the local community?" Hence, the course "Food for Thought: Health, Hunger, and Humanity" was a new approach in experiential education—designed to empower students with the confidence to learn in non-traditional ways by tackling critical global issues surrounding social justice and environmental sustainability with useful actions.

OVERVIEW OF THE COURSE

Fourteen sophomores at Simmons College in Boston, Massachusetts, lived, cooked, and worked together in teams during the two-week January intersession to work on this problem. Using a charrette and knowledge mapping, the students chose "Campus2Community: Promoting Awareness And Access To Healthy Sustainable Food Options" as their overall problem. The students then self-selected five teams to address specific aspects of the problem, conducted extensive library research, consulted with on-call faculty from multiple departments across the college, carried out interviews, and developed action plans to implement after the conclusion of the course. Several students called the course "transformative," and assessments showed that their knowledge of food safety, food production, and food distribution had increased significantly (Berger et al. 2013).

PEDAGOGY

Complex problems require interdisciplinary solutions. "Food for Thought" was chosen as the overarching topic because of its complex nature, including economics, political science, nutrition, social justice, sustainability, business, public health, and climate change. Students from a number of majors—including nutrition, nursing, English, math, management, biology/public health, and political science—were chosen for this course. The course was led by chemistry and biology professors, and the lead teaching assistant was a Registered Dietitian Nutritionist. Several other Simmons professors with expertise in different areas, such as economics, nutrition, team-dynamics, and library science were also "on-call" and available to help with the team projects.

Complex problems also require teamwork, since the staggering amount of accessible information is too extensive for one person to gather, analyze, and synthesize into a coherent action plan. Thus, faculty from the School of Management provided guidance on team skills: How to select an effective team; how to evaluate whether the team is succeeding; and how to share responsibility. These important life skills are useful well beyond the completion of the course.

As we designed the course, we were aware of the delicate balances integral to the course design that could significantly impact success for both the students and the faculty. These included: The desire for a rich process versus the delivery of a good "product" or final report; the desire for individual accomplishment and team success; the desire for intensity of the experience versus productivity; the balance of global analysis versus local action; and the desire to encourage broad exploration versus mastery of a specific subject. We aimed for a student-driven, engaging, and impactful course. Indeed, final student evaluations affirmed our goal, "I enjoyed the trust we were given to go on our own and do what we need to do. Because I was given that trust, I didn't want to violate it....Because I spent a large amount of time on the work, it had to be good. I don't think I've been as stimulated or engaged."

WHY FOOD SECURITY?

There are several reasons that food security is an ideal topic for such an experiential course. All of us think about food to some extent every day, and thus students feel "at home" or familiar with the subject as the course begins. The course content is not abstract, but is tangible—and students enter the course with some knowledge (to varying degrees) of the subject matter. Food security lends itself perfectly to this experiential course since the subject of food can be analyzed on many different levels—personally, campus-wide, locally, and internationally. "Food for Thought" is a great vehicle for going beyond the problems of everyday life, which is one of the goals of the course—making connections between global problems and local actions. Food security has become key to understanding issues that have worldwide import—for example, the connection between climate change and the "food-energy-water nexus." Food security also informs energy and economic policy as well as national and international politics.

COURSE MECHANICS

The course methodology stressed high-impact-intensive experiences that the students would not forget. Additionally, students knew that this course was a unique opportunity: We used an application process for the course, and students were given a small stipend, course credit, and housing. Students had no previous experience with such intense and compressed learning; however, they pushed themselves to excel. In two short weeks, they gained a number of new skills with support from all parts of the college: Effective team work, creation of business plans and proposals, grant writing, interviewing skills, documentary videography, library research, self-reflection and assessment, and oration.

While this was a student-centered experiential course, significant scaffolding was provided, including two three-hour orientation lectures before the two-week course introducing the students to the broad area of food security; training on how to work in teams; and access to video and published resources. Additionally, instructors arranged meetings with outside speakers from local and national organizations that provided nutritional education and food relief to the hungry.

On the second day of the course, a charrette was held. Students created a food security knowledge map based on their readings, guest lectures, and Internet resources, and they discussed what actions they could take at a local level. They developed an over-riding theme for the five different projects—"Campus2Community". The students then split up into smaller groups to tackle specific action plans that would be consistent with the overall theme.

STUDENT DELIVERABLES

Overall, the Campus2Community project provided an umbrella for five inter-connected campus projects that focused on improving health, mitigating hunger, and increasing awareness of peaceful, constructive solutions to attaining wholesome, sustainable foods—in the spirit of "thinking globally, acting locally."

An important structural component of the course was social justice and service learning. However, since the course met only for two weeks in January, it was difficult to incorporate service-learning activities during that short time period. However, the action plans developed by the teams to address the problems of access to healthy and sustainable food have in fact become sustainable service-learning projects after the completion of the course.

One group created a website with the goal of reaching out to students across the country, offering information about nutrition, food sustainability, and hunger awareness. Although none of the students had previously created a website, this course gave them the impetus to learn how, and the website was up and running by the completion of the course.

Another group created a documentary film highlighting hunger in the greater Boston area. Like the first team, these students had no experience interviewing people living on the street or with videography and video editing—but with the help of student teaching assistants they were able to create a powerful short film.

A third group created a "Slow Food" campus chapter at Simmons College in order to increase nutritional awareness among the campus community and to advocate for improved access to healthy and sustainable foods. The Slow Food chapter was formed and continued for several years at Simmons.

Another group created a plan to build a garden on the Simmons College campus that students and staff alike could utilize and experience organic gardening. Their plan was realized a few years later by other students.

The fifth project was a proposal to establish a food pantry on the Simmons College campus. These students conducted a pilot survey and found that there were students in need at many colleges, especially those who live off campus, those who do not have a meal plan, and international students who do not have access to federal and state food programs.

ASSESSMENTS AND OUTCOMES

Berger et al. (2013) described the multiple assessment tools used to evaluate the effectiveness of the project. Direct evidence of increased understanding of the course content was quantified from the results of pre- and posttests. Student peer review provided data on skills related to working in groups. Questionnaires assessed the students', faculty members', and teaching assistants' evaluation of the course. In addition, student feedback through daily journal entries and responses in a debriefing session provided additional input. "Students gained the most information about how food is related to social justice issues in the U.S. They also showed robust gains in knowledge about threats to the long-term vitality of the U.S. food system and technical issues related to food safety, production, and distribution" (Berger et al. 2013).

One goal of this course was to provide an interdisciplinary challenge. As in real life, the solutions to the most significant problems involve expertise and input from a number of different disciplines. Students responded well to the complex challenge presented by issue of food security: "I loved the interdisciplinary nature of this course. I don't think I've learned as much in a course as I have in these two weeks—about nutrition, economics, and other food-related topics." Students confirmed that the course provided the right balance of stress, engagement, and scaffolding in order to maximize student learning: "This course was a true liberal arts experiment that I will remember forever. Although it was stressful and often difficult work, I am extremely proud of the finished product—not only the physical work, but also the intangible learning." This course also motivated students for engagement in community outreach and showed them potential opportunities for making contributions. Indeed, this intangible learning outcome can be transformative and life-changing. One student noted, "This course makes me want to volunteer more. I've been making excuses and now I'm actually going to do it."

REFERENCES

Abratt, R., and S.D. Goodey. 1990 Unplanned buying and in-store stimuli in supermarkets. *Managerial and Decision Economics* 11: 111–121. DOI:10.1002/mde.4090110204.

Allen, J.E., J. Rossi, T.A. Woods, and A.F. Davis. 2017. Do community supported agriculture programmes encourage change to food lifestyle behaviours and health outcomes? New evidence from shareholders. *International Journal of Agricultural Sustainability* 15 (1): 70–82.

Anderson-Wilk, M. 2007. Does community supported agriculture support conservation? *Journal of Soil & Water Conservation* 62:126A–127A.

Barlett, P.F. 2011. Campus sustainable food projects: Critique and engagement. *American Anthropologist* 113 (2): 101–115. DOI:10.1111/j.1548-1433.2010.01309.x.

Berger, M. Scott, E., Axe, J.B., Hawkins, I.W. 2013. World Challenge: Engaging sophomores in an intensive, interdisciplinary course. *International Journal of Teaching and Learning in Higher Education* 25(3): 333–345.

Biernbaum, J.A., M. Jgouajio, and L. Thorp. 2006. Development of a year-round student organic farm and organic farming curriculum at Michigan State University. *HortTechnology*, 16 (3):432–436.

Brown, C., and S. Miller. 2008. The impacts of local markets: A review of research on farmers markets and community supported agriculture (CSA). *American Journal of Agricultural Economics* 90: 1296–1302. DOI:10.1111/j.1467-8276.2008.01220.x.

Buttel, F.H. 2003. Internalizing the societal costs of agricultural production. *Plant Physiology* 133: 1656–1665. DOI:10.1104/pp.103.030312.

Cohen, J.N., S. Gearhart, and E. Garland. 2012. Community supported agriculture: A commitment to a healthier diet. *Journal of Hunger & Environmental Nutrition* 7: 20–37.

Coker, J.S., and D.J. Porter. 2015. Maximizing experiential learning for student success. *Change: The Magazine of Higher Learning* 47: 66–72.

Clements, M.D., and B.A. Cord. 2013. Assessment guiding learning: Developing graduate qualities in an experiential learning programme. *Assessment and Evaluation in Higher Education* 38(1): 114–124.

Cullen, P. 1994. Time, tastes and technology: The economic evolution of eating out. *British Food Journal* 96: 4–9.

Curtis, K., R. Ward, K. Allen, and S. Slocum. 2013. Impacts of community supported agriculture program participation on consumer food purchases and dietary choice. *Journal of Food Distribution Research* 44: 42–51.

Dewey, J. 1938. *Experience and Education*. New York: Touchstone Publisher.

Francis, C.A., N. Jordan,, P. Porter, T.A. Breland, G. Lieblein, L. Salomonsson, N. Sriskandarajah, et al. 2011. Innovative education in agroecology: Experiential learning for a sustainable agriculture. *Critical Reviews in Plant Sciences* 30 (1–2): 226–237. DOI:10.1080/07352689.2011.554497.

Galt, R.E. 2013. The moral economy is a double-edged sword: Explaining farmers' earnings and self-exploitation in community-supported agriculture. *Economic Geography* 89: 341–365. DOI:10.1111/ecge.12015.

Galt, R.E., D. Parr, J. Van Soelen Kim, J. Beckett, M. Lickter, and H. Ballard. 2013. Transformative food systems education in a land-grant college of agriculture: The importance of learner-centered inquiries. *Agriculture and Human Values* 30: 129–142. DOI:10.1007/s10460-012-9384-8.

Hamlin, F.N. 2016. Courting the senses: Experiential learning and civil rights movement pedagogy. *Black Scholar* 46 (4): 16–32.

Harmon, A.H. 2014. Community supported agriculture: A conceptual model of health implications. *Austin Journal of Nutrition and Food Sciences* 2 (4): 1024.

Harmon, A.H., and B.L. Gerald. 2007. Position of the American Dietetic Association: Food and nutrition professionals can implement practices to conserve natural resources and support ecological sustainability. *Journal of the American Dietetic Association* 107 (6): 1033–1043.

Harmon, A.H., K. Landolfi, C. Byker Shanks, L. Hansen, L. Iverson, M. Anacker. 2017. Food insecurity experience: Building empathy in future food and nutrition professionals. *Journal of Nutrition Education and Behavior* 49 (3): 218–227. http://dx.doi.org/10.1016/j.jneb.2016.10.023.

Heinrich, W.F., G.B. Habron, H.L. Johnson, and L. Goralnik. 2015. Critical thinking assessment across four sustainability-related experiential learning settings. *Journal of Experiential Education* 38 (4): 373–393. DOI:doi/abs/10.1177/1053825915592890.

Henderson, E., and R. Van En. 1999. *Sharing the Harvest: A Guide to Community Supported Agriculture*. White River Junction, VT: Chelsea Green.

Howden, E. 2012. Outdoor experiential education: Learning through the body. *New Directory of Adult Continuing Education* 134: 43–51.

Jordan, N., J. Grossman, P. Lawrence, A. Harmon, W. Dyer, B. Maxwell, K.V. Cadieux, et al. 2014. New curricula for undergraduate food-systems education: A sustainable agriculture education perspective. *NACTA Journal* December: 302–310.

Jordi, R. 2011. Reframing the concept of reflection: Consciousness, experiential learning and reflective learning practices. *Adult Education Quarterly* 61 (2): 181–197. DOI:doi/abs/10.1177/0741713610380439.

Kolb, D.A. 1984. *Experiential Learning: Experience as a Source of Learning and Development*. Englewood Cliffs, NJ: Prentice Hall.

Kolb, D.A. 2005. *The Kolb Learning Styles Inventory, Version 3.1*. Boston, MA: Hay Resources Direct.

Koontz, S.R., D.S. Peel, J.N. Trapp, E. Clement, and C.E. Ward. 1995. Augmenting agricultural economics and agribusiness education with experiential learning. *Review of Agricultural Economics* 17 (3): 267–274.

LaCharite, K. 2016. Re-visioning agriculture in higher education: The role of campus agriculture initiatives in sustainability education. *Agriculture and Human Values* 33: 521–535. DOI:10.1007/s10460-015-9619-6.

Lass, D., G.W. Stevenson, J. Hendrickson, and K. Ruhf. 2003. *Community Supported Agriculture Entering the 21st Century: Results From the 2001 National Survey*. Amherst, MA: University of Massachusetts, Department of Resource Economics.

Malone, K., A.H. Harmon, W.E. Dyer, B.D. Maxwell, and C.A. Perillo. 2014. Development and evaluation of an introductory course in sustainable food and bioenergy systems. *Journal of Agriculture, Food Systems, and Community Development* 4 (2): 149–161. http://dx.doi.org/10.5304/jafscd.2014.042.002.

Markhart, A.H. III. 2006. Organic educational opportunities at the University of Minnesota: The role of a student-run organic farm. *HortTechnology* 16 (3): 443–445.

McFadden, S. 2003. The history of community supported agriculture, part I. Community farms in the 21st century: Poised for another wave of growth? *The New Farm*, Rodale Institute.

Merizow, J. 1991. *Transformative Dimensions of Adult Learning*. San Francisco: Jossey-Bass.

Papaoikonomou, E., and M. Ginieis. 2017. Putting the farmer's face on food: Governance and the producer-consumer relationship in local food systems. *Agriculture and Human Values* 34: 53–67. DOI:10.1007/s10460-016-9695-2.

Parr, D.M., and C.J. Trexler. 2011. Students' experiential learning and use of student farms in sustainable agriculture education. *Journal of Natural Resources and Life Sciences Education* 40: 172–180. DOI:10.4195/jnrlse.2009.0047u.

Reeve, J.R., K. Hall, and C. Kalkman. 2014. Student outcomes from experiential learning on a student-run certified organic farm. *Natural Science Educucation* 43: 16–24.

Sayre, L., and S. Clark. 2011. *Fields of Learning: The Student Farm Movement in North America*. Lexington, KY: University Press of Kentucky.

Spence, K.K., and M.A. McDonald. 2015. Assessing vertical development in experiential learning curriculum. *Journal of Experiential Education* 38 (3): 296–312. DOI:doi/abs/10.1177/1053825915571749.

Tegtmeier, E., and M. Duffy. 2005. *Community Supported Agriculture (CSA) in the Midwest United States*. Ames, IA: Leopold Center for Sustainable Agriculture, Iowa State University.

Wadsworth, L.A., C. Johnson, C. Cameron, and M. Gaudet. 2012. (Re) Focus on local food systems through service learning. *Food Culture and Society* 15 (2): 315–334. http://dx.doi.org/10.1080/15528014.2012.11422641.

Wharton, C., and A. Harmon. 2009. University engagement through local food enterprise: Community-supported agriculture on Campus. *Journal of Hunger and Environmental Nutrition* 4 (2): 112–128. http://dx.doi.org/10.1080/19320240902915235.

Worden, E.C. 2004. Grower perspectives in community supported agriculture. *HortTechnology* 14: 322–325.

14 The Road to Health Goes Through the Kitchen

Sharon Palmer

CONTENTS

14.1 INTRODUCTION

As busy commuters fight their way home through traffic at the end of their work day, many will ponder the modern question of our age: What's for dinner? This query may be quickly followed with a litany of other activities on their mental to-do lists, such as soccer practice for the kids, the dirty clothing heaped up in the laundry room, or an empty refrigerator crying out for replenishment. It's no wonder that so many people order takeout on the way home—at least that's one thing they don't have to worry about. Or is it?

This scenario is all too familiar for millions of Americans. Men and women of all ages, ethnicities, and walks of life are ditching time in the kitchen in exchange for an easier way out: A quick trip for takeout, fast food, or prepared foods in the supermarket aisle. While it may seem the best option for saving time at the moment, the losses associated with our home-cooking traditions are piling up, degrading our health (Smith et al. 2013) and the health of the planet (Cohen and Story 2014).

Today, we are in the second and third generation of people who don't know how to cook, leaving fewer people left behind to pass down the treasures of culinary knowledge and traditions acquired over the years within their families—whether it be the special way a grandmother lovingly rolled out pasta or how an aunt filled corn tamales.

Even when we do eat at home, we are increasingly eating out of packages and boxes and calling it "cooking." And more and more families are skipping meals eaten together at the dining room table for a mish-mash of quasi-meals and snacks in the car or in front of computers, phones, and television screens (Smith et al. 2013).

Our cooking practices are in decline for a number of reasons, including the lack of culinary education in the school system, distractions in the home, increased demands on our time, and more options for prepared foods (Smith et al. 2013). However, with the increasing awareness of the power of good nutrition to impact health, it is essential to bring people back to the kitchen so that they can cook meals made with healthful, sustainable, whole ingredients, including pulses, whole grains, vegetables, fruits, herbs, and spices. This is one of the most important contributions we can offer to ourselves as individuals—to the customers we serve—and for our children and family. Fortunately, there are inspiring activities along the path such as creating inventive culinary education opportunities where healthcare and food professionals use farmer's markets, classrooms, hospitals, supermarkets, farms, and communities to showcase the invaluable virtues of cooking that leads us back into our kitchens.

14.2 WHAT'S GOING ON IN THE KITCHEN?

When you think of the mid-20th century, you might conjure up an image of the perfectly coiffed, aproned mother cooking up a healthy meal for her family. Indeed, that was the heyday for contemporary home cooking, yet it also marked the beginning of America's exodus from home kitchens in the 1960s as people started reducing the amount of time they spent in the kitchen (Smith et al. 2013). Fueled by a post-war boom, more households wanted to enjoy time-savers in meal preparation (Gust 2011). This period was also the golden age for supermarkets that marketed their increasingly convenient food products (Ellickson 2015). The first frozen "television dinner" introduced by Swanson in 1953 quickly become a success in mid-century homes (Gust 2011). Kitchens also became more modern and convenient. A game-changer in cooking convenience came with the advent of the first consumer microwave in 1967 (Amana 2017).

It shouldn't be surprising that cooking declined by almost 40% in the U.S. from 1965 to 1995 (Virudachalam et al. 2013). Specifically, the largest declines of calories consumed in the home and time spent in food preparation were during the period of 1965–1992, although this downward trend has stabilized in recent years (Smith et al. 2013). In particular, women cut their time spent in food preparation substantially during the past several decades (Zick and Stevens 2010). Gender roles shifted too, with more women entering the work force and more men taking on meal preparation tasks. The proportion of men who cooked increased from 29% in 1965–1966 to 42% in 2007–2008 (Smith et al. 2013). Of those men who cooked, time spent cooking increased from 37.4 minutes per day to 45.0 minutes per day. For women, the proportion of cooking declined from 92% in 1965–1966 to 68% in 2007–2008, and those who did cook decreased the time spent cooking from 112.8 minutes per day to 65.6 minutes per day (Smith et al. 2013). However, women still spend more than twice the amount of time in food preparation then men (Smith et al. 2013).

Socioeconomics also come into play in home-cooking practices. Lower household income and educational status are linked with a higher likelihood of either always or never cooking dinner at home, compared to homes with higher incomes and educational status, which are more likely to sometimes cook dinner at home (Virudachalam et al. 2013). African-American households cook the fewest dinners at home, while households with foreign-born members cook more dinners at home (Virudachalam et al. 2013). Households with dependents cook more dinners at home (Virudachalam et al. 2013). Research also shows that lower income individuals skip cooking more often, despite consuming 72% of calories at home. This coincides with an increased reliance on foods that require little preparation (Smith et al. 2013).

Age also factors into the equation. People over 65 years of age spend more than twice the amount of time (43 minutes per day) preparing meals than those aged 18–24 years (21 minutes per day); those aged 25–64 years spend 38 minutes per day (Hamrick 2016). Survey data show that Millennials (the largest generational cohort in the U.S. born between the early 1980s and the early 2000s) enjoy speed and convenience and don't have as much interest in cooking—and thus eat out more often than non-Millennials (3.4 times versus 2.8 times per week) (Barton et al. 2012).

Simply put, there is not as much cooking in American homes today (Smith et al. 2013). On average, Americans cook five dinners per week, with 49% always cooking dinner at home, 43% sometimes cooking dinner, and 8% never cooking dinner at home, respectively (Virudachalam et al. 2013). Americans spend only 37 minutes on average per day preparing, serving, and cleaning up after meals (Hamrick 2016). We are eating more frequently in fast-food diners, cafeterias, and restaurants (Smith et al. 2013). In 1955, restaurants accounted for 25% of our food dollars, and in 2017 they accounted for 48% (National Restaurant Association 2017).

There is another message hidden in the data. Even though we still get a significant portion of our daily calories from foods consumed at home, these calories stem from prepared and packaged foods that require little meal preparation. Sixty percent (60%) of the calories in foods we buy at grocery stores comes from highly processed foods (Federation of American Societies for Experimental Biology 2015). Consumers are turning to thousands of no-prep products, ranging from microwavable pouches in the dry foods aisles to frozen wraps and pizzas in the freezer section and prepared salads and entrees in the refrigerated section. Convenient food options such as fast foods and prepared foods are widely available in supermarkets (Nielsen 2017).

14.3 WHY AREN'T WE COOKING?

Research suggests that more cooking will occur in the home if the home dynamic includes: A female cook; more time availability; one's type of employment; close personal relationships; and cooking foods of one's cultural or ethnic background (Mills et al. 2017). However, there is more to the puzzle. Getting a meal on the table may seem like a simple task, but the sequence of steps such as obtaining food, planning and preparing meals, and serving and even eating the meal may feel complicated nowadays (Jabs and Devine 2006). Many people may be challenged in one or more of these specific steps—or with cooking altogether.

Plain and simple, people don't know how to cook. In fact, the lack of culinary skills may be one of the most significant barriers getting in the way of our cooking practices. Our loss of culinary education in the school classroom can be traced back as a main detractor. Home economics courses, including meal planning, nutrition education, and cooking instruction were a fixture in public schools up until the 1960s (Lichtenstein and Ludwig 2010). The Smith-Hughes Act of 1917 provided funding for the training of teachers in home economics, with widespread provision of home economics classes in middle and elementary schools for much of the 20th century (Smith et al. 2013). However, due to tightening budgets in schools, home economics programs—considered electives in an educational system focused on core curricula—declined in most U.S. schools over recent decades (Smith et al. 2013). Many parents and caregivers never learned to cook and are unable to teach their children to prepare healthful meals. Health experts are calling for a return of comprehensive culinary education for both genders in the classroom as a strategy to help prevent childhood obesity (Lichtenstein and Ludwig 2010).

Time scarcity or the feeling of not having enough time is another barrier to cooking, leading to a decrease in home food preparation and family meals and an increase in consumption of fast foods and convenience foods (Jabs and Devine 2006). With busier lives, employed mothers are less likely to make time for food preparation, and parents may use convenient and fast food as a way to cope with stress or as a reward for handling a difficult day (Virudachalam et al. 2013). This scenario may be even more stressful for low-income adults, who have added constraints of working including multiple jobs, longer hours, shift schedules, and overtime hours (Smith et al. 2013).

Other issues may keep people from cooking, including lack of access to food (such as living in a community with limited or no access to healthful foods), money to purchase healthful ingredients, transportation, and basic cooking tools such as knives, cutting boards, and pots and pans. Furthermore, conflicting work schedules among household members, the total number of household members, caregiver relationships, and multi-generational households can impact cooking practices in a home. In addition, picky or demanding eaters may make meal preparation difficult and more stressful (Bowen et al. 2014). Even the sheer lack of enjoyment surrounding the act of cooking is a significant challenge for many who find no pleasure in the art of cooking (Wolfson et al. 2016).

The rise in distractions also translates into less time dedicated to cooking. Consider this: Cooking starting to decline just as black and white television became a fixture in American homes in the 1950s. Today the average person spends nearly two hours per day on social media while teens may spend up to nine hours that may include: YouTube—40 minutes a day; Facebook 35—minutes a day; Snapchat—25 minutes a day; Instagram—15 minutes a day; and Twitter—one minute a day) (Asano 2017). Hence, it's easy to see where people prioritize spending their time. While people clearly have enough time to spend on their phones, computers, and tablets—they don't seem to have enough time left for cooking.

The rise of food convenience has become a self-fulfilling prophecy. As people spend less time cooking, they purchase more convenient foods, and consequently spend less time cooking. Convenience reigns supreme as a top priority among consumers when making food choices. They want to save time and physical or mental energy in the kitchen, as well as reduce time spent along the stages of the meal process, such as deciding what to eat, purchasing food, preparing meals, consuming meals, and cleaning up after eating (Botonaki et al. 2017). This explains the popularity of items that reduce time along the cooking activity spectrum such as frozen stir-fry blends that cut out the step of chopping vegetables; shelf-stable pouches of cooked, seasoned rice which eliminate the need for dirtying pots and pans. Of course, food manufacturers, supermarkets, and restaurant operators are more than happy to provide convenient food options, keying into consumer desires. Why wouldn't a consumer want to stop for fast food, if they can save an average of 30 minutes of meal prep time by doing so (Hamrick 2016)?

New advances in food convenience are marching on, particularly in the area of technology. Thirty percent of consumers say technology makes them dine out or order takeout more often, and 42% say the ability to order online would make them choose a restaurant over one where you can't order online (National Restaurant Association 2017). Thirty-four percent (34%) of smartphone users have used their phones to pay for a restaurant meal (National Restaurant Association 2017).

Another alarming trend is the death of mealtime—especially family meals. People are spending less time sitting down to the table for three square meals a day and are snacking on mini-meals more than ever. People snack 30% more now than they did in the 1970s when the average American ate only one snack a day and 40% of adults and teens didn't even snack at all. Nearly all Americans (94%) snack at least once daily, and nearly half of adults snack two or three times a day (Mintel Group 2015). Forty percent of American families eat dinner together only three or fewer times a week, with 10% never eating dinner together at all (ConAgra Foods 2003).

14.4   THE FALLOUT FROM NOT COOKING

What's the net result of our national pastime of avoiding the kitchen? Unfortunately, this trend of eating out more often and choosing highly processed prepared foods as the default has made a negative impact on our health. Research indicates that consumption of convenience and away-from-home foods has been linked with increased calorie intake and decreased nutritional intake—as well as weight gain (Smith et al. 2013, French et al. 2000, Duffey et al. 2007). In contrast, the consumption of home-cooked meals is linked with an increased intake of fruits, vegetables, and whole grains; increased overall health and survival; and a decreased Body Mass Index (BMI) (Smith et al. 2013). In the end, our diets are simply less nutrient-dense today (Reedy and Krebs-Smith 2010). Less than 20% of Americans meet the USDA guidelines for healthy eating, such as intake of adequate servings of whole grains, fruits, and vegetables (Krebs-Smith et al. 2010).

A quick scan through a typical chain restaurant menu exemplifies the problem, with pasta dishes providing more than 2,300 kcal and 79 grams of saturated fat, and desserts weighing in at more than 1,700 calories per serving (Vilas-Boas 2017). Indeed, a review of the calorie content of foods in restaurant chains found that entrees averaged 674 calories (kcal), appetizers 813 kcal, side dishes 260 kcal, salads 496 kcal, drinks 419 kcal, and desserts 429 kcal, respectively. Since most people order two or more items when they dine out, most meals away from home contain more than the 640 calories the average person needs for lunch or dinner (Cohen and Story 2014).

One of the most important issues is portion size. A surfeit of prepared and away-from-home foods provide excessive portion sizes, which are often high in energy, saturated fat, sodium, and added sugars. Consumption of these foods is associated with obesity and chronic disease risk, such as cardiovascular disease, diabetes, and cancer (Jabs and Devine 2006). Foods consumed away from home are richer in calories than foods consumed at home. The calories in these large portions of foods eaten outside the home are substantially higher than what would be prepared at home (Cohen and Story 2014). This issue is of particular concern among children where eating patterns may create a lifetime of health-related problems. Thirty percent of children aged 4–19 years consume fast food on a typical day (Bowman et al. 2004).

The damage large portions of poor quality foods goes far beyond one's waistline or blood cholesterol levels. The energy input required to grow and process foods—in particular animal foods—contributes to climate change. Meat products are estimated to be responsible for 18% of all greenhouse gas emissions as well as deforestation and fossil fuel and water usage (FAO 2006). With 30–40% of all food being thrown away—especially at the consumer level, the environmental impact of producing food that will never be consumed is enormous (USDA 2018). In addition, the environmental impact of producing foods that are consumed in excess of one's energy needs further contributes to carbon emissions (Jones and Kammen 2011).

That's not factoring the impact of all of the food packaging associated with convenience food products and fast food takeout meals either. Containers and packaging contribute 23% of all materials to U.S. landfills (United States Environmental Protection Agency 2017). Litter from food packaging ends up on beaches and waterways, posing problems for wildlife, which may be harmed or killed by ingesting these materials as described in Chapter 5 (United States Environmental Protection Agency 2017).

14.5 THE BENEFITS OF COMING BACK TO THE KITCHEN

There are numerous benefits associated with cooking. When you cook meals from scratch, you can: Add more vegetables to dishes; cut out added salt and sugars; serve smaller portions; choose more healthful, sustainable ingredients; and control cooking methods. Again, studies have shown that eating foods prepared from scratch increases the intake of fruits, vegetables, and whole grains while increasing overall health including healthy weight status and survival (Smith et al. 2013).

Perhaps more importantly, when you cook at home you can bring the whole family or household together into the kitchen and around the dinner table to learn about healthful food. A family dinner together can be a way to relax and unwind and to interact with people who care for one another—advantages that are particularly important for children and adolescents. Cooking at home and engaging in family meals leads to healthier diets and lower BMIs in children and adolescents (Virudachalam et al. 2013). When children and adolescents participate in family meals at least three times per week, they have a 12% lower risk for being overweight, 20% reduced risk of eating unhealthy foods, 35% reduced risk of disordered eating, and 24% increased odds of eating healthy foods (Hammons and Fiese 2011). In addition, evidence links family meal frequency with better academic performance, decreased risk for substance use, and heightened personal and social well-being

(Story and Neumark-Sztainer 2005). Studies have even shown that people who engage in home cooking in emerging adulthood have healthier diets later on in life (Virudachalam et al. 2013).

Other benefits are important too, such as the preservation of culinary traditions and instilling the sheer joy of cooking healthful, creative, delicious meals. Some people feel that cooking brings them closer to nature. In some indigenous cultures, cooking is considered a sacred blessing. When the family chef–often the matriarch–enters the kitchen, however rustic it might be, it is a privilege and honor to possess the nourishing ingredients she now has at her fingertips to prepare a delicious meal for her family. The act of preparing these foods using time-honored traditions and techniques melded by influences of culture, religion, and geography over the millennia and passed down from generation to generation is met with humble respect. As the family cook chops the day's ingredients, simmers foods in pots, and stirs the sauces, there is joy in the process of preparing a wholesome, delicious meal that day.

Reigniting a passion for food preparation is a life-altering experience. Instead of considering it just another activity on one's long to-do list, cooking can be thought of as meditation or a joy. Cooks—men and women alike—can approach the kitchen at the end of the workday with interest and wonder, shedding their worries and stresses of the day as they chop an onion, letting the stimulating aroma of onions and garlic sautéing in olive oil wash over them. A household member—grandparent, roommate, spouse, partner, or child—can help with the culinary chores, unwinding and discussing the events of the day. They might share a remembered story of how their mother taught them to sauté onions as a child. The household members can then sit down together to enjoy a healthful meal while savoring each mouthful without the distractions of television or computer screens. This is part of the rich tapestry that cooking offers to a vibrant life beyond the sheer biometrical measurements of benefits.

14.6 INCREASING CULINARY COMPETENCE AMONG HEALTH PROFESSIONALS

It's clear that there is much to gain by getting people back into the kitchen cooking healthful meals. In today's era of lifestyle-related diseases, it is important to create new ways to teach patients about how to make behavioral changes in nutrition. Translating diet recommendations into practical advice through culinary education is at the forefront of changing and improving nutrition behavior (Eisenburg and Burgess 2015). Culinary education offers an exciting opportunity for health professionals to be part of the solution in increasing cooking self-efficacy while decreasing disease morbidity and enhancing well-being for their patients and clients.

However, health professionals may lack culinary literacy themselves. Nutrition and food-related knowledge is lacking in the current medical education, which has created a gap in physicians' ability to recognize that patients need education about health and nutrition (Polak et al. 2016). This concept is discussed in Chapter 16. And it may be no better for Registered Dietitian Nutritionists whom overlook the importance of cooking skills by focusing on the science of food and nutrition rather than asking a client about their cooking skills or demonstrating how to cook (Begley and Gallegos 2010). While dietetics education includes competence in culinary knowledge, today's students may not come to their training with cooking skills that were learned at home (Canter et al. 2007).

Thankfully, there is a new movement towards instilling culinary competence in the healthcare field. For example, "culinary nutrition" or "culinary medicine" has been proposed as a field that blends the art of food and cooking with the science of medicine (Polak et al. 2016). Many programs are incorporating culinary medicine education for healthcare professionals. Chef Coaching (The Institute of Lifestyle Medicine) provides continuing education programs in culinary health for healthcare professionals through tele-classes and practice sessions. The Goldring Center for Culinary Medicine at Tulane University is the first dedicated teaching kitchen to be implemented at a medical school. "Healthy Kitchens, Healthy Lives" is a leadership conference coordinated by the Culinary Institute of America and Harvard T.H. Chan School of Public Health aimed at bridging nutrition science, healthcare, and the culinary arts (Polak et al. 2016).

Such culinary education has been found to be effective. One study documented that attendance at the Healthy Kitchens, Healthy Lives conference increased both the clinician's self-reported diet quality as well as their ability to advise clients on nutrition and lifestyle changes (Monlezun et al. 2015). A six-week culinary nutrition program for undergraduate nutrition-related majors was found to provide significant benefits in cooking self-efficacy, self-efficacy for using basic cooking techniques, self-efficacy for using fruits, vegetables, seasonings, and the ability to use economical methods to purchase produce (Kerrison et al. 2017). In addition, some healthcare professionals are seeking chef credentials as part of their formal education.

The American Culinary Federation offers various levels of culinary certifications, and some healthcare professionals may already qualify to become certified "culinarians" based on previous knowledge (American Culinary Federation 2017). Healthcare professionals may also attend "culinary boot camps" at organizations like the Culinary Institute of America and Johnson & Wales University to further their culinary knowledge. In fact, Johnson & Wales University has a Dietetics and Applied Nutrition BS program which allows graduates to become a Registered Dietitian Nutritionist with a culinary focus (Johnson & Wales University 2017).

14.7 STRATEGIES TO INCREASE HOME FOOD PREPARATION AMONG CONSUMERS

Now that you're inspired to get consumers back into the kitchen, where do you go from here? The solutions are as exciting as they are limitless. There are numerous innovative strategies that healthcare professionals are mounting across the country to inspire healthy cooking from scratch. Research indicates that educational interventions that aim to improve culinary practices may improve short-term attitudes regarding healthy cooking, confidence in cooking, healthy food consumption, and improved health outcomes (Polak et al. 2016).

The "teaching kitchen" model—laboratory classes for nutrition, culinary, and lifestyle education—has been gaining traction even within the confines of the hospital (Eisenburg and Burgess 2015). One widely praised example is at the Henry Ford West Bloomfield Hospital, which has a Demonstration Kitchen for adults and children to explore healthy lifestyles and learn about the importance of nutrition for overall health and wellness (Henry Ford West Bloomfield Hospital 2017). A range of fun, inventive cooking and nutrition classes are offered, such as: Breast Health Boot Camp; The Art of Mindful Living; Diabetes: We Won't Sugar Coat It; and Soup's On. The classes, which are offered every month for $20 per person, include food samplings, tips, take home recipes, and guidance by hospital physicians and Registered Dietitian Nutritionists (Henry Ford West Bloomfield Hospital 2017).

The Culinary Institute of America and the Harvard T.H. Chan School of Public Health introduced the Teaching Kitchen Collaborative, in which 26 institutions are piloting teaching kitchens for select audiences in healthcare settings and universities—so that people can learn healthy living and cooking skills from healthcare and culinary professionals (Ragone 2016). These teaching kitchens range from high-end, state-of-the-art kitchens to tiny mobile stations (Ragone 2016).

It appears that these teaching kitchens may be an effective agent of change. A randomized controlled trial found that medical school-based teaching kitchens, with hands-on cooking and nutrition curriculum for patients, improved biometrics such as HbA1c, blood pressure, and cholesterol in people with Type 2 Diabetes (T2D) (Monlezun et al. 2015).

Efforts also are underway to increase healthy home-cooked foods through more culinary education in the Supplemental Nutrition Assistance Program (SNAP), and Women, Infants, and Children (WIC) Farmer's Market Nutrition program. Many initiatives are moving forward, such as cooking classes held at farmer's markets as well as budget-friendly cooking classes. Useful education resources are available at the SNAP-Ed Connection website (USDA Food and Nutrition Service 2017).

Share our Strength Cooking Matters aims to help families shop for and cook healthy meals on a budget as part of their No Kid Hungry campaign. Cooking Matters partners with programs on the local level to provide curricula, instructional materials, training, evaluation, and national leadership for hands-on, grassroots-level cooking education in the community. Some of the programs include interactive grocery store tours, cooking courses, educational tools, and online cooking programming (No Kid Hungry 2017).

School and community gardens are actively engaged in culinary education. The Edible Schoolyards in Oakland California, and New Orleans, Louisiana, offer culinary classes in the classrooms and community (The Edible Schoolyard Project 2017). The Peterson Garden Project in Chicago, Illinois, a community garden and cooking school program, created a new cooking series called "The Feasts of Resistance," which shares stories about the foods we grow and eat from places around the world impacted by social or political unrest (Peterson Garden Project 2017). Additional information about children and healthy food systems is discussed in Chapter 20.

Many Registered Dietitian Nutritionists are working in supermarkets offering grocery store tours, cooking demonstrations, tastings, and cooking classes focused on specialties such as children's nutrition, family cooking, allergies, diabetes, and heart health. For example, Giant Eagle supermarket has a Cooking With The Kids program aimed at nutrition education, healthy eating habits, and simple cooking methods (Giant Eagle 2017). Whole Foods invites Registered Dietitian Nutritionists in the community to host a variety of cooking classes such as vegetarian and vegan cooking and healthy holiday cooking for kids (Whole Foods Market 2017).

14.8 PUTTING COOKING INTO PRACTICE: FROM HOSPITAL TO FARM TO KITCHEN

Imagine this: A food and nutrition workshop hosted on a working farm on a sunny, late summer day. Cooking classes are held in the shade of the farmer's patio. A nutrition class, with samples of foods to touch, smell, and taste is assembled beneath an old citrus tree. A home-gardening workshop offers attendees practical information about growing their own vegetables. Local food artisans and farmers provide samplings of their local, sustainably grown foods in a small exhibition by the orchard. The climax at end of the day is a farm-to-table dinner, celebrated on long wooden tables ensconced by grapevines. The dinner features local wines and foods discussed in the nutrition and cooking workshops earlier that day. The farmer's family regales guests with country and gospel tunes in the balmy evening, amid the chirping of crickets. This isn't just an inspirational model for a community food and nutrition educational event–it actually happened one day in September 2017.

It all started with a request from Sutter Health Memorial Medical Center for a plant-based nutrition class for a community cancer conference in Modesto, California in 2016. The presentation provided practical information on how to choose more healthful, whole plant foods associated with lowering cancer risk. The hospital leadership as well as the community enthusiastically responded to the presentation that day and made a commitment to supporting and promoting local, wholesome, plant-based foods.

This led to teaching a plant-based food and nutrition class the following year on a farm. After a great deal of planning, 269 people attended the first annual Harvest of Hope, a community event sponsored by Sutter Health Memorial Medical Center in September 2017. The event was supported by hundreds of people in the community. La Rosa & Sons Family Farms offered their working farm as the location. The conference included a rotation of three workshops—cooking, nutrition, and gardening—where attendees cycled through the classes in small, interactive groups. This was followed by a social hour in the exhibition area, a farm-to-table dinner, and local entertainment. Marketing efforts included social media, print media, and posters in the community. The mayor of Modesto saw the poster and enjoyed attending the event. Registered Dietitian Nutritionists from the hospital hosted a booth encouraging people to eat fruits and vegetables. Local artisans offered farm fresh samplings such as fermented foods. A sustainable food organization displayed solar ovens. The evaluations signaled that the event was a success.

"The event inspired me to get back to basics, grow some of my own food, purchase locally from small-scale farms, eat more plant-based food with minimal processing, and make meals a time to relax and enjoy with family and friends," said one attendee on the evaluation form. The hospital leadership was so pleased with the event, they authorized the second annual Harvest of Hope, offering an opportunity to further expand this food and nutrition education model in their community. Can more hospitals and community health centers do something similar? Can we create these experiences in low resource communities? Imagine the power of connecting people to real, nutritious, wholesome foods while teaching the important skills of how to cook and grow food. We do have the expertise to create these experiences and to partner with diverse communities and stakeholders to make this happen.

14.9   TIPS FOR HEALTHCARE PROFESSIONALS TO COACH CLIENTS TO COOK

1. **Start small.** If people have little experience in the kitchen, take baby steps in their approach to cooking, such as teaching them how to make a simple olive oil vinaigrette, cook whole grains and pulses, or make a vegetable soup.
2. **Create a guide to local cooking resources.** Make a list of free cooking classes in your community at various organizations, supermarkets, and community centers to distribute to clients.
3. **Develop a "Top-10" recipes list.** Create a list of your best recipes divided into food categories (such as salads, side-dishes, entrees, desserts) as a resource for clients.
4. **Provide cooking tips.** If you don't have the ability to host a cooking class, share helpful tips, such as telling clients how to prepare whole grain pasta tossed with beans, tomatoes, and olive oil, for example.
5. **Teach clients to spice it up.** Some of the best ingredients to have in any kitchen are various herbs and spices that can add flavor and health benefits to foods. Teach clients how to incorporate these seasonings into their everyday meals. Herbs can be easy to grow too.
6. **Schedule a cooking demo.** You don't need a cooking facility, overhead mirrors, or fancy lighting for a cooking demonstration. A blender, hot plate, or even a cutting board will suffice. Even if you don't have a place to host a demo at work, you can volunteer to conduct one at your local community center, church, food pantry, farmers market, or after-school program.
7. **Host an ingredient tasting.** If you don't have the resources to conduct a full-on cooking demonstration, you may want to consider an ingredient tasting when people can sample and compare foods such as nut butters or leafy greens or apples.
8. **Demonstrate simple produce preparations.** Budding cooks can learn how to prepare fruits and vegetables that may seem complicated such as artichokes, mangos, and avocados or those that are unfamiliar, such as kohlrabi, bok choy, and kumquats.
9. **Discuss menu planning.** This is a fundamental tool that can help people get dinner on the table quickly after a hectic day. Meal planning education should include teaching about menus, shopping lists, pantry staples, and easy recipes.
10. **Nurture intuitive cooking.** When your grandmother cooked meals three times a day, she didn't have an iPad. She simply looked in her pantry or

kitchen garden and made something from what was available. Teach this skill by putting a bag of groceries on the counter and showing people how to make a meal out of it.

11. **Explore healthful cooking on a budget.** Dispel the myth that healthful cooking is expensive by teaching people about wholesome, economical cooking that includes grains, legumes, and seasonal produce. Encourage people to visit international markets and stores for a wider range of ethnically diverse ingredients. Suggest purchasing "ugly" fruit—produce available at farmer's markets and some supermarkets which may not appear perfectly pretty yet is nutritious and inexpensive.

14.10 CONCLUSION

People have generally lost their way around the kitchen. There is a loss of culinary skills; there is less cooking at home; and there's an increased consumption of fast food, restaurant meals, and highly processed foods. However, the opportunity is ripe for healthcare professionals to help educate people about the joys and benefits of cooking. Cooking healthful, whole foods at home is a sound nutrition strategy healthcare professionals can use to help create higher quality diets that promote a healthy weight, lowers the risk of chronic diseases, and reduces our ecological footprint. The benefits of cooking at home and sharing family meals are of particular importance for children and adolescents. Healthcare professionals are perfectly poised to play a key role in helping the public increase their culinary literacy through a number of endeavors that utilize cooking education.

REFERENCES

2017 Restaurant industry pocket fact book. *National Restaurant Association.* http://www. restaurant.org/Downloads/PDFs/News-Research/Pocket_Factbook_FEB_2017-FINAL.pdf (Accessed October 31, 2017).

Amana brand history: 80+ years of innovation. *Amana.* https://amana.com/content. jsp?pageName=amana-brand-history (Accessed October 31, 2017).

American Culinary Federation. https://www.acfchefs.org/ (Accessed October 31, 2017).

Asano, E. 2017. How much time do people spend on social media? *Social Media Today.* https://www.socialmediatoday.com/marketing/how-much-time-do-people-spend-social-media-infographic (Accessed October 31, 2017).

Barton, C., L. Koslow, J. Fromm, and C. Egan. 2012. Millennial passions. *Boston Consulting Group.* https://www.bcg.com/documents/file121010.pdf (Accessed October 31, 2017).

Begley, A., and D. Gallegos. 2010. Should cooking be a dietetic vompetency? *Nutrition and Dietetics* 67: 41–46. http://onlinelibrary.wiley.com/doi/10.1111/j.1747-0080.2010.01392.x/abstract (Accessed October 31, 2017).

Botonaki, A., D. Natos, and K. Mattas. 2017. Exploring convenience food consumption through a structural equation model. Paper prepared for presentation at the I Mediterranean Conference of Agro-Food Social Scientists. Presented April 23–25, 2017. http://ageconsearch.umn.edu/bitstream/9433/1/sp07bo06.pdf (Accessed October 31, 2017).

Bowen, S., S. Elliott, and J. Brenton. 2014. The joy of cooking? *American Sociological Association* 13 (3) http://journals.sagepub.com/doi/full/10.1177/1536504214545755 (Accessed October 31, 2017).

Bowman, S.A., S.L. Gortmaker, C.B. Ebbeling, M.A. Pereira, and D.S. Ludwig. 2004. Effects of fast-food consumption on energy intake and diet quality among children in a national household survey. *Pediatrics* 113 (1) Pt. 1: 112–118. https://www.ncbi.nlm.nih.gov/pubmed/14702458 (Accessed October 31, 2017).

Canter, D., M.E. Moorachian, and J. Boyce. 2007. The growing importance of food and culinary knowledge and skills in dietetics practice. *Topics in Clinical Nutrition* 22 (4): 313–332. http://krex.k-state.edu/dspace/handle/2097/604 (Accessed October 31, 2017).

Cohen, D., and M. Story. 2014. Mitigating the health risks of dining out: The need for standardized portion sizes in restaurants. *American Journal of Public Health* 104 (4): 586–590. https://www.ncbi.nlm.nih.gov/pmc/articles/PMC4025680/ (Accessed October 31, 2017).

Cooking classes. *Whole Foods Market.* http://www.wholefoodsmarket.com/service/cooking-classes-1 (Accessed October 31, 2017).

Duffey, K.J., P. Gordon-Larsen, D.R. Jacobs Jr., O.D. Williams, and B.M. Popkin. 2007. Differential associations of fast food and restaurant food consumption with 3-y change in body mass index: The Coronary Artery Risk Development in Young Adults Study. *American Journal of Clinical Nutrition* 85 (1): 201–208. https://www.ncbi.nlm.nih.gov/pubmed/17209197 (Accessed October 31, 2017).

Eisenburg, D.M., and J.D. Burgess. 2015. Nutrition education in an era of global obesity and diabetes: Thinking outside the box. *Academic* Medicine 90 (7): 854–860. https://www.ncbi.nlm.nih.gov/pubmed/25785680 (Accessed October 31, 2017).

Ellickson, P. 2015. The evolution of the supermarket industry: From A&P to Walmart. University of Rochester. http://paulellickson.com/SMEvolution.pdf (Accessed October 31, 2017).

FAO. 2006. Livestock a Major Threat to Environment. http://www.fao.org/newsroom/en/news/2006/1000448/index.html (Accessed January 22, 2018).

French, S.A., L. Harnack, and R.W. Jeffery. 2000. Fast food restaurant use among women in the pound of prevention study: Dietary, behavioral and demographic correlates. *International Journal of Obesity and Related Metabolic Disorders* 24:1353–1359. https://www.ncbi.nlm.nih.gov/pubmed/11093299 (Accessed October 31, 2017).

Giant Eagle. https://www.gianteagle.com/ (Accessed October 31, 2017).

Gust, L. 2011. Defrosting dinner: The evolution of frozen meals in America. *Intersect* 4 (1). http://web.stanford.edu/group/ojs3/cgi-bin/ojs/index.php/intersect/article/view/269/139 (Accessed October 31, 2017).

Hammons, A., and B.H. Fiese. 2011. Is frequency of shared family meals related to the nutritional health of children and adolescents? *Pediatrics* 127 (6): e1565–e1574. https://www.ncbi.nlm.nih.gov/pmc/articles/PMC3387875/ (Accessed October 31, 2017).

Hamrick, K. November 7, 2016. Americans spend an average of 37 minutes a day preparing and serving food and cleaning up. *United States Department of Agriculture.* https://www.ers.usda.gov/amber-waves/2016/november/americans-spend-an-average-of-37-minutes-a-day-preparing-and-serving-food-and-cleaning-up/ (Accessed October 31, 2017).

Henry Ford West Bloomfield Hospital. 2017. https://www.henryford.com/locations/west-bloomfield (Accessed October 31, 2017).

Highly processed foods dominate U. S. grocery purchases. *Federation of American Societies for Experimental Biology.* March 29, 2015. https://www.sciencedaily.com/releases/2015/03/150329141017.htm. (Accessed October 31, 2017).

Jabs, J., and C.M. Devine. 2006. Time scarcity and food choices: An overview. *Appetite* 47 (2): 196–204. https://www.ncbi.nlm.nih.gov/pubmed/16698116 (Accessed October 31, 2017).

Jones, C.M., and Kammen, D.M. 2011. Quantifying carbon footprint reduction opportunities for U.S. households and communities. *Environmental Science & Technology* 45 (9): 4088–4095.

Johnson & Wales University. 2017. https://www.jwu.edu (Accessed October 31, 2017).

Kerrison, D., M.D. Condrasky, and J.L. Sharp. 2017. Culinary nutrition education for under-graduate nutrition dietetics students. *British Food Journal* 119 (5): 1045–1051. http://www.emeraldinsight.com/doi/abs/10.1108/BFJ-09-2016-0437 (Accessed October 31, 2017).

Krebs-Smith, S.M., P.M. Guenther, A.F. Subar, S.I. Kirkpatrick, and K.W. Dodd. 2010. Americans do not meet federal dietary recommendations. *Journal of Nutrition* 140 (10):1832–1838. https://www.ncbi.nlm.nih.gov/pubmed/20702750 (Accessed October 31, 2017.).

Lichtenstein, A.H., and D.S. Ludwig. 2010. Bring back home economics education. *JAMA* 303 (18): 1857–1858. https://www.ncbi.nlm.nih.gov/pubmed/20460625 (Accessed October 31, 2017).

Mills, S., M. White, H. Brown, W. Wrieden, D. Kwasnicka, J. Halligan, S. Robalino, et al. 2017. Health and social determinants and outcomes of home cooking: A systematic review of observational studies. *Appetite* 111 (1): 116–134. http://www.sciencedirect.com/science/article/pii/S0195666316309576 (Accessed October 31, 2017).

Monlezun, D.J., E. Kasprowicz, K.W. Tosh, J. Nix, P. Urday, D. Tice, L. Sarris, et al. 2015. Medical school-based teaching kitchen improves HbA1c, blood pressure, and choles-terol for patients with type 2 diabetes: Results from a novel randomized controlled trial. *Diabetes Research and Clinical Practice* 109 (2): 420–426. https://www.ncbi.nlm.nih.gov/pubmed/26002686 (Accessed October 31, 2017).

National survey reveals nearly half of American families eat dinner together fewer than three times a week or not at all. *ConAgra Foods*. May 30, 2003. http://www.conagrabrands.com/news-room/news-national-survey-reveals-nearly-half-of-american-families-eat-dinner-together-fewer-than-three-times-a-week-or-not-at-all-1008335 (Accessed October 31, 2017).

Our priority: End child hunger in America. *No Kid Hungry*. https://www.nokidhungry.org/about-us (Accessed October 31, 2017.).

Peterson Garden Project. 2017. https://petersongarden.org/ (Accessed October 31, 2017).

Polak, R., E.M. Phillips, J. Nordgren, J. La Puma, J. La Barba, M. Cucuzzella, R. Graham, et al. 2016. Health-related culinary education: A summary of representative emerg-ing programs for health professionals and patients. *Global Advances in Health and Medicine* 5 (1): 61–68. https://www.ncbi.nlm.nih.gov/pmc/articles/PMC4756781/ (Accessed October 31, 2017).

Ragone, G. CIA, Harvard partnership gives rise to teaching kitchens. *Food Management*. Published November 3, 2016. http://www.food-management.com/management/cia-har-vard-partnership-gives-rise-teaching-kitchens (Accessed October 31, 2017).

Reducing wasted food & packaging: A guide for food services and restaurants. *United States Environmental Protection Agency*. https://www.epa.gov/sites/production/files/2015-08/documents/reducing_wasted_food_pkg_tool.pdf (Accessed October 31, 2017).

Reedy, J., and S.M. Krebs-Smith. 2010. Dietary sources of energy, solid fats, and added sugars among children and adolescents in the United States. *Journal of the American Dietetic Association* 110 (10): 1477–1484. https://www.ncbi.nlm.nih.gov/pubmed/20869486 (Accessed October 31, 2017).

Smith, L., S.W. Nu, and B.M. Popkin. 2013. Trends in US home food preparation and con-sumption: Analysis of national nutrition surveys and time use studies from 1965–1966 to 2007–2008. *Nutrition Journal* 12 (45). https://www.ncbi.nlm.nih.gov/pmc/articles/PMC3639863/ (Accessed October 31, 2017).

Snacking motivations and attitudes—US. *Mintel Group*. Published April 2015. http://store.min-tel.com/snacking-motivations-and-attitudes-us-april-2015 (Accessed October 31, 2017).

Story, M., and D. Neumark-Sztainer. 2005. A perspective on family meals: Do they mat-ter? *Nutrition Today* 40 (6): 261–266. http://journals.lww.com/nutritiontodayonline/Abstract/2005/11000/A_Perspective_on_Family_Meals__Do_They_Matter_.7.aspx (Accessed October 31, 2017).

Supplemental nutrition assistance program education. *USDA Food and Nutrition Service*. June 22, 2017. https://www.fns.usda.gov/snap/supplemental-nutrition-assistance-program-education-snap-ed (Accessed October 31, 2017).

The Edible Schoolyard Project. http://edibleschoolyard.org/ (Accessed October 31, 2017).

Think smaller for big growth: How to thrive in the new retail landscape. *Nielsen*. http://www.nielsen.com/content/dam/nielsenglobal/de/docs/Nielsen%20Global%20Retail%20Growth%20Strategies%20Report_DIGITAL.pdf (Accessed October 31, 2017).

USDA. 2018. U.S. Food Waste Challenge. https://www.usda.gov/oce/foodwaste/faqs.htm (Accessed January 22, 2018).

Vilas-Boas, E. 2017. The 8 unhealthiest Chain restaurant meals of 2017. *Thrillist*. July 31, 2017. https://www.thrillist.com/news/nation/most-unhealthy-chain-restaurant-food-2017 (Accessed October 31, 2017).

Virudachalam, S., J.A. Long, M.O. Harhay, D.E. Polsky, and C. Feudtner. 2013. Prevalence and patterns of cooking dinner at home in the USA: National Health and Nutrition Examination Survey (NHANES) 2007–2008. *Public Health Nutrition* 17 (5): 1022–1030. https://www.cambridge.org/core/services/aop-cambridge-core/content/view/S1368980013002589 (Accessed October 31, 2017).

Wolfson, J., S.N. Bleich, K.C. Smith, and S. Frattarolia. 2016. What does cooking mean to you?: Perceptions of cooking and factors related to cooking behavior. *Appetite* 97 (1): 146–154. http://www.sciencedirect.com/science/article/pii/S0195666315301070 (Accessed October 31, 2017.).

Zick, C.D., and R.B. Stevens. 2010. Trends in Americans' food-related time use: 1975–2006. *Public Health Nutrition* 13: 1064–1072. https://www.ncbi.nlm.nih.gov/pubmed/19943999 (Accessed October 31, 2017).

15 A Whole Foods Plant-Centered Diet

Monique Richard

CONTENTS

15.1 INTRODUCTION

Dietary choices profoundly influence both individual and environmental health in surprisingly parallel ways. The scientific literature reveals a growing interest related to the environmental impact of food production and the Western diet's influence on health outcomes (Aleksandrowicz et al. 2016). Concerns range from the excessive diminution of the natural environment as well as increases in: Water use, air and water pollution, greenhouse gas (GHG) emissions, and soil degradation (Eshel and Martin 2009). Dietary patterns that show optimal outcomes for good health and disease prevention at an individual level—namely diets based on minimally processed, whole plant-foods—are also associated with food production methods that are more environmentally sustainable with smaller ecological footprints (Eshel and Martin 2009). Hence, dietary recommendations that promote a wholesome plant-based diet could favorably impact environmental outcomes on a large scale.

A Whole Foods Plant-Based Diet (WFPBD) can be defined as a dietary pattern that partially or completely excludes animal products and emphasizes nutrient-dense, minimally processed plant-based foods like vegetables, fruits, whole grains, legumes, nuts and seeds, and healthy oils (Tuso et al. 2013, Lea et al. 2006). Such plant-based diets are typically low in energy density and fat and high in nutrient density, complex carbohydrates, fiber, and water (Rizzo et al. 2013, Orlich et al. 2014).

While no strict definition of the WFPBD currently exists, it generally comprises varying levels of exclusion or limitation on animal products combined with a variety of plant foods in their most natural form (legumes, lentils, fruits, vegetables, whole grains) (Tuso et al. 2013). The WFPB dietary pattern is considered a holistic approach to health and well-being.

Though the terms vegetarian or vegan may often be used interchangeably with reference to a plant-based diet, vegetarian and vegan diets are two variations in the WFPB dietary pattern. They do often contain the highest proportion of whole plant-foods and are typically the most studied (Orlich et al. 2014, Clarys et al. 2014). Additional dietary patterns often considered to be a WFPBD do focus on maximizing plant-food intake despite the inclusion of minimal amounts of animal products. These diets include (Le and Sebate 2014):

- Semi-Vegetarian or Flexitarian—includes small amounts of animal flesh less than once per week and more than once per month
- Pescetarian—the only animal flesh consumed is fish and/or other seafood, along with dairy products and eggs
- Vegetarian
  - Lacto-Ovo—no animal flesh, but includes dairy products (lacto) and eggs (ovo)
  - Vegan—no animal flesh, eggs, dairy products, or animal by-products of any kind

15.2 CHRONIC DISEASE AND ENVIRONMENTAL FOOTPRINT

As previously mentioned, about half of all American adults have one or more diet-related chronic diseases, including type 2 diabetes, high blood pressure, and cardiovascular disease (Health and Human Services, Office of Disease Prevention and Health Promotion and United States Department of Agriculture 2015). An estimated two-thirds of adults and one-third of children and youth are overweight or obese, putting them at high risk for the aforementioned chronic diseases (Health and Human Services, Office of Disease Prevention and Health Promotion and United States Department of Agriculture 2015). Chronic diseases are the most common causes of mortality around the world (World Health Organization 2011). The prevalence of these diseases and deaths are expected to increase—while cardiovascular disease is the number one killer worldwide (World Health Organization 2011).

Vegetarian and vegan dietary patterns not only demonstrate the potential for both the prevention and amelioration of chronic disease, but also offer solutions for reducing the environmental impact of food production (Burlingame 2012; Melina et al. 2016; HHS, Office of Disease Prevention and Health Promotion Scarborough et al. 2014; USDA 2015). Many health organizations endorse the benefits of vegetarian and vegan diets including: The Academy of Nutrition and Dietetics (U.S.), the largest organization of food and nutrition professionals (Melina et al. 2016); the Scientific Report of the 2015

Dietary Guidelines Advisory Committee; and the Food and Agriculture Organization (FAO) Committee on Agriculture (FAO—Committee on Agriculture 1999). These groups have also discerned that dietary patterns highest in whole plant-based foods, which are the foundation of WFPBD—vegetables, fruits, whole grains, legumes, nuts, and seeds—are associated with the least environmental impact in terms of GHG emissions, land use, water use, and energy use (Burlingame 2012; Melina et al. 2016; HHS, Office of Disease Prevention and Health Promotion (U.S.) and USDA 2015).

15.3 RESEARCH STUDIES IN ADULTS

Large prospective cohort studies along with randomized controlled trials show strong associations between higher intakes of plant-based foods and improved risk factors for, and a lower incidence of chronic diseases such as obesity, high blood pressure, cardiovascular disease, type 2 diabetes and certain cancers (Ley et al. 2014, Le and Sebate 2014, Cho et al. 2013, Mozaffarian et al. 2011). Results from the Adventist Health Studies—long term, prospective epidemiological studies of members of the Seventh-day Adventist religion, many of whom follow vegetarian, vegan, semi-vegetarian, and pescetarian diets—show that vegetarians tend to have a lower body mass index and a lower risk for coronary heart disease, hypertension, type 2 diabetes, and metabolic syndrome (Le and Sabaté 2014; Sabate and Wien 2010).

A comprehensive systematic review and meta-analysis of observational studies examining the association between vegetarian, vegan diets, risk factors for chronic diseases, risk of all-cause mortality, incidence and mortality from cardio-cerebro-vascular diseases, total cancer, and colorectal, breast, prostate, and lung cancers concluded that those with diets highest in the proportion of plant-foods—vegetarians and vegans—had significantly reduced body mass indexes, total cholesterol (TC) and low-density lipoprotein (LDL) cholesterol levels—and better glucose control compared to omnivores (Dinu et al. 2016). This included an impressive 25% reduction in the incidence and/or mortality from ischemic heart disease along with an 8% reduction in the incidence from total cancer (Dinu et al. 2016). In a systematic review and meta-analysis on the effects of diet on blood lipid levels, vegetarian diets effectively lowered blood concentrations of TC, LDL cholesterol, high-density lipoprotein (HDL) cholesterol, and non-high-density lipoprotein (non-HDL) cholesterol (Wang et al. 2015). With regard to weight reduction, further meta-analyses of randomized trials found that vegetarian diets are associated with a significant weight reduction benefit when compared to non-vegetarian diets (Huang et al. 2016), contributing to a positive outcome in addressing modifiable risk factors related to cardiovascular disease (Barnard et al. 2015).

15.4 PHYTOCHEMICALS/PHYTONUTRIENTS

A diet focused on plant-foods is rich in phytochemicals (phytonutrients) which are bioactive compounds that have demonstrated a protective influence on genetic expression and transcription at the cellular level (Thomas et al. 2015, Mierziak et al. 2014). This fact is generally overlooked and under recognized. Interestingly, the phytochemicals within plants that protect them from harm by fungi, germs, bugs, and other threats may be of great benefit when consumed by humans (Mierziak et al. 2014). Beneficial phytochemicals include many from the polyphenol category including resveratrol, carotenoids, anthocyanins, catechins, glucosinolates, flavonols and flavonoids, which have multiple functions including anti-oxidation, anti-inflammation, cancer protective mechanisms, immunity enhancement, and optimization of serum cholesterol (Hever 2016, Martin et al. 2013, Merziak et al. 2014, Thomas et al. 2015). Rich sources of phytochemicals are those found in pigmented fruits and vegetables such as onions, kale, leeks, broccoli, red grapes, berries, apples, and citrus as well as whole grains, legumes, herbs, spices, nuts, and seeds. Thus, diets based heavily on the inclusion of whole, plant-based foods are rich in these phytonutrients and can modulate the pathophysiology of diet-related chronic diseases such as diabetes, cardiovascular disease, and cancer (Orlich et al. 2014, Martin et al. 2013). However, research demonstrates that phytochemicals in the form of supplements fail to have the same effects as those found in whole foods. It is theorized that it is the synergistic effects of components not yet discovered in food that may contribute to this effect, making the focus on a WFPBD all the more important (Martin et al. 2013).

15.5 FIBER

In addition to the myriad of benefits from phytochemicals, the consumption of dietary fiber is critical to digestive health and has strong associations with reducing the risk of cardiovascular disease, obesity, prediabetes and Type 2 Diabetes (T2D) (Dahl and Stewart 2015, Melina et al. 2016). Although fiber is not considered a nutrient, it is a component of the macronutrient carbohydrate and is associated with positive health outcomes. Dietary fiber is only found in substantial quantities in plant foods. The Academy of Nutrition and Dietetics recommends 14 grams of dietary fiber per 1,000 calories (Dahl and Stewart 2015) with other health organizations recommending more. It is estimated only 3–5% of Americans meet these recommendations (Clemens et al. 2012, Dahl and Stewart 2015). Hence, dietary fiber is an under-consumed nutrient of public health concern. Those who follow plant-based diets consume significantly higher intakes of fiber compared to other dietary patterns (Davey et al. 2003, Farmer et al. 2011, Rizzo et al. 2013). The soluble, viscous fiber in plant-based foods assists in blood glucose regulation contributing to improved T2D management and the reduction of risk factors for cardiovascular disease (CVD) and obesity (Martin et al. 2013). Insoluble fiber, also known as dietary fiber, has been associated with the reduced risk of T2D, CVD, cancer, and obesity (Martin et al. 2013). Increased intakes of dietary fiber has also been inversely associated with TC concentration in both men and women (Appleby et al. 1995, Dahl and Stewart 2015).

15.6 NUTRIENTS TO NOTE

Vegetarian and vegan diets, when consumed in an eating pattern that is balanced and varied, are appropriate for all stages of life, including pregnancy, and offer numerous benefits as aforementioned (Melina et al. 2016). Vegetarians, vegans, and omnivores alike must remain cognizant about obtaining adequate nutrients such as calcium, vitamin D, etc. However, in the absence of animal flesh or animal products in the diet, certain nutrients such as vitamin B_{12} becomes extremely important for vegans. Irrespective of the type of dietary pattern consumed, if adequate amounts of nutrients cannot be obtained through a varied diet, supplements may be appropriate.

15.6.1 CALCIUM

While dairy may be the central source of calcium in a diet based heavily on animal foods, calcium is also found in a variety of plant foods (Weaver et al. 1999). Calcium-rich plant foods include bok choy, kale, collards, figs, tahini, black-strap molasses, almonds and almond butter, fortified plant-milks, calcium-set tofu, and navel oranges (Weaver et al. 1999). Vegetables containing higher oxalates such as spinach, beet greens, and Swiss chard may not be considered ideal calcium sources due to the binding properties of the oxalates in reducing ability for absorption (Weaver et al. 1999). A completely plant-based diet can provide adequate calcium for bone health (Appleby et al. 2007).

15.6.2 IODINE

Research has shown that dietary patterns with little to no animal products can lead to a risk for suboptimal iodine status, increasing the potential for thyroid dysfunction (Sobiecki et al. 2016, Leung et al. 2011). There are components in many cruciferous vegetables that when metabolized may counteract the bioavailability of iodine, affect thyroid hormone synthesis, or inhibit iodine uptake (Fenwick et al. 1983, Felker et al. 2016). Plant-based iodine sources include seaweed and iodized salt (sea salt does not contain iodine). Some vegan nutrition experts recommend that vegans who don't take a multivitamin take 75–150 µg of supplemental iodine daily or every few days (Norris and Messina 2011, Leung et al. 2011).

15.6.3 VITAMIN B₁₂

Cobalamin (vitamin B_{12}) is a vitamin synthesized by bacteria found only in animals and there are no bioactive sources found in plants (O'Leary et al. 2010). Of its many roles, B_{12} is essential to DNA synthesis, cellular renewal, and nerve transmission; long-term deficiency can lead to stroke, dementia, and impaired bone health (Melina et al. 2016, Watanabe 2007). The only reliable non-animal sources include supplements and fortified foods—including most plant-milks and some brands of nutritional yeast and cereals (Melina et al. 2016). It is recommended that those following an exclusively plant-based diet either eat at least two servings a day of B_{12} fortified foods (Melina et al. 2016, Norris and Messina 2011) or add a supplement appropriate for their age and recommended intake. When B_{12} rich whole foods are consumed as part of a WFPBD, B_{12} needs can be easily met.

15.6.4 VITAMIN D

Inadequate vitamin D is a concern for most people who don't get sufficient sunlight or do not consume enough in their diet from fortified sources (Nair and Maseeh 2012, Melina et al. 2016). The inactive form of vitamin D, 7-dehydrocholesterol, is absorbed by the body through ultraviolet B (UVB) light and then converted to the active form of vitamin D, 1,25-Dihydroxyvitamin D3 (otherwise known as calcitriol) by the liver initially then further by the kidneys (Nair and Meseeh 2012).

Unless a food is fortified or produced using irradiation such as mushrooms, adequate vitamin D may be difficult to consume within any given dietary pattern. It is recommended that 1,000–2,000 IUs of supplemental vitamin D be taken daily, although sufficient amounts of vitamin D may be already included in a multivitamin depending on the brand and ingredients (Melina et al. 2016, Norris and Messina 2011).

15.6.5 IRON

The iron found in plant foods differs from the iron in animal flesh due to its alternate molecular form (non-heme versus heme, respectively). Non-heme iron has a lower rate of absorption in the body, but it has been found that the body adapts to improve efficiency of absorption (Hunt and Roughead 2000). Due to this lower bioavailability, the recommended intake of iron for vegetarians is 1.8 times higher than the recommended 8 mg for men and 18 mg for women (Institute of Medicine (US) Panel on Micronutrients 2001). Though iron deficiency anemia is common across all dietary patterns, those consuming a plant-based diet do not have higher rates of iron deficiency, which may be attributed to the adaptation to more effectively absorb non-heme iron (Hunt and Roughead 2000, Melina et al. 2016). Specifically, vegetarians and vegan dietary patterns consist of as much or more iron than non-vegan and non-vegetarian dietary patterns (Melina et al. 2016). However, it remains important to ensure that a WFPBD include a variety of iron-rich foods (whole grains, pulses, legumes, fruits, and vegetables) consumed alongside foods high in vitamin C (i.e., citrus, tomatoes, kale, potatoes, red peppers, broccoli, cabbage, etc.) that can maximize the absorption of non-heme iron (Abbaspour et al. 2014, Melina et al. 2016).

15.6.6 PROTEIN

Protein requirements are usually met or exceeded when following a WFPBD that's calorically adequate and varied (Melina et al. 2016). The need to "combine plant-proteins" at each meal has been deemed unnecessary, as eating a variety of plant foods throughout the day supplies adequate levels of all the essential amino acids (Melina et al. 2016). However, some plant-based nutrition experts recommend eating three servings of legumes daily (e.g., beans, peanuts, dried peas, soy) to meet protein needs and fulfill the essential amino acid profile (Melina et al. 2016, Norris and Messina 2011). Protein-rich plants include nuts, seeds, pulses, quinoa, soybeans, tofu, and tempeh (Tuso et al. 2013).

Plant-based milks vary in their protein content. Protein-rich plant-based dairy alternatives include those derived from soy, pea protein, and hemp seeds. Those with lower levels of protein include cashew, almond, rice and coconut varieties.

15.6.7 OMEGA-3 AND OMEGA-6 FATTY ACIDS

All diets should include omega-3 fatty acids on a daily basis. Flaxseed, hempseed, walnuts, avocado, olive and canola oil are all rich sources of omega-3 and omega-6 fatty acids (Melina et al. 2016). More concentrated sources of omega-3 fatty acids, docosahexaenoic acid (DHA) and eicosapentenoic acid (EPA), can be found in microalgae supplements that are on par with the fatty acid profile found in fish oils. EPA and DHA can also be synthesized in the body through the metabolism of another fatty acid, alpha-linolenic acid (ALA), found in abundance in most diets (Melina et al. 2016). Although there is a slower conversion within the body, it appears to be sufficient, although some experts may recommend between 200–300 mg of supplemental DHA daily (Norris and Messina 2011). Consensus that fish or fish oil supplements are beneficial for heart health remain controversial and inconclusive; recent meta-analyses and systematic reviews show that fish oil has no effect on reducing cardiac-related death, heart attack, or stroke (Rizos et al. 2012, Myung 2012).

15.7 ENVIRONMENTAL IMPACT

Aspects of environmental quality that are impacted by livestock production include atmospheric (air quality), water (local and global reservoirs), land, and ocean health (Eshel et al. 2014; Pimentel et al. 2005). Research shows that food production associated with plant-based dietary patterns generally use less natural resources and reduce environmental damage compared to animal-based food production (Hallström et al. 2015; Ranganathan et al. 2016). The Scientific Committee of the Dietary Guidelines for Americans noted that diets rich plant foods and Mediterranean-style dietary patterns are associated with less GHG emissions as well as less energy, land, and water use than the average U.S. diet while conferring an array of health benefits (Millen et al. 2016).

A variety of sources show strong evidence regarding the negative impact livestock production has on the environment (Eshel et al. 2016, 2014, Eshel and Martin 2009). In one 2016 study by Eshel et al., the researchers revealed that replacing a beef-centered diet with a plant-based diet required an average of just 10% of the land, 4% of GHG emissions, and 6% of reactive nitrogen (Eshel et al. 2016). Switching to a plant-based diet on a nationwide scale in the United States alone would equate to a savings of 91 million cropland acres; 770 million rangeland acres; 278 million metric ton CO_2; and 3.7 million metric tons of reactive nitrogen annually (Eshel et al. 2016).

Interestingly, research suggests that those who eat a WFPBD are increasingly selecting organic plant-based foods (Baudry et al. 2016, Petersen et al. 2013). Items certified as organic by the United States Department of Agriculture (USDA) are grown and processed without the use of synthetic fertilizers, irradiation, genetic engineering, and sewage sludge (USDA-AMS 2000). Some studies indicate that conventionally grown foods contain higher levels of pesticide residue and heavy metals than their organic counterparts, hence the consumption of organic products may reduce overall exposure to pesticides, herbicides, and other synthetic products compared to those produced with conventional agricultural methods (Lu et al. 2006, Mansour et al. 2009; Johansson et al. 2014). The President's Cancer Panel Report of 2010 recommended choosing foods grown without pesticides and chemical fertilizers to decrease overall exposure to pesticides which in turn may reduce cancer risk (Reuben 2010).

15.8 CONCLUSION

As the evidenced-based research continues to document the merits of vegetarian and vegan diets for human health and that of the natural environment, it is essential for practitioners, scientists, and interdisciplinary professionals to recognize the positive outcomes associated with a WFPB dietary pattern. A collective shift to a more plant-based diet can maximize support for the regenerative processes of the natural environment while also improving human health. Action and implementation are imperative at this time due to the systematic decline in natural resources and the crisis of chronic disease across the globe. Consuming a WFPBD is a powerful step to improved human and planetary health and is an underutilized and indispensable tool.

ACKNOWLEDGMENT

The author would like to thank Eliza Mellion MS, RDN for research and formatting assistance.

VIGNETTE 15.1   Plant-Shift

A Common Denominator of Centenarians Around the Globe

Bonnie Farmer

INTRODUCTION

In 2004, researchers studied the island of Sardinia, Italy, to calculate the percentage of persons born there between 1880 and 1900 who became centenarians (Poulain et al. 2013). Areas that were identified to have the highest concentration of centenarians were highlighted on a map with a blue marker and subsequently referred to as the "Blue Zone". Later, other Blue Zones were identified with the help of Dan Buettner of the National Geographic along with anthropologists, demographers, epidemiologists, and other researchers to understand lifestyle and environmental factors that might explain why people in these regions live to be 100 years old. The additional Blue Zones identified by Buettner and colleagues are Loma Linda, California; Nicoya, Costa Rica; Ikaria, Greece; and Okinawa, Japan.

LIFESTYLE FACTORS

The lifestyle factors that were found to be common among centenarians in these areas were dubbed the "Power 9" (Buettner and Skemp 2016). Diet encompasses three of the "Power 9", with plant-based diets central to these factors:

1. **Move naturally**—walking, gardening, and working without mechanical conveniences
2. **Purpose**—having something to live for beyond work
3. **Downshift**—routine stress reduction practices like meditation or napping
4. **80% Rule**—stop eating when hunger is satisfied and before feeling full
5. **Plant Slant**—consuming a plant-based diet
6. **Wine @ 5**—1 to 2 alcoholic drinks per day with friends and/or with food
7. **Belong**—to a faith-based community
8. **Loved ones first**—committing to a life-long partner and prioritizing the care of elder family members and children
9. **Right tribe**—having social circles that support healthy behaviors

(Buettner and Skemp 2016)

THE IMPORTANCE OF WHOLE PLANT FOODS

The benefits of eating a wide variety of plant foods and their effects on mortality are widely recognized, although the physiological mechanisms associated with these benefits are still being identified. Oxidative stress is thought to contribute to diseases associated with aging, such as cardiovascular disease, Alzheimer's disease, and cancer (Liu 2013). Many plant foods are rich in antioxidants and other nutrients found only in plants (phytonutrients). Examples include vitamins C, and E, carotenoids beta-carotene and lycopene, and resveratrol—a polyphenol. Antioxidant phytonutrients can neutralize the damaging free radical compounds that are generated by oxidative stress (Rahal et al. 2014).

Plant foods commonly eaten by centenarians in Ikaria include wild greens such as purslane, dandelion, and arugula which are rich sources of minerals and antioxidants (Buettner 2015, Trichopoulou et al. 2000). Bitter melon is a vegetable consumed in Okinawa that is high in antioxidants and may also be responsible for helping to regulate blood sugar (Tan et al. 2016). The squash and papaya common to traditional Nicoyan diets provide plenty of vitamin A in the form of beta-carotene. Papaya also contains papain—an enzyme that helps to control inflammation (Pandey et al. 2016).

Saturated fat can promote cardiovascular disease, and plant-based diets are typically lower in saturated fat than dietary patterns that include meat (Kennedy et al. 2001). As a good source of protein with no saturated fat, legumes and pulses are common to the traditional diets of centenarians in the Blue Zones (Buettner and Skemp 2016). Fava beans are favored in Sardinia, while garbanzos, black-eyed peas, and lentils are enjoyed in Ikaria. In Okinawa it is soy—and in Nicoya, it's black beans (Buettner 2015). Beans and lentils are also an important source of antioxidants, and some lentils have more antioxidants than even apples, apricots, cherries, or red grapes (Carlsen 2010).

While the genes associated with heart disease and Alzheimer's disease are rare in centenarians (Schachter et al. 1994), the study of the human genome suggests that gene-nutrient interactions may also play a role in the development of chronic diseases (Kaput and Rodriguez 2004). That is, what you eat can impact your genetic makeup. In a small study comparing the effects of a Mediterranean-style meal to a high-fat meal, researchers measured the expression of genes related to oxidative stress and inflammation. The Mediterranean meal down-regulated a gene thought to play a role in obesity and diabetes as well as a gene related to leukemia (De Lorenzo et al. 2017). In another study, researchers found that consumption of extra virgin olive oil down-regulated genes related to high blood pressure (Martin-Pelaez et al. 2017).

CONCLUSION

As we continue to learn how plant-based diets interact with our genes, it is increasingly clear that we have the power to maintain health in aging. In the words of one participant in a study of centenarian perspectives on longevity, "It's quite simple. You can't do much about what you inherit, but you can change through diet and exercise and having a good spirit" (Freeman et al. 2013).

VIGNETTE 15.2 Whole Plant Foods and Optimal Gut and Host Health

Kayellen Edmonds-Umeakunne

INTRODUCTION

The gut microbiome consists of trillions of microorganisms that are involved in bowel health, digestion, and metabolism (Walter et al. 2011). A strong body of evidence identifies the role of the gut microbiome in the maintenance of host immunity and the prevention of disease (Flint et al. 2012). Dietary fiber intake provides the main substrate for gut bacteria and ensures a diverse microbiota that is key to gut homeostasis and disease prevention (Holscher 2017, Dahl et al. 2015). Populations that rely mainly on a higher fiber plant-based diet show greater gut microbial diversity (De Filippo et al. 2010). Butyrate is one of the many metabolites produced through the gut microbial fermentation of undigested foods that are primarily carbohydrates and fiber. This short chain fatty acid: (1) provides energy for colonocytes (cells in the colon) (2) helps maintain a healthy gut mucosa (3) assists in preventing pathogenic bacteria from disrupting the gut barrier known as dysbiosis (an imbalance in gut microbiota leading to pathogenesis) and (4) helps minimize inflammation and disease (Holscher 2017, Desai et al. 2016, Dahl et al. 2015).

THE ROLE OF DIET IN THE GUT MICROBIOME

Diet is instrumental in determining the type of microbiota predominate in the gut and can rapidly change microbial composition within 24 hours. While no current dietary recommendations exist for a healthy gut microbiome, mounting evidence suggests a plant-based diet is optimal for gut and host health (Klinder et al. 2016, David et al. 2014, Haro et al. 2015). Whole foods plant-based dietary patterns have been associated with a lower incidence of chronic disease and plant-foods contain large amounts of fiber (Sheflin et al. 2017; do Rosaria et al. 2016; and McMacken and Shah 2017). Plant-based diets can be defined as complex dietary patterns that emphasize foods of plant origin, particularly vegetables, grains, legumes and fruits (Hu et al. 2003). These plants provide a source of prebiotics that are non-digestible compounds that promote the growth of beneficial bacteria like bifidobacteria (Kelly 2008).

Many of the beneficial effects of a plant-based diet are mediated through the fermentation of these plant-based prebiotics to form bioactive metabolites such as butyrate. Examples of prebiotics include (1) inulin, a naturally occurring polysaccharides belonging to a class of dietary fibers known as fructans (found in leeks, garlic, onions, wheat, Jerusalem artichokes, and chicory root) (Roberfroid 2007; Kelly 2008; Slavin 2012) and (2) resistant starch, a type of starch that escapes digestion in the small intestine and is found in whole grain oats, barley, brown rice, hi-maize flour, cooked and cooled potatoes, and green bananas (Murphy et al 2008). Butyrate levels are increased by consumption of a diet high in resistance starch (McOrist et al. 2011).

The gut microbiota of vegans and vegetarians consuming higher carbohydrate/fiber diets has been shown to differ from that of omnivores by its impact on stool pH. A lower stool pH found in vegans (6.3±0.8) compared with omnivores (6.9±0.9) coincided with reduced counts of pathogenic gram negative bacteria *Escherichia coli* and Enterobacteriaceae which prefer pH ranges >6.5 (Zimmer et al. 2012, and Glick-Bauer and Ming-Chin 2014). Whole food plant-based diets may therefore produce an optimal gut pH environment to maintain homeostasis and prevent dysbiosis and disease.

BIOMARKERS OF INFLAMMATION

C-reactive protein (CRP) has gained acceptance for its usefulness as a marker of both acute and chronic inflammation (Azadbakh et al. 2011). Circulating CRP is positively correlated with cardiovascular disease (CVD), heart attack, stroke, peripheral arterial disease, diabetes mellitus, and cancer (Ridker 2003). In the case of chronic inflammatory disease, CRP levels rise due to secretion from adipose tissue as well as additional liver stimulation via cytokines and immune cells, primarily macrophages. Obesity markedly elevates the release of other inflammatory cytokines from adipose tissue, such as TNF-alpha and IL-6, further exacerbating systemic inflammation (Lumeng and Saltiel 2011).

GUT BIOMARKERS OF INFLAMMATION

Lipopolysaccharide (LPS) is an inflammatory biomarker unique to the gut microbiota. Lipopolysaccharide is found in the outer membrane of gram negative gut bacteria (Hersoug et al. 2016). If the intestinal lining is compromised, LPS can leak into the bloodstream (Manco et al. 2010). Lipopolysaccharide is a potent endotoxin which induces low grade inflammation by triggering innate immune system responses. This leads to a cascade of responses including the expression of pro-inflammatory cytokines that interfere with the modulation of glucose and insulin metabolism (Gonzalez-Quintela et al. 2013). A high-fat diet has been associated with this gut microbiota driven endotoxemia and chronic inflammation (Cani et al. 2007, De Brandt et al. 2011). Mice fed animal lard for 11 weeks showed increased receptor signaling leading to white adipose tissue inflammation through dietary fat interaction with the gut microbiota (Caesar et al. 2015). Plant-based dietary polyphenols (phytonutrients widely distributed in plant foods) have been shown to lower serum inflammatory markers such as tumor necrosis factor (TNF), interleukin (IL-6), and LPS by their modulation and promotion of gut microbial communities that are protective against diet-induced obesity (Roopchand et al 2015).

LINK BETWEEN DIET AND INFLAMMATION

Lifestyle factors such as obesity, physical inactivity, and unhealthy dietary factors have been associated with elevated CRP. Red meat and high dietary fat intake are associated with higher levels of lipopolysaccharide leading to gut barrier disruption and inflammation (Ijssennagger et al 2012, 2015 and Ahola et al 2017). Plant-based diets have been shown to reduce inflammation (Serafini and Peluso 2016, Yeon et al 2012, and Macknin et al 2014). Replacement of red meat with a legume-based diet was shown to significantly lower CRP, TNF, and inflammatory markers in overweight diabetic patients (Hosseinpour-Niazi et al. 2015). In a meta-analysis of the effect of plant-based diets on obesity-related inflammation, consumption of a plant-based diet was associated with a reduction in the mean concentrations of inflammatory biomarkers (Eichelmann et al. 2016). Sutliffe et al. 2015 determined the inflammatory response to a lifestyle intervention including a three-week vegan diet showing a significant improvement in CRP in males consuming a plant-based diet.

The beneficial effects of dietary fiber on CRP has been well documented (Ma et al. 2006, and Ning et al 2014). North et al. found that CRP levels were inversely related to total dietary fiber intake. A seven-day low-fat vegan diet reduced cardiovascular disease event risk by 27% ($p < .001$) in 1,615 participants (McDougall et al. 2014).

Other food parameters influencing inflammation have been described in the Dietary Inflammatory Index (DII) (Shivappa et al. 2014). The DII is a measurement tool created to quantify the effect of diet on inflammation using a scoring system. It was developed utilizing 929 peer-reviewed articles on population-based research investigating the effect of food parameters (dietary nutrients, bioactive food components, and whole foods, including herbs) on inflammatory markers. Food parameters are scored as pro-inflammatory (+1), anti-inflammatory (−1) or (0) if no significant effect occurred (Shivappa et al. 2014). For example, foods that are associated with low levels of inflammation include: berries, cherries, pomegranate, red grapes, grape seed extract, green tea extract, turmeric, ginger, pineapple, black currant, plums, olive oil, and citrus juice (Serafini and Peluso 2016). In a randomized control trial, adherence to a vegan and vegetarian diet resulted in improvements in DII score compared to a semi-vegetarian diet (Turner-McGrievy et al. 2015).

ROLE OF GLUTEN, PREBIOTICS, AND BUTYRATE IN GUT HEALTH

Recent findings support the role of the gut microbiome early in the development of inflammatory disorders like celiac disease in genetically predisposed individuals through its early interaction with the host environment and gluten exposure.

However, it should be noted that of the 30-40% of individuals predisposed to celiac disease, only 2-5% actually develop the condition. Reduced abundance of bifidobacteria has been linked to celiac disease (Sanz 2015). In fact, human milk oligosaccharides and prebiotic compounds found in breast milk promote bifidobacteria and establish a healthy infant gut, protected from pathogens that could cause an imbalance in gut microflora and trigger celiac disease expression (Sanz 2015; and Andreas et al. 2015).

Confusion over the difference between gluten consumption and celiac disease has led to controversies surrounding the consumption of wheat, the main dietary source of not only gluten, but fiber and prebiotic inulin, all of which stimulate the promotion of host-protective bifidobacteria throughout the lifecycle. The effect of a gluten-free diet on gut microbiota and immunity in healthy adults resulted in a significant decrease in the relative abundance of beneficial Bifidobacterium from 11.14% to 5.12%, while gram negative pathogenic *E. coli* and Enterobacteriacceae increased (De Palma et al 2009).

CONCLUSION

An impressive body of evidence-based research provides support for a whole food plant-based diet to develop and sustain a healthy diverse gut microbiome and immune system. Plants provide the necessary substrates of dietary fiber and prebiotics for gut microbial fermentation to produce butyrate which nourishes the colon epithelial cells and helps maintain gut barrier integrity. The anti-inflammatory properties of butyrate prevent high-fat diet-induced dysbiosis and chronic inflammation. Both a high-fat diet and lack of adequate dietary fiber and prebiotics results in the reduction in predominating beneficial microbiota and an increase in pathogenic bacteria. This leads to dysbiosis, gut permeability, the release of pro-inflammatory endotoxins, inflammation, and disease.

REFERENCES

Abbaspour, Nazanin, Richard Hurrell, and Roya Kelishadi. 2014. Review on iron and its importance for human health. *J Res Med SciOff J Isfahan Univ Med Sci* 19 (2): 164.

Ahola, A.J., M.I. Lassenius, C. Forsblom, V. Harjutsalo, et al. 2017. Dietary patterns reflecting healthy food choices are associated with lower serum LPS activity. *Sci Rep* Jul 26 7 (1): 6511.

Aleksandrowicz, Lukasz, Rosemary Green, Edward J.M. Joy, Pete Smith, and Andy Haines. 2016. The impacts of dietary change on greenhouse gas emissions, land use, water use, and health: A systematic review. *PloS one* 11 (11): e0165797.

Andreas N.J., B. Kampmann, and K M Le-Doare. 2015. Human breast milk: A review on its composition and bioactivity. *Early Human Develop* 91: 629–35.

Appleby, P., A. Roddam, N. Allen, and T. Key. 2007. Comparative fracture risk in vegetarians and nonvegetarians in EPIC-Oxford. *Eur J Clin Nutr* 61 (12): 1400–1406.

Appleby, P.N., M. Thorogood, K. McPherson, and J.I. Mann. 1995. Associations between plasma lipid concentrations and dietary, lifestyle and physical factors in the Oxford Vegetarian Study. *J Human Nutr Diet Off J B Diet Assoc* 8 (5): 305–314.

Azadbakht L., P.J. Surkan, A. Esmaillzadeh, and W.C. Willett. 2011. The dietary approaches to stop hypertension eating plan affects C-reactive protein, coagulation abnormalities, and hepatic function tests among type 2 diabetic patients. *J Nutr* 141 (6): 1083–88.

Barnard, Neal D., Susan M. Levin, and Yoko Yokoyama. 2015. A systematic review and meta-analysis of changes in body weight in clinical trials of vegetarian diets. *J Acad Nutr Diet* 115 (6): 954–969.

Baudry, Julia, Mathilde Touvier, Benjamin Allès, Sandrine Péneau, Caroline Méjean, Pilar Galan, Serge Hercberg, Denis Lairon, and Emmanuelle Kesse-Guyot. 2016. Typology of eaters based on conventional and organic food consumption: Results from the NutriNet-Santé Cohort Study. *B J Nutr* 116 (4): 700–709.

Buettner, Dan. 2015. *The Blue Zones Solution: Eating and Living Like the World's Healthiest People*. Washington, DC: National Geographic Society.

Buettner, D., and S. Skemp. 2016. Blue Zones: Lessons from the world's longest lived. *Am J Lifestyle Med* 10 (5): 318–321.

Burlingame, Barbara. 2012. Sustainable diets and biodiversity: Directions and solutions for policy, research and action. *Proc Int Sci Symp Biodiver Sustain Diet United Against Hunger*, November 3–5, 2010, FAO Headquarters, Rome.

Caesar R., V. Tremaroli, P. Kovatcheva-Datchary, P.D. Cani, and F. Backhed. 2015. Crosstalk between gut microbiota and dietary lipids aggravates WAT inflammation through TLR signaling. *Cell Metabol* Oct 6 22: 658–68.

Cani P.D., J. Amar, M.A. Iglesias, M. Poggi, et al. 2007. Metabolic endotoxemia initiates obesity and insulin resistance. *Diabetes* Jul 56: 1761–72.

Carlsen, M.H., B.L. Halvorsen, K. Holte, et al. 2010. The total antioxidant content of more than 3100 foods, beverages, spices, herbs and supplements used worldwide. *Nutr J* http://www.nutritionj.com/content/9/1/3.

Cho, Susan S., Lu Qi, George C. Fahey, and David M. Klurfeld. 2013. Consumption of cereal fiber, mixtures of whole grains and bran, and whole grains and risk reduction in type 2 diabetes, obesity, and cardiovascular disease. *Am J Clin Nutr*: ajcn–067629.

Clarys, Peter, Tom Deliens, Inge Huybrechts, Peter Deriemaeker, Barbara Vanaelst, Willem De Keyzer, Marcel Hebbelinck, and Patrick Mullie. 2014. Comparison of nutritional quality of the vegan, vegetarian, semi-vegetarian, pesco-vegetarian and omnivorous diet. *Nutrients* 6 (3): 1318–1332.

Clemens, R., S. Kranz, A.R. Mobley, T.A. Nicklas, M.P. Raimondi, J.C. Rodriguez, J.L. Slavin, and H. Warshaw. 2012. Filling America's fiber intake gap: Summary of a roundtable to probe realistic solutions with a focus on grain-based foods. *J Nutr* 142 (7): 1390S–1401S.

Dahl, Wendy J., and Maria L. Stewart. 2015. Position of the academy of nutrition and dietetics: Health implications of dietary fiber. *J Acad Nutr Diet* 115 (11): 1861–1870.

Dahl, W.J. et al. 2015. Position of the academy of nutrition and dietetics: Health implications of dietary fiber. *J Acad Nutr Diet*Nov 115 (11): 1861–1870.

Davey, Gwyneth K., Elizabeth A. Spencer, Paul N. Appleby, Naomi E. Allen, Katherine H. Knox, and Timothy J. Key. 2003. EPIC–Oxford: Lifestyle characteristics and nutrient intakes in a cohort of 33 883 meat-eaters and 31 546 non meat-eaters in the UK. *Public Health Nutrition* 6 (3). doi:10.1079/phn2002430.

David L.A., C.F. Maurice, R.N. Carmody, D.B. Gootenberg, et al. 2014. Diet rapidly and reproducibly alters the human gut microbiome. *Nature* 505: 559–63.

De Bandt J.P., A.J. Waligora-Dupriet, and M.J. Butel. 2011. Intestinal microbiota in inflammation and insulin resistance: Relevance to humans. *Curr Op Clin Nutr Metabol Care* 14: 334–340.

De Filippo, C., D. Cavalieri, M. Di Paola et al. 2010. Impact of diet in shaping gut microbiota revealed by a comparative study in children from Europe and rural Africa. *Proc Natl Acad Sci USA* 107: 14691–14696.

De Lorenzo, A., S. Bernardini, P. Gualtieri, et al. 2017. Mediterranean meal versus Western meal effects on postprandial ox-LDL, oxidative and inflammatory gene expression in healthy subjects: A randomized controlled trial for nutrigenomic approach in cardio-metabolic risk. *Acta Diabetol* 54: 141–149.

De Palma, G., I. Nadal, M.C. Collado, Y. Sanz. 2009. Effects of a gluten-free diet on gut microbiota and immune function in healthy adult human subjects. *B J Nutr* 102: 1154–1160.

Desai, M.S., A.M. Seekatz, N.M. Koropatkin, N. Kamada, et al. 2016. A dietary fiber-deprived gut microbiota degrades the colonic mucus barrier and enhances pathogen susceptibility. *Cell*. November 17 167 (5): 1339–53.

Dinu, Monica, Rosanna Abbate, Gian Franco Gensini, Alessandro Casini, and Francesco Sofi. 2016. Vegetarian, vegan diets and multiple health outcomes: A systematic review with meta-analysis of observational studies. *Crit Rev Food Sci Nutr*, February.

doRosario V.A., R. Fernandes, E.B.S. deTrindade. 2016. Vegetarian diets and gut microbiota: Important shifts in markers of metabolism and cardiovascular disease. *Nutr Rev*. 74(7): 444–454.

Eichelmann, F., L. Schwingshackl, V. Fedirko, K. Aleksandrova. 2016. Effect of plant-based diets on obesity-related inflammatory profiles: A systematic review and meta-analysis of intervention trials. *Obes Rev* Nov 17: 1067–1079.

Eshel, Gidon, and Pamela A. Martin. 2009. Geophysics and nutritional science: Toward a novel, unified paradigm. *Am J Clin Nutr* 89 (5): 1710S–1716S.

Eshel, Gidon, Alon Shepon, Tamar Makov, and Ron Milo. 2014. Land, irrigation water, greenhouse gas, and reactive nitrogen burdens of meat, eggs, and dairy production in the United States. *Proc Nat Acad Sci USA* 111 (33): 11996–12001.

Eshel, Gidon, Alon Shepon, Elad Noor, and Ron Milo. 2016. Environmentally optimal, nutritionally aware beef replacement plant-based diets. *Environ Sci Technol* 50 (15): 8164–8168.

FAO – Committee on Agriculture. 1999. http://www.fao.org/unfao/bodies/COAG/COAG15/X0075E.htm#P99_8218 (Accessed June 26, 2017).

Farmer, Bonnie, Brian T. Larson, Victor L. Fulgoni, Alice J. Rainville, and George U. Liepa. 2011. A vegetarian dietary pattern as a nutrient-dense approach to weight management: An analysis of the national health and nutrition examination survey 1999–2004. *J Am Diet Assoc* 111 (6): 819–827.

Felker, Peter, Ronald Bunch, and Angela M. Leung. 2016. Concentrations of thiocyanate and goitrin in human plasma, their precursor concentrations in brassica vegetables, and associated potential risk for hypothyroidism. *Nutr Rev* 74 (4): 248–258.

Fenwick, G. Roger, Robert K. Heaney, W. John Mullin, and Cecil H. VanEtten. 1983. Glucosinolates and their breakdown products in food and food plants. *CRC Crit Rev Food Sci Nutr* 18 (2): 123–201.

Flint H.J., K.P. Scott, P. Louis, S.H. Duncan. 2012. The role of the gut microbiota in nutrition and health. *Nat Rev Gastroenterol Hepatol* 9: 577–589.

Freeman, S., J. Garcia, and H.R. Marston. 2013. Centenarian self-perceptions of factors responsible for attainment of extended health and longevity. *Educ Gerontol* 39 (10): 717–728.

Hallström, Elinor, Carlsson-Kanyam Annika, and Pål Börjesson. 2015. Environmental impact of dietary change: A systematic review. *J Clean Prod* 91: 1–11.

Glick-Bauer M., M.C. Yeh. 2014. The health advantage of a vegan diet: Exploring the gut microbiota connection. *Nutrients* 6: 4822 4838.

Gonzalez-Quintela A., M. Alonso, J. Campos, L. Vizcaino, L. Loidi, F. Gude. 2013. Determinants of serum concentrations of lipopolysaccharide binding protein in the adult population: The role of obesity. *PLOS One* 8 (1): e54600.

Haro, C., S. Garcia-Carpintero, J.F. Alcala-Diaz, F. Gomez-Delgado, et al. 2016. The gut microbial community in metabolic syndrome patients is modified by diet. *J Nutr Biochem* Jan 27: 27–31.

Hersoug, L.G., P. Moller, and S. Loft. 2016. Gut microbiota-derived lipopolysaccharide uptake and trafficking to adipose tissue: Implications for inflammation and obesity. *Obes Rev* Apr 17 (4): 297–312.

Hever, Julieanna. 2016. Plant-based diets: A physician's guide. *Permanente J*. doi:10.7812/tpp/15-082.

HHS, Office of Disease Prevention and Health Promotion (U.S.), and Center for Nutrition Policy Promotion (U.S.) ̇USDA. 2015. *Dietary Guidelines for Americans 2015–2020*. Government Printing Office.

Holscher, H.D.. 2017. Dietary fiber and prebiotics and the gastrointestinal microbiota. *Gut Microbes* 8 (2): 172–184.

Hosseinpour-Niazi, S., P. Mirmiran, A.F. Fallah-Ghohroudi, and F. Azizi. 2015. Non-soya legume-based therapeutic lifestyle change diet reduces inflammatory status in diabetic patients: A randomized cross-over clinical trial. *B J Nutr* 114: 213–219.

Hu, F.B. 2003. Plant-based foods and prevention of cardiovascular disease: An overview. *Am J Clin Nutr* Sept 78 (3 Suppl): 544S–551S.

Huang, Ru-Yi, Chuan-Chin Huang, Frank B. Hu, and Jorge E. Chavarro. 2016. Vegetarian diets and weight reduction: A meta-analysis of randomized controlled trials. *J Gen Inter Med* 31 (1): 109–116.

Hunt, Janet R., and Zamzam K. Roughead. (2000). Adaptation of iron absorption in men consuming diets with high or low iron bioavailability. *Am J Clin Nutr* 71 (1): 94–102.

Ijssennagger, N., M. Derrien, G.M. van Doorn, and A. Rijnierse, et al. 2012. Dietary heme alters microbiota DND mucosa of mouse colon without functional changes in host-microbe cross-talk. *PLOS One* Dec 7 (12): 1–10.

Ijssennagger N., C. Belzer, G.J. Hooiveld, J. Dekker, et al. 2015. Gut microbiota facilitates dietary heme-induced epithelial hyperproliferation by opening the mucus barrier in colon. *PNAS* Aug 11 112 (32): 10038–10043.

Institute of Medicine (US) Panel on Micronutrients. 2001. Dietary reference intakes for vitamin A, vitamin K, Arsenic, Boron, Chromium, Copper, Iodine, Iron, Manganese, Molybdenum. Washington (DC): National Academies Press (US) Bookshelf ID: NBK222310 PMID: 25057538 DOI: 10.17226/10026

Johansson, Eva, Abrar Hussain, Ramune Kuktaite, Staffan C. Andersson, and Marie E. Olsson. 2014. Contribution of organically grown crops to human health. *Int J Environ Res Public Health* 11 (4): 3870–3893.

Kaput, J., and R.L. Rodriguez. 2004. Nutritional genomics: the next frontier in the postgenomics era. *Physiol Genomics* 16: 166–177.

Kelly G. Inulin-type prebiotics – A review: Part 1. *Alternat Med Rev* 2008; 13 (4): 315-29.

Kennedy, E.T., S.A. Bowman, J.T. Spence, et al. 2001. Popular diets: Correlation to health, nutrition, and obesity. *J Am Diet Assoc* 101: 411–420.

Kim, K.A., W. Gu, I.A. Lee, E.H. Joh, and D.H. Kim. 2012. High fat diet-induced gut microbiota exacerbates inflammation and obesity in mice via the TLR4 signaling pathway. *PLOS One* Oct 7 (10): 1–11.

Klinder, A, Q. Shen, S. Heppel, J.A. Lovegrove, I. Rowland, K.M. Tuohy. 2016. Impact of increasing fruit and vegetables and flavonoid intake on the human gut microbiota. *Food Funct*. 7: 1788–1796.

Lawrence, D.A., C.F. Maurice, R.N. Carmody, D.B. Gootenberg et al. 2014. Diet rapidly and reproducibly alters the human gut microbiome. *Nature* Jan 505: 559–563.

Le, Lap Tai, and Joan Sabaté. 2014. Beyond meatless, the health effects of vegan diets: Findings from the adventist cohorts. *Nutrients* 6 (6): 2131–2147.

Lea, E.J., D. Crawford, and A. Worsley. 2006. Public views of the benefits and barriers to the consumption of a plant-based diet. *Eur J Clin Nutr* 60 (7): 828–837.

Leung, Angela M., Andrew Lamar, Xuemei He, Lewis E. Braverman, and Elizabeth N. Pearce. 2011. Iodine status and thyroid function of Boston-area vegetarians and vegans. *J Clin Endocrinol Metabol* 96 (8): E1303–E1307.

Ley, Sylvia H., Osama Hamdy, Viswanathan Mohan, and Frank B. Hu. 2014. Prevention and management of type 2 diabetes: Dietary components and nutritional strategies. *Lancet* 383 (9933): 1999–2007.

Liu, R.H. 2013. Dietary bioactive compunds and thire health implications. *J Food Sci* 78 (S1): A18–A25.

Louis, P., and H.J. Flint. 2017. Formation of propionate and butyrate by the human colonic microbiota. *Environ Microbiol* 19 (1): 29–41.

Lu, Chensheng, Kathryn Toepel, Rene Irish, Richard A. Fenske, Dana B. Barr, and Roberto Bravo. 2006. Organic diets significantly lower children's dietary exposure to organophosphorus pesticides. *Environ Health Perspectives* 114. (2): 260.

Lumeng, C.N., and A.R. Saltiel. 2011. Inflammatory links between obesity and metabolic disease. *J Clin Invest* Jun 212 (6): 2111–2117.

Ma, Y., J.A. Griffith, L. Chasan-Taber, B.C. Olendzk, et al. 2006. Association between dietary fiber and serum C-reactive protein. *Am J Clin Nutr* Apr 83(4): 760–66.

Macfarlane, G.T., and S. Macfarlane. 2011. Fermentation in the human large intestine: Its physiologic consequences and the potential contribution of prebiotics. *J Clin Gastroenterol* Nov 45: S120–S127.

Macknin, M., T. Kong, A. Weier, S. Worley, et al. 2015. Plant-based, no-added-fat or American heart association diets: Impact on cardiovascular risk in obese children with hypercholesterolemia and their parents. *J Peds* 166 (4): 953–959.

Manco, M., L. Putignani, and G.F. Bottozzo. 2010. Gut microbiota lipopolysaccharide and innate immunity in the pathogenesis of obesity & CVD risk. *Endocr Rev* Dec 31(6): 817–844.

Mansour, Sameeh A., Mohamed H. Belal, Asem A.K. Abou-Arab, Hany M. Ashour, and Marwa F. Gad. 2009. Evaluation of some pollutant levels in conventionally and organically farmed potato tubers and their risks to human health. *Food Chem Toxicol* 47 (3): 615–624.

Martin, Cathie, Yang Zhang, Chiara Tonelli, and Katia Petroni. 2013. Plants, diet, and health. *Ann Rev Plant Biol* 64 (1): 19–46.

Martin-Pelaez, S., O. Castaner, V. Konstantinidou, et al. 2017. Effect of olive oil phenolic compounds on the expression of blood pressure-related genes in healthy individuals. *Ur Nutr* 56: 663–670.

McDougall, J., L.E. Thomas, C. McDougall, G. Moloney, et al. 2014. Effects of 7 days on an ad libitum low-fat vegan diet: The McDougall Program cohort. *Nutr J* 13 (99): 1–7.

McMacken, M., and S. Shah. 2017. A plant-based diet for the prevention and treatment of type 2 diabetes. *J Geriatr Cardiol* 14: 342–354.

McOrist, A.L., R.B. Miller, A.R. Bird, J.B. Keogh, et al. 2011. Fecal butyrate levels vary widely among individuals but are usually increased by a diet high in resistant starch. *J Nutr* 141: 883–889.

Melina, Vesanto, Winston Craig, and Susan Levin. 2016. Position of the academy of nutrition and dietetics: Vegetarian diets. *J Acad Nutr Diet* 116 (12): 1970–1980.

Micha, R., G. Michas, and D. Mozaffarian. 2012. Unprocessed red and processed meats and risk of coronary artery disease and type 2 diabetes – An updated review of the evidence. *Curr Atheroscler Rep* Dec 14 (6): 515–524.

Mierziak, Justyna, Kamil Kostyn, and Anna Kulma. 2014. Flavonoids as important molecules of plant interactions with the environment. *Molecules* 19 (10): 16240–16265.

Millen, Barbara E., Steve Abrams, Lucile Adams-Campbell, Cheryl Am Anderson, J. Thomas Brenna, Wayne W. Campbell, Steven Clinton, et al. 2016. The 2015 dietary guidelines advisory committee scientific report: Development and major conclusions. *Adv Nutr* 7 (3): 438–444.

Morrison, D.J., and T. Preston. 2016. Formation of short chain fatty acids by the gut microbiota and their impact on human metabolism. *Gut Microbes* 7 (3): 189–200.

Mozaffarian, D., T. Hao, E.B. Rimm, W.C. Willett, and F.B. Hu. 2011. Changes in diet and lifestyle and long-term weight gain in women and men. *New Eng J Med* 364 (25): 2392–2404.

Murphy, M.M., J.S. Douglass, A. Birkett. 2008. Resistant starch intakes in the United States. *J Am Diet Assoc* Jan 108: 67–78.

Myung, Seung-Kwon.. 2012. Efficacy of Omega-3 fatty acid supplements (Eicosapentaenoic acid and docosahexaenoic acid) in the secondary prevention of cardiovascular disease. *Arch Inter Med* 172 (9): 686.

Nair, Rathish, and Arun Maseeh. 2012. Vitamin D: The "sunshine" vitamin. *J Pharmacol Pharmacotherap* 3 (2): 118.

Ning, H., L. Van Horn, C.M. Shay, D.M. Lloyd-Jones. 2014. Associations of dietary fiber intake with long-term predicted cardiovascular risk and C-reactive protein levels (from the National Health and Nutrition Examination Survey Data [2005-2010]). *Am J Cardiol* Jan 15 113(2): 287–291.

Norris, Jack, and Virginia Messina. 2011. *Vegan for Life: Everything You Need to Know to Be Healthy and Fit on a Plant-Based Diet*. Boston, MA: Da Capo Lifelong Books.

North, C.J., C.S. Venter, J.C. Jerling. 2009. The effects of dietary fibre on C-reactive protein, an inflammation marker predicting cardiovascular disease. *Eur J Clin Nutr* Aug 63(8): 921–933.

O'Leary, Fiona, and Samir Samman. 2010. Vitamin B_{12} in health and disease. *Nutrients* 2 (3): 299–316.

Orlich, Michael J., Karen Jaceldo-Siegl, Joan Sabaté, Jing Fan, Pramil N. Singh, and Gary E. Fraser. 2014. Patterns of food consumption among vegetarians and non-vegetarians. *B J Nutr* 112 (10): 1644–1653.

Pandey, S., P.J. Cabot, N. Shaw, et al. 2016. Anti-inflammatory and immunomodulatory properties of Carica papaya. *J Immunotoxicol* 13 (4): 590–602.

Paul, B.P., S. Barnes, W. Denmark-Wahnefried, C. Morrow, et al. 2015. Influences of diet and the gut microbiome on epigenetic modulation in cancer and other diseases. *Clin Epigenetics* 7: 112.

Petersen, Sesilje B., Morten A. Rasmussen, Marin Strøm, Thorhallur I. Halldorsson, and Sjurdur F. Olsen. 2013. Sociodemographic characteristics and food habits of organic consumers – A study from the Danish National Birth Cohort. *Public Health Nutr* 16 (10): 1810–1819.

Pimentel, David, Paul Hepperly, James Hanson, David Douds, and Rita Seidel. 2005. Environmental, energetic, and economic comparisons of organic and conventional farming systems. *BioScience* 55 (7): 573–582.

Poulain, M., A. Herm, and G. Pes. 2013. The Blue Zones: areas of exceptional longevity around the world. *Vienna Yearb Popul Res* 11: 87–108. http://jstor.org/stable/43050798.

Rahal, A., A. Kumar, V. Singh, B. et al. 2014. Oxidative stress, prooxidants, and antioxidants: The interplay. *Biomed Res Int.* http://dx.doi.org/10.1155/2014/761264.

Ranganathan, Janet, Daniel Vennard, Richard Waite, Patrice Dumas, Brian Lipinski, and T. Searchinger. 2016. *Shifting Diets for a Sustainable Food Future*. Washington, DC: World Resources Institute.

Reuben, Suzanne H. 2010. *Reducing Environmental Cancer Risk: What We Can Do Now*. Collingdale, PA: DIANE Publishing.

Ridker PM. 2003. Clinical application of C-reactive protein for cardiovascular disease detection and prevention. *Circulation* Jan 28 107 (3): 363–369.

Riviere, A, M. Selak, D. Lantin, F. Leroy, and L. DeVuyst. 2016. Bifidobacteria butyrate-producing colon bacteria: Importance and strategies for their stimulation in the human gut. *Front Microbiol* Jun 7 (979): 1–21.

Rizos, Evangelos C., Evangelia E. Ntzani, Eftychia Bika, Michael S. Kostapanos, and Moses S. Elisaf. 2012. Association between Omega-3 fatty acid supplementation and risk of major cardiovascular disease events: A systematic review and meta-analysis. *JAMA: J Am Med Asso* 308 (10): 1024–1033.

Rizzo, Nico S., Karen Jaceldo-Siegl, Joan Sabate, and Gary E. Fraser. 2013. Nutrient profiles of vegetarian and nonvegetarian dietary patterns. *J Acad Nutr Diet* 113 (12): 1610–1619.

Roberfroid, M.B.. 2007. Inulin-type fructans: Functional food ingredients. *B J Nutr* 137: 2493–2502.

Roopchand, D.E., R.N. Carmody, P. Kuhn, K. Moskal, P. Rojas-Silva, P.J. Turnbaugh, I. Raskin. 2015. Dietary polyphenols promote growth of the gut bacterium akkermansia muciniphila and attenuate high-fat diet-induced metabolic syndrome. *Diabetes* 64: 2847–2858.

Sabate, J., and M. Wien. 2010. Vegetarian diets and childhood obesity prevention. *Am J Clin Nutr* 91 (5): 1525S–1529S.

Sanz, Y.. 2015. Microbiome and Gluten. *Ann Nutr Metab* 67 (suppl 2): 28–41.

Scarborough, Peter, Paul N. Appleby, Anja Mizdrak, Adam D.M. Briggs, Ruth C. Travis, Kathryn E. Bradbury, and Timothy J. Key. 2014. Dietary greenhouse gas emissions of meat-eaters, fish-eaters, vegetarians and vegans in the UK. *Climatic Change* 125 (2): 179–192.

Schachter, F., L. Faure-Delanef, F. Guernot, et al. 1994. Genetic associations with human longevity at the APOE and ACE loci. *Nat Genet* 6: 29–32.

Scott, K.P., J.C. Martin, S.H. Duncan, H.J. Flint. 2014. Prebiotic stimulation of human colonic butyrate-producing bacteria and bifidobacteria, in vitro. *FEMS Microbiol Ecol* 87: 30–40.

Serafini, M., and Peluso H. Functional. 2016. Foods for health: The interrelated antioxidant and anti-inflammatory role of fruits, vegetables, herbs, spices and cocoa in humans. *Curr Pharm Des* 22L6701–6715.

Sheflin, A.M., C.L. Melby, F. Carbonero, and T.L. Weir. 2017. Linking dietary patterns with gut microbial composition and function. *Gut Microbes* Mar 4 8 (2): 113–129.

Shivappa, N., S.E. Steck, T.G. Hurley, J.R. Hussey, and J.R. Hebert. 2014. Designing and developing a literature-derived, population-based dietary inflammatory index. *Public health Nutr* Aug 17 (8): 1689–1696.

Simpson, H.L., and B.J. Campbell. 2015. Review article: Dietary fibre-microbiota interations. *Aliment Pharmacol Ther* 42: 158–179.

Slavin J., Fiber. 2013. Prebiotics: Mehanisms and health benefits. *Nutrients* Apr 5 (4): 1417–1435.

Sobiecki, Jakub G., Paul N. Appleby, Kathryn E. Bradbury, and Timothy J. Key. 2016. High compliance with dietary recommendations in a cohort of meat eaters, fish eaters, vegetarians, and vegans: Results from the European prospective investigation into cancer and nutrition–Oxford study. *Nutr Res* 36 (5): 464–477.

Sutliffe, J.T., L.D. Wilson, H.D. de Heer, R.L. Foster, and M.J. Carnot. 2015. C-reactive protein response to a vegan lifestyle intervention. *Complement Therap Med* 23: 32–37.

Tan, S.P., T.C. Kha, S.E. Parks, et al. 2016. Bitter melon (Momordica charantia L.) bioactive composition and health benefits: A review. *Food Rev Int* 32 (2): 181–202.

Thomas, Robert, Elizabeth Butler, Fabio Macchi, and Madeine Williams. 2015. Phytochemicals in cancer prevention and management? *BJMP* 8 (2): a815.

Trichopoulou, A., E. Vasilopoulou, P. Hollman, et al. 2000. Nutritional composition and flavonoid content of edible wild greens and green pies: A potential rich source of antioxidants in the Mediterranean diet. *Food Chem* 70: 319–323.

Turner-McGrievy, G.M., M.D. Wirth, N. Shivappa, E.E. Wingard, et al. 2015. Randomization
to plant-based dietary approaches leads to larger short-term improvements in Dietary
Inflammatory Index scores and macronutrient intake compared with diets that contain
meat. *Nutr Res* 35: 97–106.

Tuso, Philip J., Mohamed H. Ismail, Benjamin P. Ha, and Carole Bartolotto. (2013). Nutritional
update for physicians: Plant-based diets. *Permanente J* 17 (2): 61.

U.S. Department of Agriculture, Agricultural Marketing Service. 2000. National organic
rogram; Final Rule, 7 CFR Part 205. *Federal Register*, Dec 21. www.usda.gov/nop.

Walter, J., and R. Ley. 2011. The human gut microbiome: Ecology and recent evolutionary
changes. *Annu Rev Microbiol* 65: 411–429.

Wang, Fenglei, Jusheng Zheng, Bo Yang, Jiajing Jiang, Yuanqing Fu, and Duo Li. 2015.
Effects of vegetarian diets on blood lipids: A systematic review and meta-analysis of
randomized controlled trials. *J Am Heart Ass* 4 (10): e002408.

Watanabe, F. 2007. Vitamin B12 sources and bioavailability. *Exp Biol Med* 232: 1266–1274.

Weaver, Connie M., William R. Proulx, and Robert Heaney. 1999. Choices for achieving
adequate dietary calcium with a vegetarian diet. *Am J Clin Nutr* 70 (3): 543s–548s.

World Health Organization. 2011. Global Status Report on Noncommunicable Diseases
2010. Italy ISBN 978-92-4-156422-9

Yeon, J.Y., H.S Kim, and M.K. Sung. 2012. Diets rich in fruits and vegetables suppress blood
biomarkers of metabolic stress in overweight women. *Prev Med* 54: S109–S115.

Zimmer, J., B. Lange, J.S. Frick, H. Sauer, H. Zimmermann, et al. 2012. A vegan or vegetarian diet substantially alters the human colonic faecal microbiota. *Eur J Clin Nutr* 66:
53–60.

16 Redefining Medical Practice with Lifestyle Medicine and Environmental Care

Saray Stancic

CONTENTS

16.1 INTRODUCTION: FROM INFECTIONS TO INFARCTS

In 1900, the average American could expect to live around 47 years (Linder and Grove 1947) with global estimates fairing far worse, averaging somewhere around 31 years of age (Roser 2017). Notably, the Centers for Disease Control (CDC) at the time reported the top three causes of death were consequences of an infectious disease: Pneumonia, tuberculosis, and diarrhea (Linder and Grove 1947). Public health measures were instituted to address this devastating infectious disease epidemic and during the latter half of the 20th century we witnessed remarkable advances in modern medicine with the development of vaccines, anti-infectives, improved hygiene—all of which contributed to a sharp decrease in mortality rates and extended life expectancy. The successful global eradication of small pox in 1977 which began 10 years earlier as a World Health Organization (WHO) initiative, serves as an exceptional example of the potential of the scientific community (Centers for Disease Control and Prevention 2016). To fully comprehend the enormity of this accomplishment, approximately 375 million individuals were lost to smallpox from 1900 to 1978 and since that time not one life has been lost, which is accredited to an effective vaccination campaign (Nabel 2013).

Within a few short years of this stellar public health victory, the CDC detailed a narrative of five cases of *Pneumocystis* pneumonia in homosexual men living

TABLE 16.1
Evolution from Infections to Infarcts Top Ten Causes of Death in 1900 and 2015

	Leading Causes of Death, 1900	Leading Causes of Death, 2015
1	Pneumonia & influenza	Heart disease
2	Tuberculosis	Cancer
3	Diarrhea, enteritis, & ulceration	Chronic lower respiratory disease
4	Heart disease	Accidents
5	Intracranial lesions of vascular origin	Stroke
6	Nephritis	Alzheimer's disease
7	Accidents	Diabetes
8	Cancer	Pneumonia & influenza
9	Senility	Nephritis
10	Diphtheria	Suicide

Source: Centers for Disease Control and Prevention 2015.

in Los Angeles in 1981, marking what would later be recognized as the beginning of the AIDS epidemic (Centers for Disease Control and Prevention 1981). Less than a decade later, AIDS was recognized as the number one cause of death in men in the United States (U.S.) ages 25–44 with the total number of cases surpassing 750,000 (CDC 2017, CDC 1993). In 1987, Fischl et al. published a study on azidothymidine (AZT), an antiretroviral with apparent efficacy in AIDS patients. This ushered in the era of highly active antiretroviral therapy (HAART) that when coupled with public awareness decreased the incidence and mortality rate due to AIDS (CDC 2017). Today, we have yet to achieve the exceptional accomplishments of the smallpox era in HIV medicine—but it is undoubtedly feasible considering the ongoing international efforts to expunge this viral threat. Table 16.1 delineates and contrasts the leading causes of death in the years 1900 and 2015. Overall, the U.S. has achieved great strides in life expectancy, with the most recent assessment at 78.8 years (Centers for Disease Control and Prevention 2017).

Despite critical advances, infectious diseases remain a significant source of morbidity and mortality across the globe. Infectious diseases are continuously evolving with the seemingly predictable emergence of new threats whether they be *Zika*, *Ebola* or *West Nile*.

16.2   CHRONIC DISEASES

In the 21st century, infectious diseases no longer lead the pack as the most common causes of premature death around the globe. This unfavorable distinction has been relinquished to noncommunicable or chronic diseases. These noncommunicable diseases (NCDs) are comprised primarily of cardiovascular disease (CVD), diabetes, cancer, and chronic respiratory diseases (WHO 2011). Chronic diseases bare responsibility for 70% of deaths worldwide (WHO 2011). In the WHO's 2010 Global Status Report, the authors note, "Noncommunicable diseases are the leading causes of death globally, killing more people each year than all other causes combined." Undoubtedly, these words were carefully chosen to inject a sense of grave urgency. In fact, these diseases are killing us at record rates, and in many cases in the prime of life with a quarter of these deaths occurring before age 60 (WHO 2011).

These global trends are regrettably best exemplified in the U.S. despite spending more money on healthcare than any other country when compared to sixteen other industrialized countries. The U.S. had suboptimal health outcomes for diabetes, heart disease, obesity, chronic lung disease, and disability (Kenneth et al. 2016). Further sounding the alarm, the CDC reports seven of the top ten causes of premature death are chronic diseases (Woolf and Aron 2013) with the top two contributors, heart disease and cancer, accounting for nearly 50% of all U.S. deaths (Centers for Disease Control and Prevention 2017). CVD is the number one cause of death worldwide. In 2015 alone, CVD accounted for 17.7 million deaths or 31% of global mortality (WHO 2017). Additionally, half of the American adults use 86% of national healthcare expenditures ($3.2 trillion dollars in 2015, accounting for 17.8% of Gross Domestic Product) as they are living with at least one costly chronic disease.

Are we now living longer while suffering with chronic diseases? That may be the case. Murray et al. (2015) confirm we are indeed increasing life expectancy—but we are also living more years with illness and disability. This is reflected in the measure described as HALE (Healthy Adjusted Life Expectancy), which takes into account not only the number of years people live but the years lost to premature death and illness or disability. Globally, the U.S. ranked number 49 out of 188 countries in healthy life expectancy. One of the study authors noted, "the U.S. falls behind because of factors such as socioeconomic disparities, poor healthcare access, chronic disease and behavioral risks, including obesity, inactivity, smoking, and drinking" (Yoo 2015).

Obesity is a tremendous threat to human health, fueling chronic illnesses such as CVD, stroke, diabetes, and certain cancers (Eisenberg and Burgess 2015). The CDC's Behavioral Risk Factor Surveillance System (BRFSS) which has been assessing obesity rates since the mid-1980s illustrates this point. In 1990, the BRFSS reported that no state had an obesity prevalence greater than 15%. Just twenty-five years later, that rate has more than doubled with 36.5% of all U.S. adults meeting the definition of obesity. The highest rates of obesity are reported in women ages 40–59 at an alarming rate of 42% as noted in Figure 16.1. In the U.S. today, nearly 71% of Americans are either overweight or obese, leaving those that are of normal weight in the minority (CDC 2016).

Chronic diseases fueled by obesity present devastating health consequences. The CDC has forewarned that if current trends continue, one in three Americans will have diabetes by 2050 (Centers for Medicare and Medicaid Services 2017, Centers for Disease Control and Prevention 2010). This possibility alone serves to threaten the economic viability of our current healthcare system not to mention the burden imposed on the patient. It is now indisputable that prevention and control of these NCDs must become our primary focus.

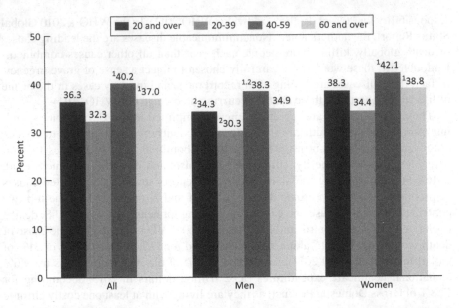

FIGURE 16.1 Prevalence of obesity among adults aged 20 and over, by sex and age: United States, 2011–2014 [1]Significantily different from those ages 20–39. [2]Significantily different from women of the same age group. (Source: From CDC/NCHS, National Health and Nutrition Examination Survey 2011–2014.)

16.3   WHAT IS FUELING THE CHRONIC ILLNESS EPIDEMIC?

In recent years we have gained a clear understanding of the variables impacting our current healthcare dilemma. Nearly a decade apart, both McGinnis et al. (1993) and Mokdad (2000) explored and reported on the root causes leading to premature death, concluding the three most prominent contributors to U.S. mortality were tobacco/smoking, poor dietary behaviors, and sedentary/subpar physical activity patterns (McGinnis et al. 1993, Mokdad 2000). While acknowledging and understanding the root cause is half the battle, we must also act to rectify unhealthy lifestyle behaviors.

Findings from the "European Prospective Investigation Into Cancer and Nutrition—Potsdam Study" assessed the role four healthy lifestyle factors could have in reducing the relative risk of developing a chronic disease. The factors studied were: never smoking; a Body Mass Index (BMI) less than 30 (a BMI of 30 denotes obesity); maintaining 3.5 hours a week of physical activity; and adhering to an ideal dietary pattern, described by the authors as high intake of fruits, vegetables, whole grains, and low meat consumption (Ford et al. 2009). A near 80% lower risk of developing a chronic disease was experienced by those participants who adhered to all four healthy lifestyle behaviors (Ford et al. 2009).

Similar findings were published by Akeeson et al. They reported impressive findings from a prospective cohort of Swedish men concluding adherence to healthy dietary and lifestyle behaviors could prevent four out of five heart attacks (Akeeson et al. 2014). Extrapolating these findings to current global CVD mortality rates equates to preventing approximately 14 million deaths per year.

TABLE 16.2

Top Ten Leading Types of Cancer for Estimated New Cases by Gender United States 2017

Male			Female		
Body System	Number	Percentage	Body System	Number	Percentage
Lung & bronchus	84,590	27	Lung & bronchus	71,280	25
Colon & rectum	27,150	9	Breast	40,610	14
Prostate	26,730	8	Colon & rectum	23,110	8
Pancreas	22,300	7	Pancreas	20,790	7
Liver & intrahepatic bile duct	19,610	6	Ovary	14,080	5
Leukemia	14,300	4	Uterine corpus	10,920	4
Esophagus	12,720	4	Leukemia	10,200	4
Urinary bladder	12,240	4	Liver & intrahepatic bile duct	9,310	3
Non-Hodgkin lymphoma	11,450	4	Non-Hodgkin lymphoma	8,690	3
Brain & other nervous system	9,620	3	Brain & other nervous system	7,080	3
All sites	318,420	100	All sites	282,500	100

Source: Adapted from data from U.S. Cancer Statistics Working Group, Centers for Disease Control and Prevention and National Cancer Institute 2017.

Optimal lifestyle choices extend beyond cardiometabolic disorders. The second most common cause of death is cancer with 600,920 deaths in 2017 (Siegel et al. 2017). Table 16.2 identifies the ten leading cancers in the U.S. by gender in 2017.

Cancer is a NCD also profoundly impacted by lifestyle behaviors. For example, breast cancer, the second leading cause of cancer deaths in American women, is methodically discussed in a revealing perspective piece published in 2015. Colditz and Bohlke conveyed that a substantial portion of breast cancer can be prevented through primary prevention and lifestyle modification with a 49% reduction in risk attributed to healthy dietary and exercise behaviors (Colditz and Bohlke 2015, Emmons and Colditz 2017).

Because we understand what is largely driving NCD rates as well as how to prevent them, we must now apply these findings in the real world setting if we are ever to effectively turn the tide of the destructive path of NCDs. When we know better, we must also do better.

16.4 PROPOSING REFORM TO MEDICAL EDUCATION

The evidenced-based data points to lifestyle choices as the root cause of many chronic diseases. However, are scientists and clinicians aware of the potential benefits of optimal lifestyle choices? The medical community, despite generating these facts, has failed to relay this extraordinary life-saving body of evidence to the general public. "Why?" is the million-dollar question. The answer is no doubt complex and multifaceted. It may be partially explained by the approach to healthcare that can also be described as "sick care" versus preventive care. That is, we wait until a disease entity is out of control instead of working to prevent the chronic disease altogether. Contemporary medical school curricula and residency training programs readily focus on pathogenesis, which is studying the mechanism by which disease is created (Eisenberg and Burgess 2015). In this pathogenesis education model, physicians are trained primarily to expeditiously diagnose (which may entail ordering a series of diagnostic studies) and treat or manage diseases by prescribing interventional strategies such as pharmaceutical medications and/or surgical procedures. In sharp contrast, Eisenberg and Burgess propose a solution by addressing the chronic illness and obesity epidemics by placing *salutogenesis* on par with pathogenesis. Salutogenesis is best defined as the processes by which health is produced and maintained. Eisenberg and Burgess proposed that future curricula include modules on nutrition and diet, exercise, sleep and rest, mindfulness, self-care, and developing superior expertise in counseling patients on behavioral change (Eisenberg and Burgess 2015).

The current day medical education model may have been appropriate for the 20th century and the management of primarily acute illnesses such as infections, but as the healthcare landscape has dramatically shifted we must modify our approach to educating medical professionals in this new millennium. We need to prepare physicians to manage a population burdened with chronic diseases that are largely a consequence of lifestyle choices. Poor dietary choices are chief contributors to chronic diseases. Logically, physicians in training would receive a solid foundation in nutrition education. However, only 27% of U.S. medical schools currently receive the recommended 25 hours of nutrition education (Adams et al. 2010) primarily dedicated to biochemistry, which is not practical for counseling patients on how to eat an optimal diet. Twenty-five hours devoted to nutrition over 4 years of medical school is simply inadequate.

Interestingly, 71% of medical students believe nutrition is clinically relevant upon entering medical school, but by the time they graduate, that number falls below 50% (Spencer et al. 2006). After graduating from medical school only 14% of physicians report they were adequately trained in nutrition (Vetter et al. 2008). The literature strongly supports lifestyle change as a key to reducing the risk of CVD, yet cardiologists have no nutrition requirements during fellowship training (Devries et al. 2014). Hence, the proposed addition of salutogenesis to the pathogenesis model offers a solution—and a physician-led movement now recognized as the practice of *lifestyle medicine*. Lifestyle medicine is an evidence-based discipline whose focus is preventing, treating, and reversing lifestyle-related chronic diseases by educating and empowering patients on the importance of consuming a plant-based diet, exercise, stress management, tobacco and alcohol cessation—as well as other non-drug modalities (American College of Lifestyle Medicine 2015).

16.5 A NEW ERA OF PHYSICIANS WHO ARE COMPETENT IN LIFESTYLE MEDICINE

Modifying lifestyle behaviors can lead to an immeasurable improvement in health outcomes. But how can medical education shift to incorporate lifestyle medicine as the core foundation of physicians today while reshaping the curricula of the next generation of medical doctors (Young et al. 2015)? Importantly, most chronic disease practice guidelines (including hypertension and diabetes management) suggest lifestyle changes as first line of therapy (Chobanian 2003, American Diabetes Association 2010). Yet most physicians in clinical practice do not relay this to their patients (Stafford et al. 2000). Doctors have failed to effectively convey this valuable prescriptive as a consequence of inadequate skills in counseling patients on lifestyle interventions (Huang et al. 2004).

In an effort to correct this lapse in physician education, a group of experts vested in creating change convened to identify solutions. The product of that gathering was summarized in a pivotal commentary published in 2010 in the *Journal of the American Medical Association* (Lianov and Johnson 2010). This paper and committee work spanned over two years with representatives from top medical organizations including the American Medical Association, the American Academy of Family Physicians, the American College of Physicians, the American Academy of Pediatrics, as well as other experts in the field of nutrition and exercise. Five core competencies for primary care physicians were delineated as the foundation of lifestyle medicine which include leadership, knowledge, assessment skills, management skills, and use of office and community support. (Lianov and Johnson 2010).

Arguably, *leadership* may be the most important of these competencies. Those working to create systematic change in the healthcare system must be willing to stand for a new culture which places the promotion of optimal lifestyle choices as the basic foundation of medical care. In order to gain mainstream acceptance, physician leaders must not only be fluent in *knowledge* but eloquent and decisive in the defense and promotion of lifestyle medicine. Next, the acquisition of effective *assessment skills* are needed to convey behavior modification to patients in the clinical setting. This involves understanding the complex interactions of social, biological, and psychological predispositions and tendencies in individual patients. Training healthcare professionals to assess patient readiness for change is a valuable tool and an integral part of lifestyle medicine. *Management* or support during treatment requires the development of a trusting relationship between the doctor and the patient (which may include the patient's family members too). This fosters sustainable and achievable patient outcomes. Finally, the last competency, *use of office and community support*, suggests a lifestyle medicine physician must serve as an exemplary captain on a team of healthcare professionals all working to support an environment that garners healthy behavioral change not only in the workplace, but also in the communities where they reside.

Physicians are gatekeepers within the healthcare system and can be powerful agents to effect changes in healthcare. Physicians need to continue to build bridges, encourage dialogue, and expand dissemination of this critically important, game-changing component of medical care. This will require an exchange of ideas from all stakeholders nationally including medical schools, medical organizations, board certification bodies, policy-makers, etc. Successful outcomes will require the incorporation of lifestyle medicine principles throughout the four years of medical school education and reinforced during residency programs and subspecialty training.

The proposed emphasis on lifestyle medicine does not mean abandoning current advances in medicines, diagnostics, and surgical interventions—all of which are important. But any healthcare service offered that fails to emphasize prevention and health maintenance will ultimately fall short.

Doctors around the country who are disenchanted and disenfranchised within the contemporary healthcare system are redefining the way they practice medicine. This new breed of medical doctors is shifting the focus of the physician visit to prevention via lifestyle modification rather than solely managing symptoms. Numerous innovative and progressive clinical practices across the country are incorporating: Shared patient health visits for efficiency; motivational enterprises such as physician-led walking groups; culinary medicine instruction as described in Chapter 14; and stress management techniques including meditation and yoga. These activities exemplify how the principles of lifestyle medicine can be used in everyday medical practice for improved patient health outcomes.

16.6 CREATING ENVIRONMENTAL SUSTAINABILITY IN MEDICINE

Lifestyle medicine will have to play a large role in the future of medicine if we hope to achieve a sustainable healthcare system. This shift is not only critical for human health but also relevant to planetary sustainability. As described by the 2015 Dietary Guidelines Advisory Committee (U.S. Department of Health and Human Services and U.S. Department of Agriculture 2015), a wholesome diet that minimizes meat intake and includes whole plant foods such as legumes and fresh produce also serves the health of the planet. Regrettably, this information was not included in the *Dietary Guidelines for Americans* because of pressure from a variety of business interests and the complicity of elected officials. As a consequence, the American public does not receive the expert committees' unadulterated, scientifically based recommendations (Nestle 1993, American Meat Institute Foundation 2014, Oldways Common Ground 2015). This is a missed opportunity to broadcast the connections between food choices and environmental degradation.

The industrialized food system contributes to deforestation, water use, and nearly a third of greenhouse gas emissions (Vermeulen et al 2012). Katz et al. remind us that reducing the consumption and production of animal products and replacing them with whole plants foods can simultaneously help to mitigate climate change while concurrently improving human health (Katz et al. 2017). Additionally, Springman et al. estimated that adopting a modest shift towards a plant-based dietary pattern could reduce global mortality by up to 10% and reduce greenhouse gas emissions by as much as 70% by 2050 (Springman et al. 2016). Over 7.3 million deaths could be prevented globally per year with the consumption of a vegetarian diet while over 8 million preventable deaths are associated with a vegan diet (Springman et al. 2016). Beyond the striking health and environmental improvements are the economic benefits, with cost savings as much as $735 billion saved in healthcare costs every year. Hence, health and environmental benefits go hand-in-hand.

The work that needs to be done to reclaim control of the current suboptimal healthcare system is clear. Physicians must charter a new course by engaging the public on all levels through multiple mechanisms and messages. Solutions to the current healthcare crisis are rooted in creating awareness (Tolle 2008).

Public education campaigns, social media, literature, and film are important avenues for delivering information to the masses so to trigger consciousness and promulgate a movement towards change. Recent documentary films have addressed lifestyle medicine for good health including the feature-length film *Forks Over Knives* (Fulkerson 2011). *Code Blue* is yet another film seeking to shed light on critical lapses in the healthcare system and hopes to catalyze the community to demand changes. *Code Blue* will be released towards the end of 2018. Leveraging enthusiasm for healthy lifestyle behaviors among the public coupled with shifts in academia and healthcare practice are key to improving the quality of life of our local and global communities. By instituting prevention in medical practice, physicians can protect and improve planetary health while upholding one of the ideals of the Hippocratic Oath, "I will prevent disease whenever I can, for prevention is preferable to cure."

16.7 CONCLUSION

The chronic disease and obesity epidemics are causing premature deaths and impaired quality of life for millions on a worldwide scale. These epidemics are fueled by poor dietary choices. The deleterious consequences of these harmful diets extend far beyond compromised health outcomes as they yield irreparable damage to the natural environment and create an immense economic burden. A powerful antidote to this destructive path is likely to be the universal adoption of a dietary pattern of whole plant foods and minimizing animal products. This will require a herculean effort on all fronts to catalyze lasting changes that are also socially and culturally acceptable. It is time to create the change required to assure we maintain the health of people now and for the generations that follow—as well as the planet.

VIGNETTE 16.1 Planning and Serving
Plant-Based Meals at Medical Conferences

John Westerdahl

OVERVIEW

Each year there are thousands of medical, nutrition, and other healthcare conferences offered throughout the United States (U.S.) and the world. These meetings range from large annual conferences at major convention centers or hotels with thousands of attendees, to small lunchtime conferences at a local hospital. Ironically, most of the meals, receptions, and break-sessions at these conferences serve foods and beverages that are not healthful (La Puma et al. 2003; Lesser et al. 2012). In fact, many of the foods served at these conferences may even promote the chronic diseases that are being discussed at that meeting. The foods served are often high in total and saturated fat, cholesterol, sugar, processed and refined grains, full-fat dairy products, and meats. Typically, there is little emphasis placed on healthy ingredients such as fruits, vegetables, whole grains, and plant sources of protein. At most big medical conferences, the financial sponsors are often major drug companies or major players in the food industry. Sponsors aim to please by leaving a positive impression on the conference attendees that may include a menu rich in animal products, alcohol, and desserts.

There are only a few medical, nutrition, and other healthcare conferences in the nation that offer plant-based meals and menus. Those conferences that provide 100% plant-based or mostly plant-based menus include the American College of Lifestyle Medicine (ACLM), The Vegetarian Nutrition Dietetic Practice Group (VN DPG) of the Academy of Nutrition and Dietetics, the Plant-Based Prevention of Disease Conference (P-POD), the University of Arizona Nutrition & Health Conference, and Loma Linda University's International Congress on Vegetarian Nutrition.

The ACLM is an organization comprised of health providers (mostly medical doctors) specializing in of lifestyle medicine (ACLM 2018). The ACLM encourages whole food, plant-based diets. As a result, the organization offers health-affirming, whole food, plant-based meals and refreshments at its conferences. This is part of the organization's strategy for educating and offering a plant-based diet experience for medical doctors attending their conferences. The meals have been well received by attendees (Katz 2015). With a growing interest in incorporating disease prevention into medical and healthcare practice, more health organizations can utilize plant-based meals as a teaching tool for food and beverages served at conferences.

SETTING THE PLANT-BASED DIETARY STANDARDS FOR THE HEALTHCARE CONFERENCE

The first step in planning plant-based menus for a conference is to set the dietary standards desired for all the foods to be served at the conference. In the case of the ACLM conferences, an example would be:

1. Only whole, plant-based foods are served; no animal products (no dairy, eggs, or animal flesh—but honey is acceptable).
2. No refined grain products (only whole grains and whole grain products are used).
3. The major emphasis is on a variety of fruits, vegetables, whole grains, legumes/beans, nuts, and seeds.
4. Little or no oil is used in recipes (if used, only healthy plant fats or oils are used such as organic extra virgin olive oil while hydrogenated or partially-hydrogenated fats as well as certain plant fats such as coconut or palm oils are avoided).
5. Only moderate use of salt and sodium-containing seasonings such as organic soy sauce are used; white sugar is avoided while unrefined sugars are used.
6. Alcohol and beverages containing refined sugar are avoided while purified water, 100% fruit juice, fruit smoothies, hot and iced caffeine-free herbal teas, organic apple cider vinegar drinks, coffee, and decaf are served.

PLANNING PLANT-BASED MENUS WITH THE FOODSERVICE STAFF

In most cases, executive chefs and/or the foodservice staff at hotels and conference centers have never prepared plant-based or vegan meals before. However, there are many chefs and staff that embrace the challenge and are enthusiastic about learning these new skills. In fact, chefs and foodservice operations are getting more requests for vegan meals and are eager to increase their repertoire of plant-based recipes (Restaurant Business 2014).

First, review the guidelines and standards with the chef. Identify overt challenges as well as solutions. Secondly, discuss all the plant-based recipes on the menu that already meet the guidelines and use as many of those recipes as possible. After that, add the custom plant-based recipes that are desired. Provide the chef with those plant-based recipes.

There are many quality plant-based resources available today as noted in Figure V16.1.

Vegetarian Nutrition Dietetic Practice Group of the Academy of Nutrition and Dietetics
www.vegetariannutrition.net

Physicians Committee for Responsible Medicine
www.pcrm.org

Vegetarian Resource Group
www.vrg.org

Forks Over Knives
www.forksoverknives.com

BenBella Vegan Books
www.benbellavegan.com

FIGURE V16.1   Plant-Based Recipe Resources

The chef can experiment with them and make the calculations to accommodate the number of people attending the conference. Developing a good rapport and communication with the chef is critical to the success of your plant-based meals. In addition to the health benefits of the plant-based menus, you may also see a cost savings associated with the use of plant-based protein foods, such as beans and legumes that replace red meat, poultry, and fish.

PLANNING FOR SUCCESS

There are two keys principles to the success and acceptance of the plant-based meals served at a conference: (1) The foods served must be visually attractive and colorful. People "eat with their eyes" first. If the foods look attractive, colorful, and appealing, they will be better accepted (The Culinary Institute of America, 1991); and (2) Foods must taste good. To win-over the skeptics, great-tasting foods must be always served. Plant-based buffet meals typically work best as attendees can select the foods of their preference from a variety of options. Examples of successful plant-based foods and meals that can be served at major conferences include:

RECEPTION FOODS

- blueberry and basil bruschetta on toasted baguette
- vegetable spring rolls with sweet chili sauce
- ratatouille stuffed cremini mushroom
- wild mushroom arancini with roasted tomato sauce
- roasted garlic and white bean hummus on cucumbers
- crispy pita with roasted piquillo and garbanzo hummus
- black bean and avocado tarts, assorted fresh fruit and berries, raw vegetable platter with hummus, sparkling apple cider juice, iced caffeine-free herbal tea

BREAKFAST FOODS

- fruit smoothies
- seasonal fresh fruit and berries
- natural nut butters (peanut butter, almond butter) on whole grain breads and whole fruit preserves
- steel cut oats with toppings (walnuts, raisins, cinnamon, dried cranberries, fresh berries)
- vegan granola
- vegan blueberry whole grain pancakes with 100 % natural maple syrup
- scrambled tofu
- quinoa porridge
- vegan breakfast burritos

BREAK TIME FOODS

- make your own trail mix
- assorted raw nuts
- unsweetened dried fruits
- raw vegetable platters with hummus
- purified water

LUNCH FOODS

- salad bar—with varieties of all types of mixed salad greens, kale, etc., and varieties of raw vegetables and beans (kidney beans, black beans, green beans, edamame)
- bulgur wheat salad
- vegan chili
- veggie burgers
- grilled portabella and veggie fajita
- black bean burritos with whole wheat tortillas
- Spanish vegetable stew with herb couscous
- vegan hot tamale
- red quinoa and roasted golden beet salad
- falafel
- split pea with barley soup
- black bean cakes with roasted tomato sauce

- spinach and kale salad
- assorted fresh fruits and berries
- vegan strawberry oat squares
- vegan chocolate black bean brownies

Dinner Banquet—Often a banquet-style plated meal is planned for the last evening of a conference. Here are some examples of items that could be included for such a meal:

- artisan greens with roasted pecans and dried berries with a fat-free berry dressing
- grilled eggplant and zucchini involtini
- roasted root vegetables mash
- roasted tomatoes
- baby vegetables
- three bean succotash
- vegan chocolate almond midnight cake

CONCLUSION

In conclusion, planning plant-based meals for medical conferences enhances the quality of the healthcare conference. They exemplify "leading by example" while emphasizing health and wellness. Beyond the health benefits, savory plant-based meals enhance the culinary experience of conference attendees. If carefully planned, the plant-based meals served become a focal point of the conference with attendees evaluating these meals with high regard that positively enhances the overall conference experience.

REFERENCES

Adams, K. M., M. Kohlmeier, and S. H. Zeisel. 2010. Nutrition education in U.S. medical schools: Latest update of a national survey. *Academic Medicine* 85: 1537–1542.
Åkesson, A., S.C. Larsson, A.Discacciati, and A. Wolk. 2014. Low-Risk diet and lifestyle habits in the primary prevention of myocardial infarction in men. *Journal of the American College of Cardiology* 64 (13): 1299–1306.
American College of Lifestyle Medicine (ACLM). 2018. https://www.lifestylemedicine.org/ (accessed January 15, 2018).
American College of Lifestyle Medicine. 2015. What is lifestyle medicine? https://www.lifestylemedicine.org/What-is-Lifestyle-Medicine.
American Diabetes Association. 2010. Standards of medical care in diabetes—2010. *Diabetes Care* 33 (suppl 1): S11–S61
American Meat Institute Foundation. 2014. Intended testimony of Betsy Booren, Ph.D., Vice President of Scientific Affairs to the Dietary Guidelines Advisory Committee. https://www.meatinstitute.org/index.php?ht=a/GetDocumentAction/i/102945 (Accessed October 7, 2016).
Centers for Disease Control and Prevention. 1981. *Pneumocystis* pneumonia—Los Angeles. *MMWR* 30 (21): 1–3.

Centers for Disease Control and Prevention. 1993. Update: Mortality attributable to HIV infection among persons aged 25–44 Years – United States, 1991 and 1992. *MMWR* 42 (45): 869–872.

Centers for Disease Control and Prevention. 2010. Number of Americans with diabetes projected to double or triple by 2050. Released October 22, 2010. https://www.cdc.gov/media/pressrel/2010/r101022.html.

Centers for Disease Control and Prevention. 2015a. Leading causes of death, 1900–1998. Last modified November 6, 2015. https://www.cdc.gov/nchs/nvss/mortality_historical_data.htm.

Centers for Disease Control and Prevention. 2016a. History of smallpox. Last modified August 2016. https://www.cdc.gov/smallpox/history/history.html.

Centers for Disease Control and Prevention. 2016b. Adult obesity facts. Last modified September 1, 2016. https://www.cdc.gov/obesity/data/adult.html.

Centers for Disease Control and Prevention. 2017a. HIV and AIDS timeline. Last modified January 10, 2017. https://npin.cdc.gov/pages/hiv-and-aids-timeline#1980.

Centers for Disease Control and Prevention. 2017b. Death and mortality. Last modified May 3, 2017. http://www.cdc.gov/nchs/fastats/deaths.htm.

Centers for Disease Control and Prevention. 2017c. Obesity and overweight. Last modified May 3, 2017. https://www.cdc.gov/nchs/fastats/obesity-overweight.htm.

Centers for Disease Control and Prevention. 2017d. Chronic disease overview. Last modified June 28, 2017. https://www.cdc.gov/chronicdisease/overview/index.htm.

Centers for Medicaid and Medicare Services. 2017. NHE fact sheet. Last modified June 14, 2017. https://www.cms.gov/research-statistics-data-and-systems/statistics-trends-and-reports/nationalhealthexpenddata/nhe-fact-sheet.html.

Chobanian, A. V., G. L. Bakris, H. R. Black, W. C. Cushman, L. A. Green, J. L. Izzo, D. W. Jones, B. J. Materson, S. Oparil, J. T. Wright, E. J. Roccella and the National High Blood Pressure Education Program Coordinating Committee. 2003. Seventh Report of the Joint National Committee on preventiond Detection, evaluation, and treatment of high blood pressure. *Hypertension* 42: 1206–1252.

Colditz, G A., and K, Bohlke. 2015. Preventing breast cancer now by acting on what we already know. *NPJ Breast Cancer* 1: 15009. Published online July 22, 2015. doi:10.1038/npjbcancer.2015.9.

Devries, S., J. E. Dalen, D. M. Eisenberg, V. Maizes, D. Ornish, A. Prasad, V. Sierpina, A. T. Weil, and W. Willett. 2014. A deficiency of nutrition education in medical training. *American Journal of Medicine* 127: 804–806.

Eisenberg, D. M., and J. D. Burgess. 2015. Nutrition education in an era of global obesity and diabetes: Thinking outside the box. *Academic Medicine* 90 (7): 854–860.

Emmons, K. M., and G. A. Colditz. 2017. Realizing the potential of cancer prevention – The role of implementation science. *New England Journal of Medicine* 376 (10): 986–970.

Fischl, M. A., D. D. Richman, M. H. Grieco, M. S. Gottlieb, P. A. Volberding, O. L. Laskin, J. M. Leedom, J. E. Groopmen, D. Mildvan, and M. S. Hirsch. 1987. The efficacy of azidothymidine (AZT) in the treatment of patients with AIDS and AIDS-related complex. A double-blind, placebo-controlled trial. *New England Journal of Medicine* 317 (4): 192–197.

Ford, E. S., M. M. Bergmann, J. Kroger, A. Schienkiewitz, C. Weikert, and H. Boeing. 2009. Healthy living is the best revenge. Findings from the European Prospective Investigation into Cancer and Nutrition–Potsdam Study. *Archives of Internal Medicine* 169 (15): 1355–1362.

Fulkerson, L. (Director). 2011. *Forks Over Knives*. United States: Monica Beach Media.

Huang, J., H. Yu, E. Marin, S. Brock, D. Carden, and T. Davis. 2004. Physicians' weight loss counseling in two public hospital primary care clinics. *Academic Medicine* 79 (2): 156–161.

Katz, D., President of the American College of Lifestyle Medicine, personal communication, November 3, 2015.

Katz, D. L., E. P. Frates, J. P. Bonnet, S. K. Gupta, E. Vartiainen, and R. H. Carmona. 2017. Lifestyle as medicine: The case for a true health initiative. *American Journal of Health Promotion*, https://doi.org/10.1177/0890117117705949. First published May 19, 2017.

Kenneth, D., Kochanek, M.A., Sherry, L., Murphy, B.S., Jiaquan, Xu, M.D., and Betzaida Tejada-Vera, M.S. Deaths: Final Data for 2014. National Vital Statistics Reports. Vol. 65(4): June 30, 2016, pp 1–122.

La Puma, J., D. Schiedermayer, and J. Becker. 2003. Meals at medical specialty society annual meetings: a preliminary assessment. *Disease Management* 6 (4):191–197.

Lesser, L. I., D.A. Cohen, and R. H. Brook. 2012. Changing eating habits for the medical profession. *JAMA* 308 (10):983–984.

Lianov, L., and M. Johnson. 2010. Physician competencies for prescribing lifestyle medicine. *JAMA* 304, (2): 202–203.

Linder, F. E., and R. D. Grove. *Vital Statistics Rates in the United States 1900–1940*. Federal Security Agency, United States Public Health Service, National Office of Vital Statistics. Washington, DC: United States Government Printing Office, 1947.

McGinnis, J. M., and W. H. Foege. 1993. Actual causes of death in the United States. *JAMA* 270 (18): 2207–2212.

Mokdad, A. H., J. S. Marks, D. F. Stroup, and J. L. Gerberding. 2004. Actual causes of death in the United States, 2000. *JAMA* 291 (10): 1238–1245.

Murray, C. J. L. and the GBD 2013 DALYs and HALE Collaborators. 2015. Global, regional, and national disability-adjusted life years (DALYs) for 306 diseases and injuries and healthy life expectancy (HALE) for 188 countries, 1990–2013: Quantifying the epidemiological transition. *The Lancet* 386 (10009): 2145–2191.

Nabel, G. J. 2013. Designing tomorrow's vaccines. *New England Journal of Medicine* 368 (6): 551–560.

National Research Council (US), Institute of Medicine (US). Woolf, S.H., and L. Aron (eds.) 2013. *U.S. Health in International Perspective: Shorter Lives, Poorer Health*. Washington, DC: National Academies Press (US), https://www.ncbi.nlm.nih.gov/books/NBK115854/doi: 10.17226/13497.

Nestle, M. 1993. Food lobbies, the food pyramid, and US nutrition policy. *International Journal of Health Services* 23 (3): 483–496.

Oldways Common Ground. 2015. Oldways common ground consensus statement on healthy living. https://oldwayspt.org/programs/oldways-common-ground/oldways-common-ground-consensus (Accessed August 22, 2016).

Restaurant Business. July 13, 2014. Vegetarianism a rising trend on menus. http://www.restaurantbusinessonline.com/food/vegetarianism-rising-trend-menus, (accessed September 24, 2017).

Roser, M. 2017. Life expectancy. *Our World in Data.* https://ourworldindata.org/life-expectancy/

Siegal, R. L., K. D. Miller, and A. Jemal. 2017. Cancer statistics. *CA: A Cancer Journal for Clinicians* 67: 7–30.

Spencer, E. H., E. Frank, L. K. Elon, V. S. Hertzberg, M. K. Serdula, and D. A. Galuska. 2006. Predictors of nutrition counseling behaviors and attitudes in US medical students. *American Journal of Clinical Nutrition* 84: 655–662.

Springmann, M., H. C. Godfray, M. Rayner, and P. Scarborough. 2016. Analysis and valuation of the health and climate change co-benefits of dietary change. *Proceedings of the National Academy of Sciences of the United States of America* 113 (15): 4146–4151.

Stafford R. S., J. H. Farhat, B. Misra, and D. A. Schoenfeld. 2000. National patterns of physician activities related to obesity management. *Archives of Family Medicine* 9 (7): 631–638.

The Culinary Institute of America, 2014. *The New Professional Chef*, Fifth Edition. New York, NY: Van Nostrand Reinhold, p. 46.

Tolle, Eckhart. *A New Earth; Awakening to Your Life's Purpose*. New York: Penguin, 2008.

US Department of Health and Human Services and US Department of Agriculture. 2015. Scientific Report of the 2015 Dietary Guidelines Advisory Committee. https://health. gov/dietaryguidelines/2015-scientific-report/pdfs/scientific-report-of-the-2015-dietary-guidelines-advisory-committee.pdf (Accessed June 7, 2016).

Vermeulen S. J., B. M. Campbell, and J. S. I. Ingram. 2012. Climate change and food systems. *Annual Review of Environment and Resources* 37 (1):195–222.

Vetter, M. L., S. J. Herring, M. Sood, N. R. Shah, and A. L. Kalet. 2008. What do resident physicians know about nutrition? An evaluation of attitudes, self-perceived proficiency and knowledge. *Journal of the American College of Nutrition* 27 (2): 287–298.

World Health Organization. 2011. Global status report on noncommunicable diseases 2010. http://www.who.int/nmh/publications/ncd_report_full_en.pdf.

World Health Organization. 2017. Cardiovascular diseases. http://www.who.int/mediacentre/ factsheets/fs317/en/.

Yoo, S. 2015. Study: Americans living longer, but also sicker. *Statesman Journal*, August 31, 2015. http://www.statesmanjournal.com/story/news/health/2015/08/31/study-americans-living-longer-also-sicker/71485782/.

Young, A., H. J. Chaudhry, X. Pei, K. Halbesleben, D. H. Polk, and M. Dugan. 2015. A census of actively licensed physicians in the United States. *Journal of Medical Regulation* 101 (2): 8–23.

17 Too Many Prescriptions, Too Few Plants

Lessons on Diabetes Care from a Nurse Practitioner

Caroline Trapp

CONTENTS

17.1 INTRODUCTION

Type 2 diabetes (T2D) is epidemic in the United States and around the world. It is more common among people consuming a Western dietary pattern which is high in animal products, saturated fat, and cholesterol and low in fiber, antioxidants, and other nutrients found in plants. Diabetes "management" is an example of a medical-model phenomenon in chronic disease care where symptoms or biomarkers are aggressively treated and medications, products, and services have multiplied—but the underlying lifestyle-related causes of the disease are not adequately addressed, resulting in a perceived need for more medications, products, and services.

Nurses and nurse practitioners, with expertise in patient education and counseling, are well-suited to help shift the paradigm in the care of people at risk for or diagnosed with T2D. This chapter will consider concepts of biomedical ethics to explore the overuse of pharmaceutical interventions and the underuse of meaningful

299

lifestyle changes in the prevention and treatment of T2D. A new paradigm is proposed, encouraging a plant-based dietary pattern as the centerpiece of care.

17.2   THE SCOPE OF THE PROBLEM

The Center for Disease Control and Prevention (2017) estimates that in 2015 more than 30 million—or roughly 12% of U.S. adults had diabetes. Approximately 90–95% of all cases are T2D are largely amenable to lifestyle interventions (Center for Disease Control [CDC] 2017). Among adults who are 65 years of age or older, more than 25% were estimated to have diabetes (CDC 2017). An additional 84 million people, or almost 34% of all U.S. adults, were estimated to have prediabetes, a condition defined as mildly elevated blood glucose levels, increasing the risk of developing T2D (CDC 2017). Nearly half (more than 48%) of adults over the age of 65 had prediabetes. If current trends continue, almost 15% of the U.S. population (around 53 million people) will have diabetes by the year 2025 (Rowley and Bezould 2012), and by the year 2050, one in three adults will have diabetes (Boyle et al. 2010).

People with diabetes are at increased risk for stroke, blindness, heart disease, kidney disease, peripheral vascular disease, nerve damage, and lower extremity amputations. In addition, people with T2D are more likely to develop certain cancers, cognitive impairment/dementia, fatty liver disease, fractures, hearing impairment, obstructive sleep apnea, periodontal disease, depression, and disordered eating behavior (American Diabetes Association [ADA] 2017). Diabetes was the seventh leading cause of death in the United States in 2015 (CDC 2017).

Diabetes and prediabetes are usually diagnosed with either elevated fasting blood glucose or a glycosolated hemoglogin (A1c) level. In the absence of symptoms of hyperglycemia, results should be confirmed by repeat testing (ADA 2017). Common symptoms of T2D include thirst, frequent urination, nocturia, and blurred vision. Sometimes these symptoms are subtle, and an individual may attribute them to other causes, delaying diagnosis. While T2D was once rare among people under the age of 40, it is now being diagnosed in teens and even children, most of whom are overweight (CDC 2017).

17.3   CURRENT TREATMENT OF T2D

A diagnosis of T2D comes with many responsibilities: Routine medical care, daily self-care, and education. The American Diabetes Association (2017) recommends a formal education program for the patient and a family member, which encourages lifestyle changes related to physical activity and meal planning, adherence to medication(s), self-monitoring of blood sugars (for some), and close medical follow-up for detection of complications and comorbidities. A healthy lifestyle is encouraged, but in primary care settings, few receive meaningful counseling or ongoing support for nutritional interventions (Nutrition and Weight Status 2017).

Much of the care centers on medication. It is common for the person with diabetes to be prescribed one or more oral or injectable medications to treat or protect against hyperglycemia. An estimated 88.2% of adults with diabetes are treated with oral medications, non-insulin injectables, insulin of one or more types—or some combination of these medications (Saydah et al. 2014). In addition, many also have been prescribed medications for hypertension, cholesterol, and antiplatelet therapy (such as aspirin) while some may also receive prescriptions for the treatment of depression and sexual dysfunction. Monitoring of blood glucose levels was until recently recommended for nearly all patients (Society of General Internal Medicine 2017). This test involves pricking a finger and placing a drop of blood on a test strip (with a cost of as much as $1 per test) one or more times a day. Monitoring is especially important for people who are at risk for hypoglycemia, which can result from too much medication, too much exercise, too little food, or a combination of these factors.

People with diabetes incur more medical expenses than those without. Medical care includes eye exams, podiatry care, dental care, and specialty care, such as cardiology. It is estimated that annual medical expenditures for the person with diabetes were about $13,700 per year in 2012, with about $7,900 attributed to diabetes (CDC 2017). For the person with diabetes and a BMI of 35 kg/m^2 or higher (ADA 2017), metabolic surgery (previously called bariatric surgery) for weight loss may be recommended. The cost of this surgery is now covered by many insurance plans, although there are associated risks and a large percentage of patients (estimated to be 37–70%) do not experience sustained diabetes remission within one to five years (Rubino et al. 2016).

Despite significant expenditures on pharmaceutical and surgical interventions that incur significant monetary expenditures, diabetes remains a tremendous public health burden. Compared to 17 countries of similar economic status, the death rate in the United States from diabetes is among the highest (National Research Council [US] and Institute of Medicine [US] 2013). Thus, there is room for improvement in our approach to the disease.

17.4 THE ROOT(S) OF TYPE 2 DIABETES

Effective treatment of any disease requires knowledge of its pathogenesis. The American Diabetes Association (2017) classifies T2D as a progressive loss of insulin secretion that stems from insulin resistance, which results in hyperglycemia. The understanding of what causes these conditions has evolved, as have treatment options. Though diabetes was rare, clinicians first observed two types of diabetes in the late 1800s. Early nomenclature of "early" and "maturity onset," based on age at diagnosis and changed in the 1930s to "insulin-dependent" and "non-insulin dependent" before being changed to the current "type 1" and "type 2" between 1980–1990 (Gale 2014). It was in the 1920s that the treatment of children and young adults with diabetes was transformed with the discovery of insulin. In 1957, tolbutamide and other oral agents were introduced, which led to population-wide screening and the treatment of asymptomatic hyperglycemia. However, high cardiovascular mortality persisted (Gale 2014).

Defronzo (1988) first proposed that hyperglycemia in T2D resulted from a "triumvirate" of deficits in three organs: impaired insulin secretion by the pancreas, impaired suppression of glucose production by the liver, and decreased glucose uptake in the muscle. In 2009, he described a new paradigm, called the "ominous octet," which added five more organs or systems to target, and concluded that "multiple drugs used in combination will be required to correct the multiple pathophysiological defects" (DeFronzo 2009). Building on this model, Schwartz et al. (2016) recently described a constellation they named the "egregious 11" of physiologic pathways involved in hyperglycemia, and for each, one or more classes of appropriate pharmaceutical treatments. T2D is often described as multifactorial and heterogenic, and now another classification system is being considered based on the degree of beta-cell failure and involvement of mediating pathways (Schwartz 2016).

These increasingly more complicated descriptions of pathogenesis often distract clinicians and people with diabetes from the best target for treatment, which could be called the "ominous one." Through patterns of food consumption, the human mouth mediates not just weight, but many of the pathways identified in the "egregious 11" that lead to hyperglycemia in susceptible individuals, such as insulin resistance, inflammation, immune dysregulation, and changes in the gut microbiota (Greger 2015). Consuming unhealthful foods over time may also contribute to hypertension, hyperlipidemia, and other diabetes comorbidities. Thus, the increased consumption of unhealthy foods alters the course of the disease for a large percentage of the population. Additionally, medications that suppress appetite are generally ineffective and/or unsafe (Padwal and Majumdar 2007; Derosa and Maffioli 2012).

17.5 DIET AND DIABETES

Food environments as well as dietary patterns have changed dramatically over the past century and are a significant matter of public health concern. Diet is one of the primary factors to explain the high incidence and prevalence of obesity and diabetes in the United States compared to 17 countries of similar economic standing (National Research Council and the Institute of Medicine 2013). Consumption of calorically dense foods including meat, fish, poultry, cheese, added oils, frozen dairy products, and sweetened beverages has risen dramatically along with more advertising and more meals eaten outside the home (Barnard 2010). Animal products have become inexpensive and affordable due to subsidies to agribusinesses. Meat and cheese are conveniently available in fast-food restaurants, and are included in federally funded school meals and food-assistance programs to economically vulnerable populations.

Large observational studies have shown that as intake of animal products rises, so do rates of obesity and diabetes (Tonstad et al. 2009; Chiu et al. 2014; Satija et al. 2016). Even when controlled for differences in body weight and other confounding variables, meat consumption raised the risk of T2D (Tonstad et al. 2013). In studies with large populations that engage in healthier eating behaviors than the general population such as cohorts of Seventh-day Adventists or Taiwanese Buddhists, study participants who regularly consumed as little as three to four servings a month of red meat, fish, or poultry had higher rates of diabetes when compared to those who abstained (McMacken and Shah 2017). For those diagnosed with T2D, a meta-analysis showed that plant-based diets are effective for glycemic control, reducing and sometimes eliminating the need for medications (Yokoyama et al. 2014). The American Diabetes Association (2017) and American Association of Clinical Endocrinologists (Garber et al. 2016) have included a plant-based dietary pattern in their clinical practice recommendations.

An exclusively whole foods plant-based diet is made up vegetables, whole grains, fruits, and legumes such as beans, peas, and lentils as noted by the Power Plate in Figure 17.1. When plant foods replace animal products in the diet, such as beans instead of beef—and whole grains, such as oatmeal replacing unrefined grains, such as corn flakes—the diet is higher in fiber, and requires fewer calories for satiety. Barnard et al. (2006) found that even without limiting carbohydrates or total calories, individuals with T2D naturally ate less and lost more weight with further reductions in blood glucose than those following a portion-controlled diet that included but restricted amounts of meat and dairy. Carbohydrates such as those in starchy vegetables, whole grains, beans, and fruits are beneficial for T2D. Unfortunately, many people with diabetes have often been told to avoid these foods. It is important to make the distinction between refined and unrefined carbohydrates, as the former are low in nutritional value and fiber.

Meat, cheese, and added oils are substantial sources of fat in the Western dietary pattern. Saturated and trans-fat (Wang et al. 2003) along with excess fat from plant sources (Vessby et al. 2001) have been shown to increase insulin resistance due to the accumulation of fat particles in skeletal muscle and liver cells (Peterson et al. 2004). Whole food, plant-based diets that proscribe added fats have been shown to reverse advanced heart disease (Ornish et al. 1998; Esselstyn et al. 2014) which is the leading cause of death among people who have diabetes.

Plant-based diets have ample protein—even enough to sustain endurance athletes—and protein-deficiency does not occur with plant-based diets as long as adequate calories are consumed (Melina et al. 2016). Long thought to be a superior source of protein and iron, red meat contains heme iron, which is stored in the body and can contribute to insulin resistance (Wolk 2017). Plant sources of iron such as beans and green leafy vegetables have non-heme iron that does not accumulate in excess. Also, there is no need to combine certain plant foods to obtain adequate protein intake (Melina et al. 2016).

There is one cause for concern regarding plant-based dietary patterns for people with T2D. Patients who are on medications that can cause hypoglycemia, such as

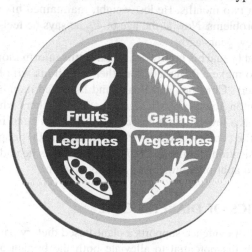

FIGURE 17.1 Physician's Committee for Responsible Medicine (PCRM) "Power Plate"

sulfonylureas or insulin, or who are on antihypertensive medications, may find their medications are too strong. These patients should be instructed in symptoms to watch for along with proactive medication monitoring and reduction. Those who make a diet change who already have normal or near-normal blood glucose or blood pressure readings may need reduced medication(s) before they start. This is especially true in elderly patients.

17.6 CASE STUDY: MEET MARC RAMIREZ

Marc Ramirez was diagnosed with T2D at the age of 34 in 2002. He was told by his doctor that his Mexican heritage increased his risk (Personal communication, August 6, 2017). He had been well aware of his risk, as his mother and six of his seven siblings had the disease. He lost his mother to diabetes, watching her suffer vision loss, heart disease, and kidney failure. Among his siblings, there was a death from pancreatic cancer and others experienced amputations, kidney disease, transplants, dialysis, and blindness. His twin brother suffered a heart attack.

A successful college athlete while attending the University of Michigan on a football scholarship and now a happily married father of two, Marc saw himself following the same path as his mother and siblings. In addition to T2D, he developed high cholesterol, high blood pressure, erectile dysfunction, heartburn, and psoriasis. He was on four different medications and required 80 units of insulin a day. For Marc, the turning point came in 2011, when his in-laws gave him a copy of *Forks Over Knives*, a documentary which concludes that a low-fat, whole-food, plant-based diet can prevent or reverse many chronic diseases, including T2D. Marc and his wife Kim learned of the work of Neal Barnard, M.D. from the film, and purchased his book *Dr. Neal Barnard's Program for Reversing Diabetes*. Using these two resources, they decided that they would start a plant-based diet.

The results were almost immediate. Within three days, he needed less insulin and was able to stop it completely in 15 days. He was able to discontinue all of his medications within two months. He lost weight, maintained his weight loss, and is free of all health problems. Now at the age of 49, he says he feels 20 years younger than he did just a few years ago.

Marc regrets that he and his family did not have this information sooner. However, he is determined to make a difference for others. With his wife Kim, he founded a support group called "Chickpea and Bean" and launched monthly meetings in his community of Clinton Township, Michigan to support others who want to improve their health through a low-fat plant-based diet. Marc has been invited to give presentations around the country, and now has more than 3,000 people on his email list (Personal communication, August 6, 2017). The resources he and his wife have created may be viewed at http://www.chickpeaandbean.com/.

17.7 THE ETHICS OF DIABETES CARE

A substantial body of evidence supports a plant-based dietary pattern to prevent and treat diabetes, with the potential to alleviate both the burden and expense of the disease. In fact, T2D may be less of a complicated, multi-organ/multi-system disease and more of an expected response to excess caloric intake of obesogenic foods. This information is now making its way into some practice guidelines, medical practices, and even some medical and nursing schools. However, history shows that when medical practice habits are entrenched, change comes slowly. It has been estimated to take an average of 10 years for clinicians to shift from disproven therapies (Tatsioni et al. 2007). The current prevention and treatment paradigm for T2D generally fails to sufficiently empower people with the option of a plant-based dietary pattern, and remains medication-focused. Clinical guidelines recommend that medications are initiated at the time of diagnosis (Inzucchi et al. 2012). Very little has been written about when and how to reduce diabetes medications, or how to "activate" lifestyle interventions.

Overreliance on diabetes medications is problematic for many reasons, including ethical concerns. People with diabetes need accurate information, and expect their healthcare professionals to have their best interests at heart. Viewing the over-reliance on diabetes medications through the lens of biomedical ethical principles offers the opportunity to improve the quality of care. It invites nurses and other healthcare professionals to use an improved paradigm for T2D management.

17.8 BIOMEDICAL ETHICAL PRINCIPLES OF BENEFICENCE AND NONMALEFICENCE

The intertwined concepts of beneficence and nonmaleficence describe the clinician's duty to act in the best interest of the patient. To do good and to do no harm, clinicians must first be current in their knowledge of T2D treatment options, including the efficacy and implementation of specific lifestyle interventions as well as the side effects of medications. Since 1995, many new medications for the management of hyperglycemia have emerged, and there are now nine additional classes of medications in addition to the two that were available prior to 1995 (White 2014). Clinicians are responsible for seeking out and completing continuing education, accessing clinical practice guidelines, and critically analyzing and translating research into practice. Nurses are bound by a Code of Ethics (Lachman et al. 2015). Some barriers to knowledgeable prescribing may include the overall quantity of information, lack of time for reading, and limited access to published research.

The role of the pharmaceutical industry in impacting clinicians' ability to act with beneficence deserves special mention. While some medications are lifesaving such as antibiotics for bacterial infections, medications for T2D should be considered differently than they currently are. Patients and clinicians may reasonably think that using a diabetes medication as prescribed provides protection against diabetes related micro- and macrovascular complications. However, U.S. Food and Drug Administration (FDA) regulations for diabetes medications only require that they lower blood glucose levels (Gandhi et al. 2008) and do not cause cardiovascular compromise (Goldfine 2008). While the use of medications has been shown to help patients achieve A1c levels close to normal levels known as "tight control" and other improvements in clinical markers, they have not been found to translate into the prevention of kidney failure/dialysis, blindness, stroke, or death from heart disease or any other cause (Rodríguez-Gutiérrez and Montori 2016). Hence, some believe the benefits of medication for diabetes may have been exaggerated (Makam and Nguyen 2017).

Over the past 14 years, a number of diabetes medications have been removed from the market or received a black box warning due to safety concerns. These include but are not limited to troglitazone (liver failure) (Graham et al. 2003), inhaled insulin (lung cancer) (Kling 2008), rosiglitazone (myocardial infarction and cardiovascular death) (Nissen and Wolski 2007), pioglitazone (bladder cancer) (U.S. FDA 2011), and exenatide and sitagliptin (acute pancreatitis) (U.S. FDA 2013). Incidentally, pharmaceutical companies realized tremendous profits before these problems became evident.

Significant safety concerns are not limited to newer agents. The quest for tight control of blood glucose has led to many people with T2D being prescribed insulin. However, Lebovitz (2011) showed no protective effect of early insulin use, and lowering A1c with medication to achieve tight control is associated with increased risk of severe hypoglycemia and other concerns. Another study of approximately 48,000 patients found an increased risk of all-cause mortality with an A1c below 7.5% (Currie et al. 2010). A retrospective cohort study of more than 84,000 patients showed insulin therapy was associated with an increased risk of diabetes-related complications, cancer, and death (Currie et al. 2013). The elderly are especially vulnerable to a poor risk/benefit ratio for medications used to prevent or treat hyperglycemia (Finucane 2012).

Pharmaceutical marketing is ubiquitous and has been shown to influence Advanced Practice Registered Nurse (APRN) prescribing (Ladd et al. 2010). Marketing includes full-page journal advertisements, face-to-face conversations and luncheons offered by sales representatives, distribution of samples, booths and sponsored lectures at professional meetings, and electronic or postal promotions (Gagnon and Lexchin 2008; Sufrin and Ross 2008). Prescribers are more likely to choose more expensive and not necessarily more effective medications as a result of these efforts (Gagnon and Lexchin 2008; Sufrin and Ross 2008).

In Standard 4 of the Code of Ethics for Nurses (Winland-Brown et al. 2015), the nurse is called upon to be responsible for individual nursing practice. However, accessing unbiased and accurate information is challenging. Some studies published in reputable medical journals have used deceptive practices to skew and slant conclusions in favor of new medications. Author John Abramson, M.D. describes methods that may obfuscate the truth in the book *Overdosed America: A Broken Promise of American Medicine* (2008). For example, expensive brand-name medications may be tested against placebo. Studies comparing two or more medications may not compare equivalent doses. Patients in studies may be younger and healthier than the patients who are most likely to receive the medication. Studies may be too short in duration or stopped prematurely to avoid showing long-term risks. Abstracts, conclusions, and recommendations may not reflect the actual outcomes. Determining what is true can be a challenge for even the most diligent clinician.

Systematic analyses such as the *Cochrane Reviews* are considered the most reliable source of information, but are only as good as the quality and freedom from industry influence of the studies they aggregate. Clinical practice guidelines, another trusted clinician resource, are often based on drug-company-funded studies. Guideline authors may have financial ties to the companies that produce the medications they are recommending and have been shown to be at risk for bias (Norris et al. 2013). Ethical clinicians must maintain a healthy skepticism for industry-influenced studies along with a strong desire for unbiased information before writing any prescriptions. Clinicians are challenged to increase their skills in critical appraisal in order to assess the reliability and usefulness of publications (Ionnidis et al. 2017).

What is not marketed and should be are older medications that may be more affordable and have a sound safety profile. For blood glucose control, metformin, an inexpensive, generic medication, is the rare pill where the risks may have been exaggerated. A *Cochrane* systematic review of 347 trials with 70,490 patient-years of metformin treatment (mean length 1.3 years, range 1 month to 10.7 years) found zero cases of lactic acidosis (Salpeter et al. 2010). Metformin may confer some protection against atherosclerotic heart disease in comparison to other agents (Maruther et al. 2016). As metformin can interfere with vitamin B12 absorption (Aroda et al. 2016), patients on metformin should be instructed to supplement with vitamin B12.

17.9 JUSTICE AND ETHICS

In bioethics, justice is described as the fair distribution of healthcare resources and services (Beauchamp and Childress 2013). Injustice can occur when expensive pharmaceutical agents are prescribed as first-line therapy over more affordable and effective older medications or lifestyle interventions. Clinicians may also unknowingly promote injustice by providing free medication samples, under the mistaken belief that companies provide these as charity rather than marketing expenditures to increase the utilization of newer patented brand-name agents (Ladd et al. 2010). A third example of injustice from overreliance on medication is that of "opportunity cost" as defined by John Abramson, M.D. (2013) as the missed opportunity that occurs when a patient is provided a prescription instead of being effectively encouraged or supported to make the lifestyle changes. This results in an increased financial burden on patients and the society overall.

17.10 ENVIRONMENTAL CONCERN

A discussion of ethical considerations in diabetes care would be incomplete without mention of the impact on non-human animals and the natural environment. Pharmaceuticals contribute to the pollution of air, land, and water in unexpected ways. For example, metformin, the most widely prescribed medication worldwide for T2D, was found in water samples taken from the Great Lakes due to incomplete filtration of waste water that negatively impacted the reproductive systems of fish (Niemuth 2015). Furthermore, extensive resources go into the production and disposal of the plastic pill bottles and injectable pens required to supply the ~88% of adults with diabetes on one or more medications. Plastics pollution is reviewed in detail in Chapter 5.

While hidden from view of the public, millions of animal carcasses, along with animal excrement, bedding, needles, syringes, and hazardous chemicals are discarded each year for pharmaceutical research and testing (Groff et al. 2014). Recommendations for people with diabetes to choose "healthier" low-fat dairy products and leaner cuts of meat may still increase demand for these products, contributing to the slaughter of more than 50 billion land animals a year globally (Kineswaran and Nierenberg 2008; Food and Agriculture Organization of the United Nations 2014). The impact of animal agriculture on the natural environment is concerning as recognized by the Food and Agriculture Organization of the United Nations (Steinfeld 2006). While these concerns are new to prescribers, it is essential to recognize that care of the individual patient is inextricably related to the natural environment and animal welfare. For some patients and clinicians, these profound concerns provide additional incentives to recommend and consume a plant-based dietary pattern.

17.11 INADEQUATE EDUCATION

Every clinical encounter with a person with diabetes should emphasize the importance of diet. The primacy of nutrition was recognized in the earliest days of the nursing profession. In the words of Florence Nightingale, "The most important office of the nurse, after she has taken care of the patient's air, is to take care to observe the effect of his food…" (Nightingale 1860). The first nurses were instructed in food preparation and service. Didactic nursing education expanded in the early 1900s to include principles of nutrition and diet with nearly 100 hours of instruction over three years (Hassenplug 1969). The period from 1950–1970 saw a transition from separate nutrition courses totaling about 65 classroom hours to content that was integrated into classes as a thread throughout programs as other academic content requirements emerged. In the 1950s (Leitch 1956), many State Boards of Nursing dropped the requirement of a specified number of hours devoted to nutrition though nutrition was (and continues to be) tested on licensure exams for Registered Nurses (DiMaria-Ghalili et al. 2013). The growth of the dietetics profession resulted in changes in nurses' responsibilities related to nutrition, too.

National surveys of nursing schools regarding nutrition preparation and competence were conducted in 1985 (Stotts et al. 1987) and 1997 (Touger-Decker et al. 2001), but are now outdated. A 2011 survey of nurse practitioners found nutrition was the number one topic of interest. Specifically, nurse practitioners identified the need for nutrition skills training for everyday clinical practice (DiMaria-Ghalili et al. 2014).

Registered Dietitians Nutritionists (RDNs) with expertise in plant-based dietary patterns are key team members in the care of the person with T2D. Many dietitians, physicians, and nurses have become experts through their own efforts. Clinicians should seek out RDN's for patient referrals and continue to reinforce the importance of diet with patients. See Table 17.1 for a list of educational resources for clinicians.

TABLE 17.1

Resources for Nutrition Continuing Education

American College of Lifestyle Medicine (www.LifestyleMedicine.org)

Center for Nutrition Studies (www.NutritionStudies.org)

Nutrition CME (www.NutritionCME.org)

Nutrition Facts (www.NutritionFacts.org)

Physicians Committee for Responsible Medicine (www.PhysiciansCommittee.org)

Plant-Based Prevention of Disease (www.P-POD.org)

The Plantrician Project (www.plantricianproject.org)

17.12   TOWARD A NEW PARADIGM

Given the limitations of medication and the power of a plant-based dietary pattern to benefit people with T2D or those at risk, how can nurses and other clinicians use this knowledge in practice? What would a nutrition-centered clinical practice model of diabetes prevention and reversal look like? Food would be the primary intervention tool used to address T2D, with medication used as a last resort. Posters of delicious plant-based meals and cooking videos would welcome patients and family members. Healthy lifestyle habits, including physical activity and smoking cessation would be strongly encouraged through interactions and effective programs. A nutrition-centered practice would recommend healthful eating patterns immediately while offering advice on practical skills: Cooking, adapting recipes, label reading, meal planning, eating out, and handling interpersonal and social situations. Classes would be offered at times that are convenient for patients, and families would be welcome to participate in sessions that may include field trips to grocery stores or restaurants. Group medical visits may be used to increase the number of people reached by clinicians and to offer additional support. Nutrition myths such as the need for animal products or the risks of starchy vegetables would be addressed.

Area businesses would appreciate new marketing opportunities and could create plant-based menu items or offer discounts to shoppers on their plant-based purchases. Local employers can lower healthcare expenses by partnering with a plant-based healthcare practice to provide education and care to their employees. Farmer's markets would be incorporated into healthcare facilities. "Prescriptions" for fruit and vegetable boxes can be offered through area food-assistance programs.

Individuals successful in implementing a plant-based diet can serve as ambassadors to newcomers and can organize support groups and become liaisons to community businesses and other potential partners—all with an eye towards creating a sustainable community of plant-based eaters. Plant-centered practitioners would educate future healthcare professionals in schools and universities where course content would go beyond the classroom—offering real-world experiences to students. Clinicians themselves would eat plant-based diets, leading by example.

Is this framework difficult to implement? It's already a burgeoning area of healthcare. One example is the Barnard Medical Clinic (Barnard Medical Center 2015) in Washington, D.C. Every patient has access to physicians, nurse practitioners, and Registered Dietitian Nutritionists with expertise in plant-based nutrition, along with classes that teach cooking skills. A bowl of fresh fruit is always available in the waiting room where posters, books, and videos demonstrate the importance a plant-based lifestyle. Other examples include Rochester Lifestyle Medicine (Rochester, NY) that has trained a large and exclusively plant-based team of clinicians to provide medical nutrition assessment, classes, and support groups to individuals and employers. Kaiser Permanente, one of the country's largest health plans and medical service providers, encourages their physicians to offer plant-based nutrition education (Tuso et al. 2013).

Strategies for individual practitioners to effectively support patients to make and sustain plant-based eating are becoming more readily available (Karlsen and Pollard 2017). Registered Dietitian Nutritionist Matt Ruscigno (2017) has outlined 10 key considerations for counseling patients transitioning to a plant-based diet. One of his recommendations is to "keep it simple." While plant-based cooking can seem complicated, he recommends creating vegan bowls with a mix-and-match template of whole grains, beans, greens, and a flavorful sauce. Breakfast foods are easy: Overnight oats with blueberries, walnuts, and plant milk, or peanut butter and strawberries on toasted whole wheat bread. Again, practitioners may also consider group medical visits to teach plant-based nutrition to patients (Patel-Saxena 2016).

17.13 CONCLUSION

As the predominant food environment contributes to unhealthful dietary patterns, an epidemic of T2D has emerged. An important solution for prevention and treatment lies in addressing diet in clinical practice and throughout the larger society. Pharmaceutical interventions may not prevent untoward outcomes, raising numerous bioethical concerns. Promoting healthy plant-based diets is in the scope of practice of nurses, doctors, and dietitians so to ameliorate diet-related chronic diseases. Routine referrals to Registered Dietitian Nutritionists are also recommended, as are the use of plant-based classes, books, websites DVDs, and other supportive resources. Clinicians are encouraged to become experts by adopting a plant-based dietary pattern themselves, and exploring ways to transform practice settings and communities so they are health promoting.

REFERENCES

Abramson, John. 2008. *Overdosed America: The Broken Promise of American Medicine*. 3rd edition. Harper Perennial.

Abramson, John. 2013. Why cholesterol-lowering statins fail to save lives. Presented at the McDougall Advanced Study Weekend, Santa Rosa, CA.

American Diabetes Associaiton. 2017. Standards of medical care in diabetes-2017. *Diabetes Care* 40 (Supplement 1): 1–142.

Aroda, Vanita R., Sharon L. Edelstein, Ronald B. Goldberg, William C. Knowler, Santica M. Marcovina, Trevor J. Orchard, George A. Bray, David S. Schade, Marinella G. Temprosa, Neil H. White and Jill P. Crandall. 2016. Long-term metformin use and vitamin B12 deficiency in the Diabetes Prevention Program Outcomes Study. *The Journal of Clinical Endocrinology & Metabolism* 101 (4): 1754–1761.

Barnard Medical Center. 2015. Barnard Medical Center. Text. *The Physicians Committee.* July 20. http://www.pcrm.org/barnard-medical-center.

Barnard, Neal D. 2010. Trends in food availability, 1909–2007. *The American Journal of Clinical Nutrition*, 91(5), pp.1530S–1536S.

Barnard, Neal D., Joshua Cohen, David J. A. Jenkins, Gabrielle Turner-McGrievy, Lise Gloede, Brent Jaster, Kim Seidl, Amber A. Green, and Stanley Talpers. 2006. A low-fat vegan diet improves glycemic control and cardiovascular risk factors in a randomized clinical trial in individuals with Type 2 diabetes. *Diabetes Care* 29 (8): 1777–1783. doi:10.2337/dc06-0606.

Beauchamp, Tom L., and James F. Childress. 2014. *Principles of Biomedical Ethics, 7th edition.* Oxford University Press, USA.

Boyle, James P., Theodore J.Thompson, Edward W. Gregg, Lawrence E. Barker, David F. Williamson. 2010. Projection of the year 2050 burden of diabetes in the U.S. adult population: Dynamic modeling of incidence, mortality, and prediabetes prevalence. *Population Health Metrics* 8 (29). http://www.pophealthmetrics.com/content/8/1/29.

Centers for Disease Control and Prevention. 2017. National diabetes statistics report, 2017 estimates of diabetes and its burden in the United States. *U.S. Department of Health and Human Services.* https://www.cdc.gov/diabetes/pdfs/data/statistics/national-diabetes-statistics-report.pdf.

Chiu, Tina H. T., Hui-Ya Huang, Yen-Feng Chiu, Wen-Harn Pan, Hui-Yi Kao, Jason P. C. Chiu, Ming-Nan Lin, and Chin-Lon Lin. 2014. Taiwanese vegetarians and omnivores: Dietary composition, prevalence of diabetes and IFG. *PloS One* 9 (2): e88547. doi:10.1371/journal.pone.0088547.

Currie, Craig J., John R. Peters, Aodán Tynan, Marc Evans, Robert J. Heine, Oswaldo L. Bracco, Tony Zagar, and Chris D. Poole. 2010. Survival as a function of HbA(1c) in people with Type 2 diabetes: A retrospective cohort study. *Lancet (London, England)* 375 (9713): 481–489. doi:10.1016/S0140-6736(09)61969-3.

Currie, Craig J., Chris D. Poole, Marc Evans, John R. Peters, and Christopher Ll Morgan. 2013. Mortality and other important diabetes-related outcomes with insulin vs other antihyperglycemic therapies in Type 2 diabetes. *The Journal of Clinical Endocrinology and Metabolism* 98 (2): 668–677. doi:10.1210/jc.2012-3042.

DeFronzo, R. A. 1988. Lilly lecture 1987. The triumvirate: Beta-cell, muscle, liver. A collusion responsible for NIDDM. *Diabetes* 37 (6): 667–687.

DeFronzo, Ralph A. 2009. Banting lecture. From the triumvirate to the ominous octet: A new paradigm for the treatment of type 2 diabetes mellitus. *Diabetes* 58 (4): 773–795. doi:10.2337/db09-9028.

Derosa, Giuseppe, and Pamela Maffioli. 2012. Anti-obesity drugs: A review about their effects and their safety. *Expert Opinion on Drug Safety* 11 (3): 459–471. doi:10.1517/1 4740338.2012.675326.

DIA_Ch39.pdf. 2017. https://www.niddk.nih.gov/about-niddk/strategic-plans-reports/Documents/Diabetes%20in%20America%203rd%20Edition/DIA_Ch39.pdf (Accessed September 19).

DiMaria-Ghalili, Rose Ann, Marilyn Edwards, Gerald Friedman, Azra Jaferi, Martin Kohlmeier, Penny Kris-Etherton, Carine Lenders, Carole Palmer, and Judith Wylie-Rosett. 2013. Capacity building in nutrition science: Revisiting the curricula for medical professionals. *Annals of the New York Academy of Sciences* 1306 (December): 21–40. doi:10.1111/nyas.12334.

DiMaria-Ghalili, R.A., Mirtallo, J.M., Tobin, B.W., Hark, L., Van Horn, L. and Palmer, C.A. 2014. Challenges and opportunities for nutrition education and training in the health care professions: intraprofessional and interprofessional call to action. *American Journal of Clinical Nutrition*, 99(5): 1184S–1193S.

Esselstyn, Caldwell B., Gina Gendy, Jonathan Doyle, Mladen Golubic, and Michael F. Roizen. 2014. A way to reverse CAD? *The Journal of Family Practice* 63 (7): 356–364b.

Finucane, Thomas E. 2012. 'Tight Control' in geriatrics: The emperor wears a thong. *Journal of the American Geriatrics Society* 60(8): 1571–1575. doi:10.1111/j.1532-5415.2012.04057.x.

Food and Agriculture Organization of the United Nations. FAOSTAT. FAOSTAT (Database). Latest update: 07 Mar 2014. http://data.fao.org/ref/262b79ca-279c-4517-93de-ee3b7c7cb553.html?version=1.0 (Accessed October 5, 2017).

Gagnon, Marc-André, and Joel Lexchin. 2008. The cost of pushing pills: A new estimate of pharmaceutical promotion expenditures in the United States. *PLoS Medicine* 5 (1): e1. doi:10.1371/journal.pmed.0050001.

Gale, E.A.M. 2014. Historical aspects of Type 2 diabetes (Revision Number 28). *Diapedia*. Diapedia.org. doi:10.14496/dia.3104287134.28.

Gandhi, Gunjan Y., M. Hassan Murad, Akira Fujiyoshi, Rebecca J. Mullan, David N. Flynn, Mohamed B. Elamin, Brian A. Swiglo, William L. Isley, Gordon H. Guyatt, and Victor M. Montori. 2008. Patient-important outcomes in registered diabetes trials. *JAMA* 299 (21): 2543–2549. doi:10.1001/jama.299.21.2543.

Garber, Alan J., Martin J. Abrahamson, Joshua I. Barzilay, Lawrence Blonde, Zachary T. Bloomgarden, Michael A. Bush, Samuel Dagogo-Jack, et al. 2016. Consensus statement by the American Association of Clinical Endocrinologists and American College of Endocrinology on the Comprehensive Type 2 Diabetes Management algorithm–2016 Executive summary." *Endocrine Practice: Official Journal of the American College of Endocrinology and the American Association of Clinical Endocrinologists* 22 (1): 84–113. doi:10.4158/EP151126.CS.

Goldfine, Allison B. 2008. Assessing the cardiovascular safety of diabetes therapies. *The New England Journal of Medicine* 359 (11): 1092–1095. doi:10.1056/NEJMp0805758.

Graham, David J., Carol R. Drinkard, and Deborah Shatin. 2003. Incidence of idiopathic acute liver failure and hospitalized liver injury in patients treated with troglitazone. *The American Journal of Gastroenterology* 98 (1): 175–179. doi:10.1111/j.1572-0241.2003.07175.x.

Greger, Michael and Gene Stone. 2015. *How Not to Die*. New York, NY: Flatiron Press.

Groff, Katherine, Eric Bachli, Molly Landsdowne and Theodora Capalda. 2014. *Environments* I: 14–30. Doi:10.330/environments1010014.

Hassenplug, L. W. 1969. The expanding role of the nurse. *The Oklahoma Nurse* 44 (9): 1–5.

Ioannidis, John, Michael E. Stuart, Shannon Brownlee, and Sheri A. Strite. How to survive the medical misinformation mess. *European Journal of Clinical Investigation* (2017).

Inzucchi, S. E., R. M. Bergenstal, J. B. Buse, M. Diamant, E. Ferrannini, M. Nauck, A. L. Peters, A. Tsapas, R. Wender, and D. R. Matthews. 2012. Management of Hyperglycaemia in Type 2 Diabetes: A Patient-Centered Approach. Position Statement of the American Diabetes Association (ADA) and the European Association for the Study of Diabetes (EASD). *Diabetologia* 55 (6): 1577–1596. doi:10.1007/s00125-012-2534-0.

Karlsen, M.C. and K.J. Pollard. 2017. Strategies for practitioners to support patients in plant-based eating. *Journal of Geriatric Cardiology* 14:338–341. doi:10.11909/j.issn.1671-5411.2017.05.006.

Kling, Jim. 2008. Inhaled insulin's last gasp? *Nature Biotechnology* 26 (5): 479–480. doi:10.1038/nbt0508-479.

Koneswaran, G., and Nierenberg, D. (2008). Global farm animal production and global warming: Impacting and mitigating climate change. *Environmental Health Perspectives*, 116 (5): 578–582. http://doi.org/10.1289/ehp.11034.

Lachman, Vicki D., Elizabeth O'Connor Swanson, and Jill Winland-Brown. 2015. The new 'Code of Ethics for Nurses with Interpretative Statements' (2015): Practical clinical application, part II." *Medsurg Nursing: Official Journal of the Academy of Medical-Surgical Nurses* 24 (5): 363–366, 368.

Ladd, Elissa C., Diane Feeney Mahoney, and Srinivas Emani. 2010. 'Under the Radar': nurse practitioner prescribers and pharmaceutical industry promotions. *The American Journal of Managed Care* 16 (12): e358–e362.

Lebovitz, Harold E. 2011. Insulin: Potential negative consequences of early routine use in patients with Type 2 diabetes. *Diabetes Care* 34 Suppl 2 (May): S225–S230. doi:10.2337/dc11-s225.

Leitch, M. A. 1956. Educational standards for student nurses in the dietary department. *Journal of the American Dietetic Association* 32 (4): 337–340.

Makam, Anil N., and Oanh K. Nguyen. 2017. An evidence-based medicine approach to anti-hyperglycemic therapy in diabetes mellitus to overcome overtreatment. *Circulation* 135 (2): 180–195. doi:10.1161/CIRCULATIONAHA.116.022622.

Maruthur, Nisa M., Eva Tseng, Susan Hutfless, Lisa M. Wilson, Catalina Suarez-Cuervo, Zackary Berger, Yue Chu, Emmanuel Iyoha, Jodi B. Segal, and Shari Bolen. 2016. Diabetes medications as monotherapy or metformin-based combination therapy for type 2 diabetes: A systematic review and meta-analysis. *Annals of Internal Medicine* 164 (11): 740–751.

McMacken, Michelle, and Sapana Shah. 2017. A plant-based diet for the prevention and treatment of Type 2 diabetes. *Journal of Geriatric Cardiology: JGC* 14 (5): 342–354. doi:10.11909/j.issn.1671-5411.2017.05.009.

Melina, Vesanto, Winston Craig, and Susan Levin. 2016. Position of the Academy of Nutrition and Dietetics: Vegetarian diets. *Journal of the Academy of Nutrition and Dietetics* 116 (12): 1970–1980. doi:10.1016/j.jand.2016.09.025.

National Research Council (US), and Institute of Medicine (US). 2013. *U.S. Health in International Perspective: Shorter Lives, Poorer Health,* edited by Steven H. Woolf and Laudan Aron. The National Academies Collection: Reports Funded by National Institutes of Health. Washington, DC: National Academies Press, US). http://www.ncbi.nlm.nih.gov/books/NBK115854/.

Niemuth, Nicholas J., Renee Jordan, Jordan Crago, Chad Blanksma, Rodney Johnson, and Rebecca D. Klaper. 2015. Metformin exposure at environmentally relevant concentrations causes potential endocrine disruption in adult male fish. *Environmental Toxicology and Chemistry* 34 (2): 291–296. doi:10.1002/etc.2793.

Nightingale, Florence. 1860. Notes on nursing. http://digital.library.upenn.edu/women/nightingale/nursing/nursing.html.

Norris, Susan L., Haley K. Holmer, Lauren A. Ogden, Brittany U. Burda, and Rongwei Fu. 2013. Conflicts of interest among authors of clinical practice guidelines for glycemic control in Type 2 diabetes mellitus. *PloS One* 8 (10): e75284. doi:10.1371/journal.pone.0075284.

Nissen, Steven E., and Kathy Wolski. 2007. Effect of rosiglitazone on the risk of myocardial infarction and death from cardiovascular causes. *New England Journal of Medicine* 356(24): 2457–2471.

Nutrition and weight status | Healthy people 2020. 2017. *U.S. Department of Health and Human Services.* https://www.healthypeople.gov/2020/topics-objectives/topic/nutrition-and-weight-status/objectives.

Ornish, D., L. W. Scherwitz, J. H. Billings, S. E. Brown, K. L. Gould, T. A. Merritt, S. Sparler, et al. 1998. Intensive lifestyle changes for reversal of coronary heart disease. *JAMA* 280 (23): 2001–2007.

Padwal, Raj S., and Sumit R. Majumdar. 2007. Drug treatments for obesity: Orlistat, Sibutramine, and Rimonabant. *Lancet (London, England)* 369 (9555): 71–77. doi:10.1016/S0140 6736(07)60033 6.

Patel-Saxena, Shilpa.2016. Leveraging time with lifestyle-based group visits. *American Journal of Lifestyle Medicine*10 (5): 330–337.

Petersen, Kitt Falk, Sylvie Dufour, Douglas Befroy, Rina Garcia, and Gerald I. Shulman. 2004. Impaired mitochondrial activity in the insulin-resistant offspring of patients with Type 2 dDiabetes. *The New England Journal of Medicine* 350 (7): 664–671. doi:10.1056/NEJMoa031314.

Rodríguez-Gutiérrez, René, and Victor M. Montori. 2016. Glycemic control for patients with Type 2 diabetes mellitus: Our evolving faith in the face of evidence. *Circulation. Cardiovascular Quality and Outcomes* 9 (5): 504–512. doi:10.1161/CIRCOUTCOMES.116.002901.

Rowley, William R., and Clement Bezold. 2012. Creating public awareness: State 2025 diabetes forecasts. *Population Health Management* 15 (4): 194–200. doi:10.1089/pop.2011.0053.

Rubino, Francesco, David M. Nathan, Robert H. Eckel, Philip R. Schauer, K. George, M. M. Alberti Paul Z. Zimmet, Stefano Del Prato, et al. 2016. Metabolic surgery in the treatment algorithm for Type 2 diabetes: A joint statement by International Diabetes Organizations. *Surgery for Obesity and Related Diseases: Official Journal of the American Society for Bariatric Surgery* 12 (6): 1144–1162. doi:10.1016/j.soard.2016.05.018.

Ruscigno, Matt. 2017. *Today's Dietitian* 19(10): 20. http://www.todaysdietitian.com/newarchives/1017p20.shtml.

Saenz, A., I. Fernandez-Esteban, A. Mataix, M. Ausejo, M. Roque, and D. Moher. 2005. Metformin monotherapy for Type 2 diabetes mellitus. *The Cochrane Database of Systematic Reviews*, no. 3 (July): CD002966. doi:10.1002/14651858.CD002966.pub3.

Salpeter, Shelley R., Elizabeth Greyber, Gary A. Pasternak, and Edwin E. Salpeter Posthumous. 2010. Risk of fatal and nonfatal lactic acidosis with metformin use in Type 2 diabetes mellitus. *The Cochrane Database of Systematic Reviews*, no. 1 (January): CD002967. doi:10.1002/14651858.CD002967.pub3.

Saydah, Sharon H. 2014. Medication use and self-care practices in persons with diabetes. *Insulin*, 15(14.5), 11–8.

Satija, Ambika, Shilpa N. Bhupathiraju, Eric B. Rimm, Donna Spiegelman, Stephanie E. Chiuve, Lea Borgi, Walter C. Willett, JoAnn E. Manson, Qi Sun, and Frank B. Hu. 2016. Plant-based dietary patterns and incidence of Type 2 diabetes in US men and women: Results from three prospective cohort studies. *PLoS Medicine* 13 (6): e1002039. doi:10.1371/journal.pmed.1002039.

Schwartz, Stanley S., Solomon Epstein, Barbara E. Corkey, Struan F. A. Grant, James R. Gavin, and Richard B. Aguilar. 2016. The time is right for a new classification system for diabetes: Rationale and implications of the β-Cell-centric classification schema. *Diabetes Care* 39 (2): 179–186. doi:10.2337/dc15-1585.

Scientific Report of the 2015 Dietary Guidelines Advisory Committee. 2017. https://health.gov/dietaryguidelines/2015-scientific-report/pdfs/scientific-report-of-the-2015-dietary-guidelines-advisory-committee.pdf (Accessed September 19).

Society of General Internal Medicine. 2017. Don't recommend daily home finger glucose testing in patients with Type 2 diabetes mellitus not using insulin. *Choosing Wisely*. http://www.choosingwisely.org/clinician-lists/society-general-internal-medicine-daily-home-finger-glucose-testing-type-2-diabetes-mellitus/.

Standards of Medical Care in Diabetes 2017. 2017. https://professional.diabetes.org/sites/professional.diabetes.org/files/media/dc_40_s1_final.pdf (Accessed September 19).

Steinfeld, H., Food and Agriculture Organization of the United Nations., & Livestock, Environment and Development (Firm). 2006. *Livestock's Long Shadow: Environmental Issues and Options*. Rome: Food and Agriculture Organization of the United Nations.

Stotts, N. A., D. Englert, K. S. Crocker, N. W. Bennum, and M. Hoppe. 1987. Nutrition education in schools of nursing in the United States. Part 2: The status of nutrition education in Schools of Nursing. *JPEN. Journal of Parenteral and Enteral Nutrition* 11 (4): 406–411. doi:10.1177/0148607187011004406.

Sufrin, Carolyn B., and Joseph S. Ross. 2008. Pharmaceutical industry marketing: understanding its impact on women's health. *Obstetrical & Gynecological Survey* 63 (9): 585–596. doi:10.1097/OGX.0b013e31817f1585.

Tatsioni, Athina, Nikolaos G. Bonitsis, and John P. A. Ioannidis. 2007. Persistence of contradicted claims in the literature. *JAMA* 298 (21): 2517–2526. doi:10.1001/jama.298.21.2517.

Tonstad, S., K. Stewart, K. Oda, M. Batech, R. P. Herring, and G. E. Fraser. 2013. Vegetarian diets and incidence of diabetes in the adventist health study-2. *Nutrition, Metabolism, and Cardiovascular Diseases: NMCD* 23 (4): 292–299. doi:10.1016/j.numecd.2011.07.004.

Tonstad, Serena, Terry Butler, Ru Yan, and Gary E. Fraser. 2009. Type of vegetarian diet body weight, and prevalence of Type 2 diabetes. *Diabetes Care* 32 (5): 791–796. doi:10.2337/dc08-1886.

Touger-Decker, R., J. M. Barracato, and J. O'Sullivan-Maillet. 2001. Nutrition education in health professions programs: A survey of dental, physician assistant, nurse practitioner, and nurse midwifery programs. *Journal of the American Dietetic Association* 101 (1): 63–69.

Tuso, P.J., M.H. Ismail, B.P. Ha, and C. Bartolotto. 2013. Nutritional update for physicians: Plant-based diets. *The Permanente Journal* 17 (2): 61–66.

U.S. Food and Drug Administration (FDA). 2011. Drug safety and availability – FDA drug safety communication: Updated drug labels for pioglitazone-containing medicines. *The U.S. Food and Drug Administration (FDA).* https://wayback.archive-it.org/7993/20170112005525/http://www.fda.gov/Drugs/DrugSafety/ucm266555.htm.

U.S. Food and Drug Administration (FDA). 2013. Drug safety and availability – FDA drug safety communication: FDA Investigating reports of possible increased risk of pancreatitis and pre-cancerous findings of the pancreas from Incretin Mimetic Drugs for Type 2 diabetes. *The U.S. Food and Drug Administration (FDA).* https://www.fda.gov/Drugs/DrugSafety/ucm343187.htm.

Vessby, B., M. Uusitupa, K. Hermansen, G. Riccardi, A. A. Rivellese, L. C. Tapsell, C. Nälsén, et al. 2001. Substituting dietary saturated for monounsaturated fat impairs insulin sensitivity in healthy men and women: The KANWU study. *Diabetologia* 44 (3): 312–319.

Wang, Lu, Aaron R. Folsom, Zhi-Jie Zheng, James S. Pankow, John H. Eckfeldt, and ARIC Study Investigators. 2003. Plasma fatty acid composition and incidence of diabetes in middle-aged adults: The Atherosclerosis Risk in Communities (ARIC) study. *The American Journal of Clinical Nutrition* 78 (1): 91–98.

White, John R. 2014 A brief history of the development of diabetes medications. *Diabetes Spectrum* 27 (2): 82–86.

Winland-Brown, Jill, Vicki D. Lachman, and Elizabeth O'Connor Swanson. 2015. The new 'Code of Ethics for Nurses With Interpretive Statements' (2015): Practical clinical application, Part I. *Medsurg Nursing: Official Journal of the Academy of Medical-Surgical Nurses* 24 (4): 268–271.

Wolk, A. 2017. Potential health hazards of eating red meat. *Journal of Internal Medicine* 281 (2): 106–122. doi:10.1111/joim.12543.

Yokoyama, Yoko, Neal D. Barnard, Susan M. Levin, and Mitsuhiro Watanabe. 2014. Vegetarian diets and glycemic control in Diabetes: A systematic review and meta-analysis. *Cardiovascular Diagnosis and Therapy* 4 (5): 373–382. doi:10.3978/j.issn.2223-3652.2014.10.04.

18 A Global Network of Environmental Stewardship in Healthcare

Stacia Clinton

CONTENTS

18.1 INTRODUCTION

Hospitals have the potential to improve public and environmental health and to strengthen the economic vitality of their communities. As "anchor" institutions, they are rooted in place and often explicitly oriented toward supporting community health. They hold significant investments in real estate and social capital and may serve as the largest employers in their communities (Initiative for a Competitive Inner City 2011). Hospitals have the opportunity to evaluate where their purchasing clout can create local jobs and where their investments with other institutions can help weave together healthy regional food systems, clean energy, healthier housing, and low carbon transportation systems that build equitable, sustainable, and resilient communities. It was the recognition of the paradox that many of the operations and procurement practices of these anchor institutions were directly contributing harm to the environment and subsequently human health, which launched the formation of Health Care Without Harm (HCWH) in 1996.

18.2   HEALTH CARE WITHOUT HARM (HCWH)

Twenty-eight organizations from across the globe formed HCWH largely in response to the U.S. Environmental Protection Agency (EPA) identifying medical waste incineration as the leading source of dioxin emissions (U.S. EPA 1995)—one of the most potent carcinogens (U.S. EPA 2010a; National Research Council 2006). The coalition is based on the belief that healthcare has a mission-driven interest to "first, do no harm," and therefore a responsibility to address its own environmental footprint and become leaders to support a sustainable economy and healthy communities. Since its founding, HCWH has grown into a broad-based international coalition of hundreds of organizations and thousands of hospitals and health partners in more than 50 countries, with offices in the United States, Europe, Latin America, and the Philippines with strategic partners located on every continent.

The coalition is driving the healthcare sector away from a focus on treating individual patients with acute and chronic diseases to addressing the social, economic, and environmental conditions that are the major underlying contributors of good or bad health. Efforts to address these upstream conditions can be mutually reinforcing when they are woven together toward a vision of healthy individuals residing in sustainable, equitable, and resilient communities on a planet whose biodiversity and natural resources are preserved for future generations.

18.3   GLOBAL GREEN AND HEALTHY HOSPITALS

The Global Green and Healthy Hospitals community was formed by HCWH in 2010 as a vehicle for networking and peer learning. The Global Green and Healthy Hospitals online social platform serves to facilitate communication and networking among hospitals around the world to accelerate innovation and the scaling up of solutions. As of 2017 the GGHH network includes 797 members in 47 countries on six continents who represent the interests of over 25,600 hospitals and health centers globally.

Leveraging the collective clout of this network, the 2020 Health Care Climate Challenge was launched in 2015 to mobilize healthcare institutions around the globe to protect public health from climate change. HCWH has played a leading role in depicting climate change as a public health issue and working with the healthcare sector to "lead by example" in reducing their carbon footprint by beginning the transition to renewable energy sources and other carbon mitigation solutions. As of 2017, leading hospitals and health systems from more than 20 countries have joined the Health Care Climate Challenge and have committed to taking meaningful action based on three main pillars:

1. Mitigation—Reducing healthcare's carbon footprint and/or fostering low carbon healthcare.
2. Resilience—Preparing for the impacts of extreme weather and shifting the burden of disease.
3. Leadership—Educating staff and the public while promoting policies to protect public health from climate change.

18.4 THE IMPACT OF GLOBAL SECTOR ACTION

Since inception, HCWH and its partners have achieved previously insurmountable challenges through collective action. More than 50 medical societies, cities, and states have passed resolutions to reduce polyvinyl chloride (PVC), dioxin, mercury or medical waste incineration. The number of medical waste incinerators in the United States has been reduced by 99% since 1998 (U.S. EPA 1988, 2010b; Stringer 2011). The Philippines passed a national ban on incineration (Republic of the Philippines 1998) and hundreds of incinerators have closed throughout Europe. Globally, HCWH has worked with the United Nations Development Programme and the World Health Organization to demonstrate the safety (Farshad et al. 2014; Lee et al. 2004; Nguyen 2017), efficacy, and cost effectiveness of non-burn medical waste treatment technologies and has developed training programs on medical waste management for hospitals and clinics all over the world (Rafiee et al. 2016; Chartier 2014).

As a result of HCWH's campaign to address the environmental and human concerns with mercury waste, the market for mercury thermometers has been virtually eliminated in the United States, as almost all hospitals and all major pharmacies have switched to safer non-mercury devices. Under the Minamata Treaty signed in October 2013, mercury-based measuring devices will be phased out of global production and use by 2020 (United Nations Environmental Programme 2013).

Major public health associations have promulgated the elimination of PVC in medical devices due to health concerns that phthalates leaching out of the devices may cause harm (American Medical Association 2001; Republic of the Philippines Department of Health 2008; Tickner et al. 2001). The healthcare industry's demand for non-toxic products has driven the innovation of PVC-free flooring and wall protection products while driving down the price of latex-free, vinyl-free nitrile gloves.

HCWH and other partners developed the first health-based green building system for hospitals, the Green Guide for Health Care, which became the catalyst and foundation for the U.S. Green Building Council's Leadership in Energy and Environmental Design for Health Care. Over 265 major healthcare projects representing over 30 million square feet of healthcare construction have adopted the Green Guide for Health Care as their framework for design and construction (GGHC 2017).

Global collective action within the HCWH network starts with a few leadership facilities willing to set a new benchmark for purchases and practices that support greater protection of human and environmental health and ultimately, biodiversity.

18.5 U.S. HEALTHCARE: A DRIVER FOR GLOBAL HEALTHCARE TRANSFORMATION

The U.S. healthcare sector has a prominent role to play in driving change that impacts the global sector. Healthcare accounts for 17.8% of the United States GDP as of 2015 (Centers for Medicare & Medicaid Services 2016). On a global scale, U.S. healthcare is more than double that of other developed countries and has the highest per-capita healthcare spending in the world (Peter G. Peterson Foundation 2016; Squires and Anderson 2015). With $340 billion spent on goods and services annually, the U.S. healthcare system is in a position to drive market change in favor of preserving and restoring public health (Howard and Norris 2016).

Despite this, the United States maintains relatively poor health outcomes (Blumenthal et al. 2015) along with significant racial, ethnic, and socioeconomic disparities in health and access to quality healthcare services (Agency for Healthcare Research and Quality 2010). This has prompted policy makers and healthcare providers to re-envision their approach to population health from an upstream prevention-based strategy in order to reverse the trajectory of poor health and unsustainable costs.

The role of the environment as a determinant of health is often absent from the conversation when exploring the drivers of health outcomes. Similar to social factors, it is well documented that exposures to environmental toxins such as pesticides or endocrine disrupting chemicals such as those found in our food system impact not only the health of individuals but that of future generations (Manikkam et al. 2014; Anway and Skinner 2006). HCWH continues to champion the inclusion of environmental factors in the evaluation of health and implementation of upstream strategies.

18.5.1 Practice Greenhealth

Recognizing that the U.S. healthcare sector is a driving force globally, HCWH focused efforts on building a network and stimulating change within the nation's hospitals. The Hospital for a Healthy Environment program launched in 1998 based on a commitment by the American Hospital Association and the U.S. EPA aimed at advancing pollution prevention efforts in U.S. healthcare facilities. In 2008, under the direction of HCWH, Hospital for a Healthy Environment was renamed Practice Greenhealth and reorganized as a non-profit organization. Practice Greenhealth remains as the nation's leading membership and networking organization for healthcare facilities that have committed to environmentally preferable practices. The tools, resources, peer-learning, technical assistance, and measurable outcomes set the sector benchmark for sustainable operations.

In 2012, Practice Greenhealth, HCWH, and a steering committee of leaders from a select number of hospitals throughout the country launched the Healthier Hospitals

Initiative as a three-year challenge to the sector to collectively track and benchmark their progress towards common operational goals that improve environmental and human health outcomes. Through the collective action of over a 1,000 participating hospitals and subsequent reporting by a subset of participants, the Healthier Hospitals Initiative achieved in just three years:

- Elimination of 73,600 metric tons of greenhouse gas emissions or the equivalent of removing 15,600 vehicles from U.S. roads annually.
- Diversion of 445,722 tons of materials from landfills.
- Spent $6,745,284 on certified cleaning agents that do not contain chemicals of concern representing 46.3% of monies spent for these products.
- Reduced meat purchases by 1,359,009 lbs. equating to the prevention of 21,093 metric tons of carbon dioxide release into the atmosphere (Quint 2015).

The initiative has now become a formal program of Practice Greenhealth.

18.5.2 GREENHEALTH EXCHANGE

Hospitals within the HCWH and the Practic Greenhealth network are forging new models and leveraging their aggregated demand to prompt a transformation of the healthcare supply chain in the United States. However, evaluations of progress indicate that the rate at which the healthcare supply chain is responding to demand for environmentally sound products is too slow to address urgent public health threats. In 2016, HCWH and Practice Greenhealth launched Greenhealth Exchange as a green purchasing cooperative designed to accelerate the adoption of environmentally superior products and technologies in the marketplace. Evolving from the group-purchasing model that dominates the healthcare supply chain, Greenhealth Exchange leverages the aggregated demand and commitment of its member hospitals to prioritize only products meeting the environmentally preferable purchasing standards of HCWH. In addition, an objective of Greenhealth Exchange is to assist hospitals in localizing their purchases to bring economic vitality to the communities the hospitals serve.

18.6 HEALTHY FOOD IN HEALTH CARE

Acknowledging that current global and U.S. food and nutrition policies favor a consolidated food marketplace where access to fresh, health-promoting foods comes at a premium, HCWH launched the Healthy Food in Health Care program to harness the purchasing power, expertise, and voice of the healthcare sector to advance the development of a sustainable food system. HCWH maintains a vision of a global food system comprised of a diverse network of local food systems that are transparent, health and wealth promoting, resilient, sustainable, fair, and economically just. Since 2005, the work of this national program has brought the sector's clout and perspective to bear on critical food systems issues, such as the overuse and misuse of antibiotics in animal agriculture, aligning dietary guidelines with health and sustainability principles, strategies to reduce the impact of food production on climate, and opportunities for healthcare to make upstream investments in public health. This program works with over 1,000 hospitals across North America to source and serve foods that are produced, processed, and transported in ways that are protective of public and environmental health. In collaboration with thousands of health professionals, HCWH has assisted in the creation of sustainable food purchasing policies; the development of environmental health curricula; and advocacy for healthy food policy at the federal, state, and local levels.

18.6.1 The Environmental Nutrition Approach-Redefining Healthy Food for Health Care

At the foundation of the Healthy Food in Health Care program is the concept of environmental nutrition. Environmental nutrition is the understanding that "healthy food cannot be defined by nutritional quality alone, rather it is the end result of a food system that conserves and renews natural resources, advances social justice and animal welfare, builds community wealth, and fulfills the food and nutrition needs of all eaters now and into the future" (Tagtow and Harmon 2009). While nutrition quality and environmental impact varies within food groups depending upon the methods of production used (Ghebremeskel and Crawford 1994; Health Care Without Harm 2017), it is well documented that food production practices both directly and indirectly impact environmental and public health (Casey et al. 2015). Therefore, HCWH argues that nutrition recommendations must take into account agricultural production practices and the potential health risks generated by agricultural decisions in order to adequately guide the public towards food that will optimize health.

This new approach to food and nutrition policy is controversial, as exemplified by the dialogue following the release of the 2015 Dietary Guidelines Scientific Advisory Committee Report which suggested national dietary recommendations focus not only on nutritional composition but also follow "sustainable diet" principles. As a result, agriculture, nutrition, and health professionals were for the first time at the same table discussing the trajectory of our nation's food and nutrition policy. Ultimately, sustainable diet principles were not embraced, reaffirming the need for additional advocacy by the healthcare community to emphasize the critical connection between agriculture and health.

18.6.2 The Healthy Food in Health Care Pledge

To guide hospitals in championing this broader concept of environmental nutrition in their operations, the Healthy Food in Health Care Pledge was initiated in 2006. By signing this non-binding pledge of principles, it has prompted over 550 healthcare facilities to date to align with their peers and work toward a vision of a food system that supports human and environmental health. As a next step, hospitals are urged to set a strategic plan towards implementing strategies in their own operations in order to support this collective vision. A HCWH Menu of Options is provided and includes activities such as: Articulating an internal food policy; setting purchasing criteria that prioritize verifiable sustainable production; hosting a farmer's market on hospital grounds; creating a hospital garden; or reducing and composting food waste. This "Menu" allows facilities to initiate activities that prompt a shift internally while also impacting the broader food marketplace by creating greater access to foods produced sustainably.

To augment the virtual peer-learning network, the Healthy Food in Health Care program employs far-reaching, on-the-ground work in designated "innovation regions" throughout the country. Active regions include: California, the Pacific Northwest, the Southwest, Michigan, the Northeast, and the Mid-Atlantic with new relationships underway in the Southeast. Central to the success of innovation region activities is an active and engaged set of healthcare facilities that form HCWH Hospital Leadership Teams. These hospitals are dedicated to implementing new models of food purchasing, forging community connections with otherwise unlikely partners, and applying strategies that place their hospitals as drivers for local food system growth and viability. As momentum for the Healthy Food in Health Care program grows, leadership facilities drive innovative strategies and models that are then elevated and replicated throughout the Practice Greenhealth and HCWH networks.

18.7   PARTNER ALIGNMENT AND COLLECTIVE ACTION

An essential component to the success of HCWH and the Healthy Food in Health Care program is the development and maintenance of key partnerships including those with allied non-profit organizations, governmental entities, health professional associations, and other institutional sectors. Each hospital within the network has the individual power to motivate change, but their individual power is amplified in collaboration with other hospitals, health systems, and even allied anchor institutions such as schools and colleges. Anchors in Action, formed in 2016, is a first-of-its-kind, national cross-sector partnership with the Center for Good Food Purchasing, HCWH, Real Food Challenge, and School Food Focus. Together these groups represent a collective network of hospitals, elementary and secondary schools, municipal agencies, and colleges and universities. These founding organizations aim to shape the public conversation about food systems change; clarify priority food system standards among institutions; pilot and prove models of food system change at a cross-sector and a multi-institutional level; and leverage public and institutional monies to localize food economies and open pathways for equitable food access.

By joining forces, Anchors in Action creates a cohesive voice to the food marketplace prompting swift action through the collective demand of multi-sector institutions.

Whether it is collective action facilitated by cross-sector collaboration, a national cohort of hospitals—or discrete partnerships with agriculture, health, and community organizations—Healthy Food in Health Care embraces the opportunity to maximize the impact of programs and strategies through these relationships. The following examples of Healthy Food in Health Care's "innovation in action" showcase the multi-level scale and focus of programs and strategies undertaken to stimulate progress towards a sustainable food system.

18.8   INNOVATION IN ACTION: RESILIENT COMMUNITIES

Several provisions of the Patient Protection and Affordable Care Act (ACA) which was signed into law in 2010 sought to promote an important shift in the U.S. healthcare community—from treating sickness and disease to promoting prevention and wellness. In particular, the December 2014 changes in the IRS regulations governing the community benefit regulations of tax-exempt hospitals under the ACA allowed greater flexibility for health industry leaders to promote population health interventions. This includes upstream environmental health interventions such as food access investments, substandard housing remediation, toxin reduction, and a variety of climate-related interventions. This affords a powerful opportunity for non-profit hospitals to collaborate with other stakeholders to implement community health improvement plans that address the social determinants of health such as the availability of high quality, affordable food.

In addition to community benefit funds, many hospitals have access to investment funds as well as hospital-affiliated foundations—or public and private grants that may amplify the impact of their investments. Many U.S. hospitals are self-insured too, providing the impetus to invest funds in the health of their staff to reduce health insurance expenditures. HCWH promotes widespread adoption of upstream investment strategies by hospitals as an opportunity to improve community health and reduce healthcare costs. In particular, hospital community benefit programs that strengthen food system resilience and sustainability, improve physical and economic access to healthy foods, and promote healthier dietary patterns hold the greatest promise. Shifting healthcare facilities to rely on a regional food system has the opportunity to instill a fundamental shift in ownership in promoting good health by revitalizing our communities through job training, land preservation and stewardship, and equitable reimbursement of labor and goods.

18.8.1   ANCHORS IN RESILIENT COMMUNITIES

Anchors in Resilient Communities (ARC) is a multi-sector collaborative initiated by Emerald Cities Collaborative and HCWH that applies an upstream approach to community health and wealth with emphasis on the San Francisco Bay Area communities of Oakland and Richmond. Each organization brings its unique strategies, partners, and long-term relationships with anchor institutions and the community to the table to deliver the outcomes articulated in the ARC mission: A strategy for long-term anchor institution engagement with community partners which will leverage their economic, political, community benefit, and investment assets to support and create resilient, equitable, and sustainable communities.

Despite a thriving technology-fueled economy in San Francisco, income and health inequities in the San Francisco Bay Area are prevalent and on the rise (Reidenbach et al. 2016; Ilton et al. 2008). Attempts at addressing these inequities nationally have often failed to include the communities most impacted in the architecture of solutions and therefore, have not been successful in reversing the trends of food insecurity, chronic disease, and other social determinants of health. With community engagement as a primary pillar of the ARC project, community members participate together with anchor institutions in articulating a common mission, common values, and a commitment to equity while being active in the design and implementation of the project. This important program design element is a new orientation for how hospitals interact with the communities they serve, placing decision-making in the hands of those most affected.

Comprised of representatives from key anchor institutions in the health and education sectors, non-profit organizations, lenders, foundations, community leaders, and city and county government, ARC focuses on expanding community wealth and ownership, improving health outcomes, and strengthening the capacity of communities of color and low and moderate-income residents to be resilient in the face of climate and economic disruption. An initial assessment of the collective procurement of goods and services of anchor institutions in the East Bay corridor totaled $6.8 billion dollars per year (Dubb and Rudzinski 2016). If even a small percentage of this wealth was shifted to the local economy, improvements to community health and wealth could be profound.

After a robust analysis that included community stakeholder interviews to assess the needs of the East Bay community, fostering healthy regional food systems was identified as a realistic and attainable strategy to help improve health outcomes and build community wealth in the Bay Area. This was based on factors including the existing agricultural productivity of the region and the vibrant urban "good food" and food justice movements in the underserved communities of Oakland and Richmond.

18.8.2 MyCultiver

The Anchors in Resilient Communities planning team recognized that directing the purchasing of East Bay anchor institutions to regional farm and food businesses has the opportunity to create market access and stimulate local economic growth. However, prioritizing the purchase of regionally produced and processed foods by institutions has many imbedded challenges such as: Lack of processing infrastructure, garnering enough supply, and processing whole foods to the institutions' specifications. However, this also presents opportunities for infrastructure investments and local job growth that can localize the food economy and transition the ownership of a regional food system back to the community. A localized, sustainable food system can stimulate increased sustainable food production in the urban neighborhoods and beyond, preserve agricultural land, and provide greater control by purchasers over food product development. Sustainable food production can create the co-benefit of mitigating climate impact from the dominant food system reliant on industrial-scale conventional food production (Rodale Institute 2014).

One of the first proposed projects of ARC, MyCultiver, was launched in 2017 with the aim of producing up to 200,000 healthy, locally-sourced meals per day to distribute to institutions in the region, including large health systems and hospitals. These meals will be comprised mostly of fresh, seasonal, locally produced sustainable ingredients and will be delivered ready-to-eat to institutions all over the region. The project includes the development of a 100,000-square-foot food processing and meal preparation/distribution center secured in Richmond, California. Within a single program, MyCultiver will create jobs and business ownership opportunities for residents; support urban and regional sustainable food production; and increase access to healthy food for community residents in Oakland and Richmond. Jobs generated by MyCultiver will pay a minimum of $15/hour, with training and transportation to the jobsite provided for the first six months.

Anchor in Resilient Communities sets in motion a series of four working groups, which provide engagement opportunities for community partners, food producers, and anchor institutions in the region:

1. Economic/Workforce Development Work Group—Focused on the creation of career pathways through relationships with non-profit partners in Oakland and Richmond and the Department of Economic Development of both cities.
2. Food Production and Distribution Work Group—Focused on the development of a producer's cooperative that will allow both urban and regional sustainable food producers to participate as suppliers for the MyCultiver meal preparation and food product development facility.
3. Microbusiness Development Work Group—MyCultiver is developing relationships with several small food businesses in Oakland and Richmond that are interested in scaling up their production to enter into institutional markets. The MyCultiver processing facility in Richmond will have capacity for large-scale processing of local products that can open potential markets for the smaller processors.
4. Healthy Food Access Work Group—A focus on exploring potential expansion of meal delivery programs in the East Bay communities of Oakland and Richmond by developing strategies to increase access to healthy foods through neighborhood distribution.

18.8.3   INSTITUTION-SUPPORTED AGRICULTURE

The success of MyCultiver is dependent upon the ability to aggregate food products from local food producers both in urban communities and in the surrounding 250-mile foodshed (the foods produced in a specific region). To produce the volume of food needed to meet institutional demand, both urban and regional food producers need up-front support in the form of committed purchase volumes and other investment. Traditionally, farmers hold great risk at the beginning of a growing season as they plant what they think they can sell and hope that enough can be sold to cover their costs. A growing market for local foods is helping to absorb some of that risk, but institutional buying agreements take this support to a whole new level. Since ARC includes participation and a pre-commitment to purchase from MyCultiver by local institutions, MyCultiver can determine how many millions of pounds of local food products are needed for institutional contracts on an annual basis, making pre-planning and contracting with farmers possible. This includes anything from raw foods such as carrots, beets, potatoes, onions to finished value-added products such as pasta sauce and salsa.

18.9 INNOVATION IN ACTION: TRANSFORMING MEAT PRODUCTION AND DRIVING LESS RESOURCE INTENSIVE DIETS

In recognition of the well-documented human and environmental health concerns associated with intensive animal production, HCWH launched a Less Meat, Better Meat strategy in 2010 challenging hospitals to deliver an important preventive health message to patients, staff, and communities by reducing the amount of meat and poultry they serve and prioritizing the purchase sustainably produced meat. Active today, the challenge prompts hospitals to reduce their meat purchases by 20% while transitioning remaining meat purchases to those from production systems that are judicious with our natural resources and important human medicines (such as antibiotics). By participating, hospitals change the composition of their menus and purchases to drive changes in meat production to reduce their respective environmental footprint while improving nutritional quality. By transitioning to sustainable meat purchases and reducing meat procurement altogether, hospitals can improve human health outcomes while transforming and conserving agricultural resources that foster biodiversity.

In assessing the current meat production system, HCWH identified the overuse of antibiotics—critical medicines important for the health of human populations—as a fundamental problem of industrial-scale confined animal production. Raising livestock to emphasize efficiency by confining a large number of animals in close quarters prompts a higher risk for disease and the transmission of antibiotic resistance between animals—and from animals to their surrounding environment. In 2011, 13.8 million kg of antimicrobials were attributed to sales and distribution in food-producing animals; this translates to approximately 70% of the overall tonnage of antimicrobial agents sold in the United States (Food and Drug Administration 2015). While antibiotic use is only one concern attributed to the dominant conventional meat production system, efforts to curb its use has pressured the food marketplace to reform their production practices while also raising public awareness about the broader human and environmental health concerns associated with intensive animal agriculture production systems.

18.9.1 FOOD MARKET TRANSFORMATION—AGGREGATING AND COMMUNICATING DEMAND

Consumption rates drive demand and therefore agricultural production. Americans eat more than twice the global average of meat per capita (Organisation for Economic Co-operation and Development 2015). Global consumption of meat is projected to rise alongside economic growth (Tilman et al. 2011). Hospital food service operations often mirror food trends placing meat at the center of the plate amounting to nearly a quarter of hospital food budgets. As a result, hospital food purchases reinforce the demand for food produced from a system that negatively impacts human health and the associated healthcare costs.

To reverse this trend, a growing leadership network of 17 health systems representing over 350 hospitals in the United States joined forces in the formation of the Market Transformation Group (MTG)—a working group convened by HCWH and PGH. The goal of MTG is to leverage the aggregate buying power of participating health systems to accelerate the transformation of the healthcare supply chain towards more sustainable products, technologies, and services. Target initiatives are carefully chosen based on factors such as the potential for broad supplier engagement and market impact. The MTG has prioritized meat sourcing as a first focus with the goal of collectively communicating to the healthcare supply chain their preference for meat and poultry products raised without routine antibiotics. To understand their collective power, MTG member hospitals calculated their food purchases amounted to approximately $200 million on food and beverages annually, including an estimated $40 million on meat and poultry alone.

Suppliers, distributors, group-purchasing organizations, contracted food service management companies, and other relevant parties are invited to meet with MTG members to set goals toward increasing the accessibility of requested meat products. This has assisted in driving a transformation of the institutional food marketplace and the meat production system more broadly. At the end of 2016, the production of U.S. broiler chicken verified as No-Antibiotics-Ever (NAE) grew to nearly 33% of total production (O'Keefe 2017). By 2016, hospitals in the MTG noted upward of 60% of their meat and poultry purchases qualified under HCWH standards for judicious antibiotic use. The impacts of this focused group of hospitals has rippled throughout the sector with 54% of hospital respondents to the annual Practice Greenhealth sector survey reporting the purchase of sustainable meats.

18.9.2 POLICY AND CULTURE TRANSFORMATION—CLINICIAN ENGAGEMENT

While hospital purchasing is driving market changes, clinicians remain on the front lines driving public health behaviors. Clinicians are often faced with the health consequences of our food production decisions, which challenges their ability to provide effective care. The respected voice of clinicians is a powerful vehicle for motivating local and national legislative action in favor of public health. Clinicians have long demonstrated their capacity to shape health by influencing policies. This type of advocacy encourages clinicians to step beyond clinical practice into an often less familiar arena of policy and politics. This has been especially important in conversations surrounding strategies to address antibiotic resistance.

In 1998, the National Academy of Sciences noted that antibiotic-resistant bacteria generate a minimum of $4 billion to 5 billion in costs to U.S. society and individuals yearly. In 2009, Cook County Hospital (Chicago, Illinois) and the Alliance for Prudent Use of Antibiotics estimated that the total healthcare cost of antibiotic-resistant infections in the United States was between $16.6 billion and $26 billion annually. Evidence has demonstrated that hospital-based Antibiotic Stewardship Programs (ASPs) significantly reduce hospital rates of antibiotic-resistant infections. However, most existing programs fail to address the upstream causes of to antibiotic-resistant bacteria such as animal agriculture (DiazGranados 2012; Elligsen et al. 2012).

To address this gap in knowledge and focus within the health professional community, the Clinician Champions in Comprehensive Antibiotic Stewardship (CCCAS) collaborative was formed as a joint committee of HCWH, the Pediatric Infectious Disease Society, and the Sharing Antimicrobial Reports for Pediatric Stewardship group. Led by a steering committee of clinician representatives from the founding organizations, membership is open to any medical health professional invested in increasing the knowledge within the clinical community of the link between antibiotic resistance and antibiotic use in agriculture and in promoting policy action that supports judicious use.

Since its founding in 2015, CCCAS has prompted action within the healthcare community during the annual Centers for Disease Control and Prevention (CDC) Antibiotics Awareness Week in November. In 2015, the CCCAS Antibiotics Awareness Week activity garnered national media attention when they called on clinicians to commit to changing their own purchasing behavior by selecting a turkey raised without routine antibiotics for their holiday meals. In 2016, the Collaborative prompted clinicians to submit a written request to their local or affiliate hospital requesting a commitment for the hospital to phase out the purchase of these meats. In 2017, CCCAS released guidance for clinicians on formulating a science-based narration of their personal experiences with antibiotic resistance for use in advocacy and social media.

Aside from this annual week of action, CCCAS offers the tangible application of a comprehensive approach to antibiotic stewardship by way of creating tools such as the *Antimicrobial Stewardship Through Food Animal Agriculture Toolkit Module: Guidance For Health Care Facilities And Health Professionals* released in 2017. The toolkit follows the CDC Core Principles of Antibiotic Stewardship to guide hospital-based clinicians in incorporating strategies of food procurement and tracking into their Antimicrobial Stewardship Programs. A primary aim of the toolkit is to increase the uptake of hospital purchasing resolutions to phase out the use of meat raised without routine antibiotics and activate clinicians as advocates for important federal policies that mandate the judicious use and monitoring of these important medicines in agriculture. Additionally, in 2017 the group sponsored a Health Care Culinary Contest where participating facilities were encouraged to "reimagine hospital food" and encouraged showcasing vegetarian and vegan meals alongside the reduction in meat-based meals.

18.10 CONCLUSION

The work of HCWH and its many programs and affiliations has forged an important bridge between the health professional community and that of the food and agriculture sector. Often seen as separate in their focus and impact, the need to address this disconnect is urgent. Agricultural decisions such as the use of synthetic pesticides, the loss of community wealth through food system consolidation, and the increased production of meat globally directly impacts human and environmental health. This impact can be seen through variations in the quality of our food and the safety of the air, water, and land where we live, work, eat, and play. Agricultural decisions are public health decisions and, therefore, it is essential that the healthcare community promotes sound and healthy agricultural practices and policies as primary stewards of public health. Healthcare facilities and health professionals connected to the HCWH network have made this important connection that affirms the inextricable link between the health of our environment and that of the public. Through changes in their practices, these facilities have modeled to the broader global health community that change can and must take place.

REFERENCES

Agency for Healthcare Research and Quality. 2010. Disparities in healthcare quality among racial and ethnic minority groups. U.S. Department of Health & Human Services. https://archive.ahrq.gov/research/findings/nhqrdr/nhqrdr10/minority.html.

American Medical Association. 2001. AMA resolution 506: Use of antimicrobials in consumer products. https://www.ama-assn.org/sites/default/files/media-browser/public/mss/a16-mss-proceedings-032017.pdf.

Anway, M., and M. Skinner. 2006. Epigenetic transgenerational actions of endocrine disruptors. *Endocrinology* 147(6 Suppl.): S43–S49, doi: 10.1210/en.2005-1058.

Belaich, A., and J.P. Belaich. 1976. Microcalorimetric study of the anaerobic growth of Escherichia Coli: Growth thermograms in a synthetic medium. *Journal of Bacteriology* 125(1): 14–18.

Blumenthal, D., M. Abrams, and R. Nuzum. 2015. The affordable care act at 5 years. *New England Journal of Medicine* 372(25): 2451–2458, doi: 10.1056/NEJMhpr1503614.

Casey, J., B. Kim, J. Larsen, L. Price, and K. Nachman. 2015. Industrial food animal production and community health. *Current Environmental Health Reports* 2(3): 259–271, doi: 10.1007/s40572-015-0061-0.

Centers for Medicare & Medicaid Services. December 6, 2016. The national health expenditure accounts government. *Centers for Medicare & Medicaid Services.* https://www.cms.gov/research-statistics-data-and-systems/statistics-trends-and-reports/national-healthexpenddata/nationalhealthaccountshistorical.html.

Chartier, Y. 2014. *Safe Management of Wastes from Health-Care Activities: A Practical Guide.* World Health Organization. http://site.ebrary.com/id/10931321.

DiazGranados, C. 2012. Prospective Audit for antimicrobial stewardship in intensive care: Impact on resistance and clinical outcomes. *American Journal of Infection Control* 40(6): 526–529, doi: 10.1016/j.ajic.2011.07.011.

Dubb, S., and A. Rudzinski. 2016. Building resilient communities summary report. The democracy collaborative. https://noharm-global.org/sites/default/files/documents-files/4284/Building%20Resilient%20Communities%20Summary%20Report.pdf.

Elligsen, M., S. Walker, R. Pinto, A. Simor, S. Mubareka, A. Rachlis, V. Allen, and N. Daneman. 2012. Audit and feedback to reduce broad-spectrum antibiotic use among intensive care unit patients: A controlled interrupted time series analysis. *Infection Control and Hospital Epidemiology* 33(4): 354–361. doi: 10.1086/664757.

Farshad, A., H. Gholami, M. Farzadkia, R. Mirkazemi, and M. Kermani. 2014. The safety of non-incineration waste disposal devices in four hospitals of Tehran. *International Journal of Occupational and Environmental Health* 20(3): 258–263. doi: 10.1179/2049396714Y.0000000072.

Food and Drug Administration. 2015. FDA summary report on antimicrobials sold or distributed for use in food-producing animals, September 2014. *Food and Drug Administration Department of Health and Human Services.* https://www.fda.gov/downloads/ForIndustry/UserFees/AnimalDrugUserFeeActADUFA/UCM476258.pdf.

Ghebremeskel, K., and M.A. Crawford. 1994. Nutrition and health in relation to food production and processing. *Nutrition and Health* 9(4): 237–253, doi: 10.1177/026010609400900401.

Green Guide for Health Care. 2017. Green guide for health care – About GGHC: development history. Toolkit. *Green Guide for Health Care*. https://www.gghc.org/about.history.php.

Health Care Without Harm. 2017. Redefining protein: Adjusting diets to protect public health and conserve resources. https://noharm-uscanada.org/RedefiningProtein.

Howard, T., and T. Norris. 2016. *Can Hospitals Heal America's Communities*. Retrieved from Democracy Collaborative: www. democracycollaborative.org. http://democracy-collaborative.org/content/can-hospitals-heal-americas-communities-0.

Ilton, T., S. Witt, and D. Kears. 2008. Life and death from unnatural causes: Health and social inequity in Alameda County, Oakland, CA. *Alameda County Public Health Department*. http://www.acphd.org/media/53628/unnatcs2008.pdf.

Initiative for a Competitive Inner City. 2011. Initiative for a competitive inner city. V.1.2. Nonprofit. *Inner City Insights*. http://icic.org/research/anchor-initiatives/.

Lee, B., M. Ellenbecker, and R. Moure-Ersaso. 2004. Alternatives for treatment and disposal cost reduction of regulated medical wastes. *Waste Management* 24(2): 143–151, doi: 10.1016/j.wasman.2003.10.008.

Manikkam, M., M. Haque, C. Guerrero-Bosagna, E. Nilsson, and M. Skinner. 2014. Pesticide methoxychlor promotes the epigenetic transgenerational inheritance of adult-onset disease through the female germline. *PLoS One* 9(7): e102091, doi: 10.1371/journal.pone.0102091.

National Research Council. 2006. *Health Risks from Dioxin and Related Compounds: Evaluation of the EPA Reassessment*. Washington, DC: National Academies Press. http://www.nap.edu/catalog/11688.

Nguyen, A. 2017. Vietnam - Hospital waste management support project: P119090 - Implementation status results report : Sequence 12. ISR27092. *The World Bank*. http://documents.worldbank.org/curated/en/463421488967364394/Vietnam-Hospital-Waste-Management-Support-Project-P119090-Implementation-Status-Results-Report-Sequence-12.

O'Keefe, T. March 14, 2017. One-third of US broilers raised antibiotic free. *WATTAgNet.com*. http://www.wattagnet.com/articles/30116-one-third-of-us-broilers-raised-antibiotic-free?v=preview.

Organisation for Economic Co-operation and Development. 2015. Agricultural output - Meat consumption - OECD data. *Organisation for Economic Co-Operation and Development*. http://data.oecd.org/agroutput/meat-consumption.htm.

Peter G. Peterson Foundation. October 17, 2016. Per capita healthcare costs – International comparison. Nonprofit. *Peter G. Peterson Foundation*. http://www.pgpf.org/chart-archive/0006_health-care-oecd.

Quint, C. May 11, 2015. Healthier hospitals initiative's 2014 milestone report caps three years of sustainability achievement among hospitals nationwide. *Healthier Hospitals Initiative*. http://healthierhospitals.org/media-center/press-releases/healthier-hospitals-initiatives-2014-milestone-report-caps-three-years.

Rafiee, A., K. Yaghmaeian, M. Hoseini, S. Parmy, A. Mahvi, M. Yunesian, M. Khaefi, and R. Nabizadeh. May 2016. Assessment and selection of the best treatment alternative for infectious waste by modified sustainability assessment of technologies methodology. *Journal of Environmental Health Science and Engineering* 14. doi: 10.1186/s40201-016-0251-1.

Reidenbach, L., M. Price, E. Sommeiller, and E. Wazeter. 2016. The growth of top incomes across California. *California Budget & Policy Center*. http://calbudgetcenter.org/wp-content/uploads/The-Growth-of-Top-Incomes-Across-California-02172016.pdf.

Republic of the Philippines. 1998. An act providing for a comprehensive air pollution control policy and for other purposes. http://www.lawphil.net/statutes/repacts/ra1999/ra_8749_1999.html.

Republic of the Philippines Department of Health. 2008. Medical devices containing DEHP plasticized PVC advisory. http://portal.doh.gov.ph/sites/default/files/advisory_medical_devices_20080603.pdf.

Rodale Institute. 2014. Regenerative organic agriculture and climate change a down-to-earth solution to global warming. Rodale Institute. http://rodaleinstitute.org/assets/WhitePaper.pdf.

Squires, D., and C. Anderson. 2015. U.S. health care from a global perspective. http://www.commonwealthfund.org/publications/issue-briefs/2015/oct/us-health-care-from-a-global-perspective.

Stringer, R. 2011. Medical waste and human rights: Submission to the UN human rights council special rapporteur. *Health Care Without Harm*. https://noharm-europe.org/documents/medical-waste-and-human-rights-report.

Tagtow, A., and A. Harmon. 2009. Healthy land, healthy food & healthy eaters dietitians cultivating sustainable food systems. http://www.uwyo.edu/winwyoming/pubs/healthyland%20healthyfood%20healthyeaters.pdf.

Tickner, J.A., T. Schettler, T. Guidotti, M. McCally, and M. Rossi. 2001. Health risks posed by use of Di-2-Ethylhexyl Phthalate (DEHP) in PVC medical devices: A critical review. *American Journal of Industrial Medicine* 39(1): 100–111.

Tilman, D., C. Balzer, J. Hill, and B. Befort. 2011. Global food demand and the sustainable intensification of agriculture. *Proceeding of National Academy of Sciences of the United States of America* 108(50): 20260–20264, doi: 10.1073/pnas.1116437108.

United Nations Environmental Programme. 2013. Minamata convention on Mercury. http://www.mercuryconvention.org/Portals/11/documents/Booklets/Minamata%20Convention%20on%20Mercury_booklet_English.pdf.

U.S. Environmental Protection Agency. 1988. Hospital waste combustion study-data gathering phase. https://nepis.epa.gov/Exe/tiff2png.cgi/2000MKHN.PNG?-r+75+-g+7+D%3A%5CZYFILES%5CINDEX%20DATA%5C86THRU90%5CTIFF%5C00001012%5C2000MKHN.TIF

U.S. Environmental Protection Agency. 1995. Science advisory board dioxin reassessment review. https://yosemite.epa.gov/sab/sabproduct.nsf/0D86745602ADB6C68525719B006B0260/$File/ec95021.pdf.

U.S. Environmental Protection Agency. 2010. Summary of requirements for revised or new section 111(d)/129 state plans following amendments to the emission guidelines. https://nepis.epa.gov/Exe/tiff2png.cgi/P1009ZW6.PNG?-r+75+-g+7+D%3A%5CZYFILES%5CINDEX%20DATA%5C06THRU10%5CTIFF%5C00001066%5CP1009ZW6.TIF

19 Creating Biodiversity-Friendly Healthcare Institutions

Chin-Lon Lin and Tina H.T. Chiu

CONTENTS

19.1   INTRODUCTION

Healthcare institutions strive to treat or prevent illness and to improve the general health of the population. While the basic tenet of healthcare practice is "Do no harm," the practice of healthcare itself causes a major impact on the natural environment and, consequently, negatively impacts biodiversity and public health. Healthcare institutions such as a general hospital not only use large amounts of a vast array of resources such as electric power, gas, water, and so forth—they generate greenhouse gases. In addition, hospitals produce a large amount of waste that may be potentially hazardous, radioactive, or infectious. The healthcare sector impacts the environment in three different ways: (1) direct effects (2) upstream effects (the manufacturing of medical equipment and pharmaceuticals) and (3) downstream effects (the disposal of waste). This first section discusses the environmental impacts arising from the unique activities of the healthcare industry, while the following sections demonstrate solutions.

19.2   HOSPITALS' IMPACT ON THE NATURAL ENVIRONMENT

19.2.1   ENERGY

Healthcare buildings are intensive energy consumers. They perform energy-intensive activities that include sophisticated heating, cooling, and ventilation systems; computing; medical and laboratory equipment use; sterilization; refrigeration; laundry services; as well as foodservice (U.S. Energy Information Administration 2016). Also contributing to this high-energy consumption is a vast array of medical equipment including high-air exchange rate systems to minimize airborne infections. Hospitals and long-term care facilities operate around the clock, 24 hours a day, seven days a week, all year-round. They most often have cafeterias with cooking equipment; use fuels for emergency electricity generation; and have high-volume laundering facilities. In addition, disposable medical supplies are commonly used in the industry to prevent disease transmission between and among patients and healthcare employees. The manufacturing and disposal of these items are energy intensive (Davies and Lowe 1999).

19.2.2   WATER

According to U.S. Energy Information Administration, inpatient healthcare facilities are the most intensive water users of large commercial buildings (U.S. Energy Information Administration 2016). The water used in hospitals and other healthcare facilities comprises 7% of the total water use in commercial and institutional facilities in the United States (Dziegielewski et al. 2000). The largest uses of water in hospitals are for cooling equipment; the direct use from plumbing fixtures; landscaping; and medical processing/rinsing. Implementing water-efficient practices in commercial and institutional facilities can decrease operating costs by approximately 11% and energy and water use by 10% and 15%, respectively (Water Use in Buildings SmartMarket Report 2009).

19.2.3 MEDICAL WASTE MANAGEMENT

The majority of solid waste (approximately 85%) from healthcare facilities is typical of commercial solid waste streams: Office paper, cardboard, plastics, metals, glass, and food wastes (U.S. Environmental Protection Agency [U.S. EPA] 1994). The other 15%, often referred to as "red bag" or "regulated medical waste" is handled as potentially infectious (U.S. EPA 1994). Radiological and chemical wastes are also generated in the medical sector. A number of chemically hazardous wastes are generated including: Chemotherapy wastes, spent formaldehyde from dialysis membrane disinfection, waste anesthetic gases, photographic processing chemicals, and pharmaceuticals. Additionally, there are uniquely complex and difficult to dispose of wastes. These include multi-hazard wastes that have some combination of infectious, radiological, chemical, or physical hazards which have a significant impact on the environment (U.S. EPA 1994).

19.2.4 AIR EMISSIONS

In 2013, the U.S. healthcare sector was responsible for a significant percentage of national air pollution emissions including acid rain, greenhouse gas emissions, smog formation, criteria air pollutants (oxone, particulate matter, lead, carbon monoxide, sulfur oxides, and nitrogen oxides), stratospheric ozone depletion, and carcinogenic and non-carcinogenic air toxins (Eckelman and Sherman 2016). A study by Chung and Meltzer (2009) found the total effects of healthcare activities contributed to 8% of total U.S. greenhouse gas (7150 million metric tons CO_2 equivalents) and 7% of total carbon dioxide emissions (6103 million metric tons CO_2 equivalents), respectively. In England, the healthcare sector is also a major contributor to carbon emissions. According to data published by National Health Services (NHS) of England, the NHS has a carbon footprint of more than 18 million tons of CO_2 each year—25% of total public sector emissions (NHS 2009). Most of these emissions come from (1) Procurement (60%) and the embodied emissions in the manufacturing and transportation of NHS purchased goods and services, with the two largest categories being pharmaceuticals and medical equipment; (2) building energy (22%) that includes heating, hot water, electricity consumption, and cooling; and (3) travel (18%) that includes the movement of people (i.e., patients, visitors and staff). In Australia, the health sector is responsible for 7% of carbon emissions from all buildings (The Australian Healthcare and Hospital Association 2012).

19.2.5 INCINERATORS

Incineration used to be the predominant disposal method for regulated medical waste. As mentioned in Chapter 18, medical incinerators were found to be significant sources of airborne mercury and dioxin. Since 1997, the number of licensed Hospital, Medical, and Infectious Waste Incinerators (HMIWI) units in the United States dropped from 2400 in 1997 to only 111 by 2004; this 95% reduction is attributed to increasing environmental awareness among healthcare facilities, stricter clean air regulations, and the availability of alternative treatment technologies that eliminate combustion (Healthcare Environmental Resources Center 2017). Since 2013, the U.S. EPA has delineated stricter emission guidelines to reduce mercury by 89%, hydrogen chloride by 85%, lead by 74%, and dioxin/furans by 68%, respectively (U.S. EPA 2013 April). Alternative disposal methods with less impact on the environment such as autoclave, microwave, chemical, and mechanical treatment have been developed and approved for use in a number of states in the United States and other countries (Rafiee et al. 2016; Kühling and Pieper 2012).

19.2.6 DIOXIN

Dioxins and their related compounds are extremely toxic substances, producing negative effects in humans and animals at extremely low doses (Thornton et al. 1996). Of particular concern are dioxin's effects on reproduction, development, immune system function, and carcinogenesis (Thornton et al. 1996). Medical waste incineration is a major source of dioxins (U.S. EPA 2013 August). Polyvinyl chloride (PVC) plastic is the dominant source of organically bound chlorine in the medical waste stream and is the primary source of iatrogenic dioxin produced by the incineration of medical wastes (Thornton et al. 1996). Medical waste incinerators are also responsible for over 10% of nationwide air emissions of mercury and other airborne toxicants such as ethylene oxide that comes from sterilizing medical instruments (U.S. EPA 1997).

19.2.7 PHARMACEUTICAL WASTE MANAGEMENT

Thousands of tons of pharmacologically active substances are used yearly to prevent and treat illness (Kosjek et al. 2005). Pharmaceuticals are ingested or absorbed and then excreted via urine and feces. Many ingested pharmaceuticals are excreted in the original state or are slightly transformed. They are a source of sewage and water contamination as these compounds are not treated in wastewater treatment plants (Tauxe-Wuersch et al. 2005). As mentioned in Chapter 17, pollution by pharmaceutical effluent is an important environmental problem (Fatta-Kassinos et al. 2011). The most common method for the disposal of unused medications for households is putting them in the garbage (Paut Kusturica et al. 2017). Additionally, the practice of flushing drugs into the sewage system still takes place in many countries. However, both Sweden and Germany promote the practice of returning drugs to pharmacies for proper disposal, also known as reverse distribution (Paut Kusturica et al. 2017). The lack of adequate information and clear instructions on the disposal of phamaceuticals is a common problem in most countries around the globe (Paut Kusturica et al. 2017).

19.2.8 WATER DISCHARGES

Hospital wastewater can contain hazardous substances, such as pharmaceutical residues, chemical hazardous substances, pathogens, and radioisotopes. Because of these substances, hospital wastewater can represent significant risks for public and environmental health (Carraro 2016).

19.2.9 SILVER

The large volume of silver-based photographic films used in medical x-ray imaging accounts for over 15% of the domestic silver consumption in the United States (Davies and Lowe 1999). The city of San Francisco's Regional Water Quality Control Board identified wastewater discharges from silver derived from the spent photographic processing chemicals as one of the major sources of silver in San Francisco Bay (Interagency Workgroup on Industrial Ecology, Material and Energy Flows, Materials 1998). The vast majority of these discharges are from small medical offices such as dentists, chiropractors, and orthopedists. The new technology of filmless digital imaging and PACS (Picture Archiving and Communication Systems) eliminated the need for photographic processing and should reduce silver content in medical waste.

19.2.10 MERCURY

Mercury-containing products are common in healthcare settings and include thermometers, blood pressure devices, dental amalgam, saline solutions, batteries used to power medical equipment, reagents, stains, and fixatives in clinical laboratories (Davies and Lowe 1999). Efforts are being made to eliminate or reduce the use of mercury-containing products in healthcare institutions as mentioned in Chapter 18.

19.2.11 IONIZING RADIATION

X-ray imaging, or radiography, is used to assist in the diagnosis of a wide variety of specializations such as chiropracty, oncology, dentistry, orthopedics, and surgery. Nuclear medicine requires the use of radioisotopes in diagnostic and therapeutic medical procedures. When averaged across the entire U.S. population, half of the total ionizing radiation received by U.S. residents comes from man-made sources (US Nuclear Regulatory Commission 2014). Medical x-ray imaging (36%) and nuclear medicine procedures (12%) are the major sources of anthropogenic radiation (US Nuclear Regulatory Commission 2014).

19.2.12 NOSOCOMIAL INFECTIONS

Patients visiting medical facilities are at risk of gaining an infection during their stay, referred to as nosocomial infections. In hospitals alone, 5%–10% of patients contract an infection while under medical care (Wenzel and Edmond 2001; Weinstein 1998). The most common are pneumonia, bloodstream, urinary tract, central catheter, and surgical site infections. (Wenzel and Edmond 2001; Weinstein 1998). Infection control remains an important challenge to the healthcare industry. Many infection control measures have significant environmental ramifications, such as natural rubber latex gloves and gaseous and liquid chemical sterilants.

The negative impact of emissions from the healthcare sector and the related burden of disease is largely unrecognized by the healthcare sector. Interestingly, it is similar in magnitude to the number of annual deaths stemming from preventable medical errors reported (44,000–98,000 each year) in the United States (Eckelman and Sherman 2016; Kohn et al. 2000). In addition to increasing the regulation of safety procedures to prevent medical errors, regulating and ultimately decreasing the healthcare industry's impact on the natural environment is urgent in an era of unprecedented environmental degradation and biodiversity loss.

19.3 HEALTH INSTITUTIONS THAT PROTECT THE NATURAL ENVIRONMENT

19.3.1 THE TZU CHI FOUNDATION: HISTORY AND COMMUNITY OUTREACH

"Working from the source to reduce our carbon footprint, mitigate climate change, and protect the natural environment"

Master Cheng Yen, Tzu Chi Sustainability Report, 2010

Founded in 1966 by Buddhist Dharma Master Cheng Yen, the Buddhist Tzu Chi Foundation started as a small-scale charity. Thereafter, the Master soon found that poverty is often coupled with illness and thus started a free medical mission inviting local doctors and nurses to volunteer. Because that was not enough, she decided to build a modern hospital in Hualien, a remote town on the eastern coast of Taiwan. The hospital opened its doors in 1986, but the Master soon realized great obstacles in staffing the hospital because of difficulties in recruiting doctors and nurses. She built a nursing school and then a medical school to educate these providers. Then came monthly newsletters, a radio program, and a television station. Hence, charity, medicine, education, and humanity became the four major missions of the Tzu Chi Foundation. Because of the dire needs of people around the globe, the Foundation branched out into international disaster relief, a bone marrow donor registry, environmental protection, and community volunteerism. Together these form the pillars of the Foundation.

Out of love for the remarkable beings on the planet and also for planet Earth itself, the Tzu Chi Foundation began promoting recycling in 1990. Poor waste management plagued the country. An article in *Time* that year described Taiwan as "greedy with garbage everywhere" (Branegan 1990). The industrialization of the 1950s and 1960s produced so much waste that the country's waste management system couldn't handle the volume. The rapid buildup of waste in the streets, factories, and homes earned Taiwan the nickname, "Garbage Island" (Chen 2016).

Master Cheng Yen gave a lecture at a high school in Taichung on August 23, 1990. Her talk was received with warm applause from the audience. While she appreciated the positive reception, Master Cheng Yen asked the audience to "use their clapping hands to do recycling." What transpired that day was a massive mobilization of spirit inspired to build a cleaner and greener society. After listening to Master Cheng Yen's talk, Tzu Chi volunteer Shun-Ling Yang, who lived in Taichung, immediately turned her own living room into the first recycling station in Taiwan and encouraged her neighbors to do the same. Many Tzu Chi volunteers have followed her lead since then and diligently promote recycling and environmental protection in neighborhoods, businesses, schools, and on the busy streets (Tzu Chi Foundation 2009).

Tzu Chi volunteers also actively show how to reduce one's carbon footprint and use of resources by carrying their own dining set; using bicycles or push carts to collect recyclables—and implent the 5 R's:

> *Refuse* non-environmentally friendly products.
> *Reduce* the use of materials so to minimize waste.
> *Reuse* anything that still has salvage value. Do not replace casually.
> *Repair* anything that is repairable so to reduce waste and minimize recycling activities.
> *Recycle* things that have salvage value. Do not dump them randomly.

Now understanding the importance of recycling, many residents offered vacant space in their homes or in other suitable sites in the neighborhood for the collection and storage of recyclables. Recyclable items being sent to collecting sites will be sorted before shipping to Tzu Chi's recycling station for further processing. Tzu Chi now has over 300 recycling stations and 8,000 collection sites in Taiwan. More than 80,000 volunteers devote their time in upholding the organization's environmental mandate. But Tzu Chi Foundation's recycling activities are not limited to Taiwan. Tzu Chi volunteers recycle in many countries around the world. It's not enough that people know about recycling—they have to adapt it into their lives. However, our approach to recycling makes the task enjoyable. Tzu Chi's "Eco-Movement" engages the whole family in the green living lifestyle. Children are often invited to volunteer at recycling stations with their family, promoting family bonding.

The Tzu Chi Environmental Protection Stations serve not only as the recycling awareness center, but also as a multi-purpose center for communities. While serving as a place to showcase environmental protection, they offer volunteers a place to gather and socialize while also receiving medical care and meals—especially older adults and those who are handicapped. Because the majority of the volunteers at the centers are older adults, the Tzu Chi Foundation pulls together its resources from the Tzu Chi University and the Tzu Chi hospitals to form a "Silver Age" service project aimed at health monitoring and health promoting services.

Between 1995 and 2015, the amount of paper recycled by the Tzu Chi centers in Taiwan was equivalent to sparing as many as 25 million big trees from the chainsaw (Tzu Chi Foundation 2016). Trees reduce greenhouse gas emissions as they take in carbon dioxide and produce breathable oxygen, preserve biodiversity, and anchor the Earth to prevent the threat of landslides amongst other ecosystem services.

In 2010, Tzu Chi volunteers had seen an increased level of environmental awareness across Taiwan. The campaign reminds people to reduce or refuse plastic products. Our recycling effort has become a national campaign supported by the general public in Taiwan. Consequently, Taiwan has emerged as a world leader in recycling over the past 17 years (Taiwan News 2017). Tzu Chi has played a prominent although seemingly inconspicuous role in leading the effort.

19.3.2 BEYOND RECYCLING

In 2008, Dharma Master Cheng Yen emphasized the idea of "Blessing comes from a simple and frugal life." By seeking fewer material items, we embrace the virtues of diligence and frugality, which are the basis for helping reduce our carbon footprint and preserving biodiversity. As the world faced a food shortage crisis in 2011, Tzu Chi launched an 80/20 Program, which urged people to "eat until 80 percent full and give the other 20 percent to the needy." The program urged people to buy just enough food for themselves, reduce food waste, and use the savings to help the needy of the world. Master Cheng Yen also encourages applying this philosophy not only for food but also in other ways that include water, electricity, etc.

Another way Tzu Chi tackles the problem of food insecurity is by adopting a vegetarian diet. According to The World Population Prospects Report, the global population will reach eight billion by 2025 (United Nations Population Fund (UNFPA) 2013). Thus, denuding more land will occur for food production. Clearing forests contributes to biodiversity loss, climate change, and other environmental maladies. As fruits and vegetables generally require less land, the need to clear huge swathes of land that support biodiversity is diminished. Additionally, a simple vegetable garden at home cuts food costs as well as transportation emissions from traveling to the supermarket.

A vegetarian diet is also a good way to reduce carbon dioxide emissions to mitigate climate change. One vegetarian meal can save up to 780 g of carbon dioxide emissions, 780 g $= 0.06$ kg (daily meat intake) $\times 13$ kg (CO_2-equivalents per kilograms of meat) (Bellarby et al. 2008).

As a Buddhist organization, Tzu Chi respects all living beings right to life, including animals raised for food. The first of Tzu Chi's Ten Precepts, which are also the first of Buddhism's Five Precepts, is abstaining from harming or killing living beings. Upholding this precept involves abstaining from meat and subsequently adopting a vegetarian diet.

In 2010, while the Foundation celebrated the 20th anniversary of its environmental protection advocacy, Tzu Chi launched a series of "Veggies Save Your Health and Brings Auspices to Complete Your Life" events by inviting private and public organizations to experience the vegetarian diet as an action in protecting our planet. In unison with World Environmental Day on June 5, we encouraged simplicity to reduce carbon emissions. The "Savings in 5" campaign promoted water conservation, reducing electricity use, and consuming less gasoline by driving less and walking more. This campaign drew attention to saving our natural resources while increasing physical activity for improved human health.

In 2015, the Tzu Chi Foundation was invited to the United Nations Climate Change Conference (COP21) held in Paris. Thereafter, Tzu Chi USA launched the "Earth Ethical Eating Day" campaign that connects dietary choices to climate

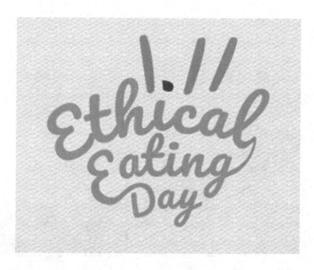

FIGURE 19.1 With the slogan "Eating means everything," Tzu Chi USA uses their annual January 11th Ethical Eating Day campaign to draw attention to the link between diet and climate change, encouraging people to choose vegetarian meals. (Photo courtesy of the Tzu Chi Medical Foundation.)

change mitigation. Every January 11, Tzu Chi invites people to go vegetarian on this auspicious day and spread the word about ethical eating. The campaign collected over 1 million participants around the world by January 11, 2018 (Figure 19.1).

19.3.3 BUDDHIST TZU CHI HOSPITALS, TAIWAN

The Buddhist Tzu Chi Foundation now operates six hospitals on the island of Taiwan, offering high-quality medical care in a compassionate and patient-centered manner where the natural environment is considered every step of the way.

19.3.4 LEADERSHIP

Hospital leadership is critical to championing environmental sustainability. Environmentally conscious leadership provides a vision and incentives that transform the infrastructure to make environmental care convenient and effortless (Figure 19.2). Employees are empowered to "go green" in both their professional and personal lives. Exhibits are also set up to promote the green hospital concept to patients, family, and visitors. All Tzu Chi hospitals are members of the International Health Promoting Hospitals Network as well as the Global Green and Healthy Hospitals.

19.3.5 GREEN BUILDING DESIGN

The Tzu Chi hospitals were built with the vision of reducing resource consumption. The buildings are designed using large skylights and wide corridors between

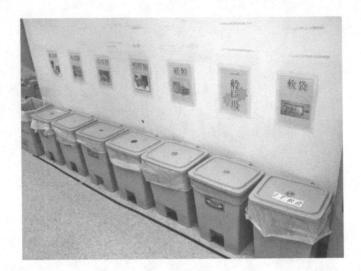

FIGURE 19.2 Recycling stations at Buddhist Dalin Tzu Chi General Hospital. These bins represent the organized recycling system at the nursing stations, labeled in different languages. (Photo courtesy of Chin-Lon Lin, M.D.)

buildings, offering ample natural light and fresh air. This also reduces electricity use and creates a healthy indoor air environment. The hospitals have rainwater collecting systems to reduce fresh water needs. Rainwater is collected on roof tops and from the pavement with permeable bricks which help prevent flooding and soil erosion. In addition, the hospital "skyline garden" creates more green space, increasing oxygen levels, reducing noise, and creating an ecosystem that fosters biodiversity. The architectural design of Taipei Tzu Chi Hospital received the "Health Facilities of The Year" Award by The American Institute of Architects, 1999.

19.3.6 Energy Efficiency

At Taipei Tzu Chi Hospital energy consumption was reduced by turning off the power at night; shutting it off whenever feasible; and by elevating the standard target temperature of the building to reduce air-conditioning needs. Additionally, old light fixtures were replaced with energy-efficient bulbs wherever feasible. Street lamps on the hospital campus were replaced with solar lamps. At the Taichung Tzu Chi Hospital, huge solar panels that follow the direction of sun were installed on the roofs. These photovoltaic systems provide electricity for the hospital. The system provides up to 5% of the hospital's total power needs.

19.3.7 Water Conservation and Recycling

Our hospitals use water-saving devices such as electronic sensor water taps, dual flush toilets, reduced water pressure, and reduced flow volume on each faucet. Buckets of water are collected during a shower to flush the toilet. Water-permeable bricks allow rainwater to filter through to the ground instead of gushing into storm drains. Rainwater reclamation systems and graywater recycle systems were installed wherever feasible to capture and recycle water in order to conserve this precious natural resource. The amount of recycled water at the Dalin Tzu Chi Hospital accounts for approximately 30% of total water usage.

19.3.8   Waste Management

Our hospitals use an "E-hospital" concept by eliminating hard copies of paper or films altogether. This is achieved by using modern information technology such as an Electronic Medical Record (EMR), Hospital Information System (HIS), Laboratory Information System (LIS), and the PACS. These systems aid in the goal of becoming a complete paper and film-free hospital. Additionally, our general waste over the past few years has decreased from 2.05 to 1.92 kg per hospital bed per month while the amount of materials recycled has increased significantly.

19.3.9   Eliminating Disposable Food-Serving Waste

By eliminating disposable tableware while both offering and mandating the use of reusable items whenever possible, it is estimated that solid waste has been reduced by 1,728 kg per year in the Dalin Tzu Chi Hospital alone. Upon employment in all Tzu Chi hospitals, new employees are given a set of dining utensils that includes a bowl, a pair of chopsticks, a cup, and a handbag to store these utensils. Washing stations are readily available.

19.3.10   Managing Plastics Waste

For the recycled plastics, the hospital partners with the company DA.AI Technology, our foundation's subsidiary company founded in December 2008. It is Taiwan's first non-profit company dedicated to producing eco-friendly products, and is one of the world's first non-profit companies that donates 100% of its net proceeds to charity. DA.AI Technology adheres to Dharma Master Cheng Yen's concept of "coexist with the Earth" by using recycled plastic PET bottles as a raw material to manufacture upcycled products, creating a new lifecycle for the PET bottles and reducing the consumption of natural resources altogether.

DA.AI Technology has created recycled raw textile materials such as recycled poly chips, recycled polyester fibers, and recycled fabrics. These recycled raw materials are then upcycled to produce items such as clothing, bedding, and other everyday textile products. DA.AI Technology's production process has earned a "Global Recycling Standard" (GRS) certification from the Netherland's Peterson Control Union. In order to gain GRS process certification, all stages of production from obtaining raw materials to manufacturing and trade have to be in compliance with the GRS standard. Our fleece blankets made with 100% recycled polyester has also received the Carbon Footprint Certification from both the U.S. EPA and the German TÜV Rheinland Group (an internationally recognized provider of testing, inspection, and certification founded in 1872).

DA.AI Technology works with over 8,000 Tzu Chi recycling stations in Taiwan. Each year, nearly 2,000 tons of post-consumer PET bottles are collected and recycled

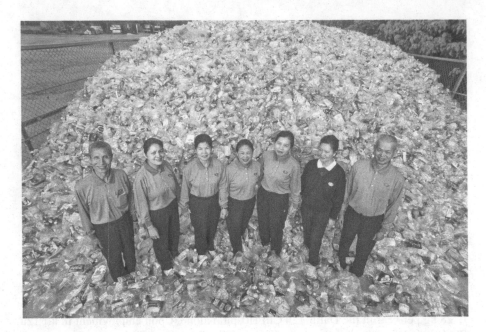

FIGURE 19.3 DA.AI Technology, Tzu Chi's subsidiary non-profit recycling entity. All of DA.AI's profits are directed to charity. Photo courtesy of Chin-Lon Lin, M.D.

with the help of more than 200,000 recycling volunteers. The recycling volunteers carefully sort and clean PET bottles, and remove caps and bottle rings to ensure the quality of raw materials. As of 2016, over 536 million (536,263,228) PET bottles have been recycled and then upcycled (Figure 19.3).

19.3.11 ALTERNATIVE TRANSPORTATION

Buddhist Tzu Chi hospitals encourage staff to take the stairs instead of elevators. The stairways are decorated with beautiful pictures of the natural environment and health promotion tips. Free bicycles are provided to staff, encouraging active living over using cars and motorcycles (Figure 19.4). Furthermore, free shuttle buses are provided between villages and the hospital to encourage people to take public transportation. These measures not only promote an active lifestyle, but reduces 1.2 billion kg of carbon emissions per year.

19.3.12 CREATING LOW-IMPACT FOOD SERVICES

Food service is an area within hospitals where environmental stewardship can be accomplished most often without major changes in infrastructure. Food service is a critically important area of environmental care and in the prevention of biodiversity loss. In aiming for an environmentally friendly foodservice operations, hospitals may work on reducing or preventing food waste, reducing or eliminating disposable food-serving waste, reducing animal product procurement, etc. The vegetarian diet served in all Tzu Chi hospitals have the following characteristics: (1) provide

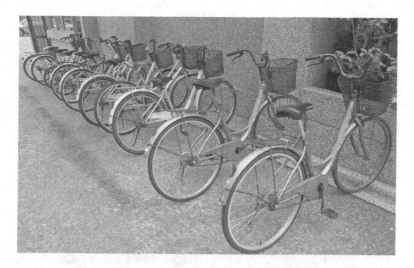

FIGURE 19.4 Free bicycles are offered to Tzu Chi to encourage cycling over driving cars. (Photo courtesy of Chin-Lon Lin, M.D.)

a vegetarian diet that may include dairy and eggs (2) follow the recommendation of the Dietary Reference Intakes (DRIs) which is formulated by the Department of Health, Taiwan (3) provide seasonal fresh food and fruits (4) serve at least 200g of vegetable per meal (5) serve a variety of complex carbohydrates such as unpolished rice, noodles, porridge, steamed buns, etc. and (6) serve meals in accordance with the appropriate medical nutrition therapy regimen.

19.3.13 REDUCING FOOD SYSTEMS IMPACT ON THE NATURAL ENVIRONMENT

Food services influence not only the nutritional and therapeutic aspects of patient care, but also the environmental footprint and biodiversity. Food services may affect the environment in three ways: Direct effect, upstream effect, and downstream effect. The direct effect includes the use of energy and natural resources in the transportation, storage, and the preparation of food. Hence, the use of fresh local food that are grown sustainably and in harmony with the environment not only enhances biodiversity, but also fosters a sense of community that strengthens the relationships between healthcare professionals and the local community.

19.3.14 DIRECT IMPACT OF THE FOOD SYSTEM

As a way to reduce the amount of miles food travels from point of origin to the plate, the Buddhist Dalin Tzu Chi Hospital in Chia-Yi runs an organic farm next to the hospital. The 15-acre farm includes a rice patty, vegetable garden, and an orchard featuring pineapple, mango, guava, bananas, and other seasonal fruits. The hospital hires local farmers to operate the farm, stimulating the local economy while ensuring a reliable supply of fresh produce free of pesticides and other agrichemicals. Additionally, a unique rice species that is smaller in size and softer in texture than

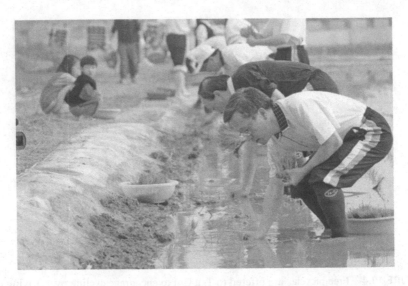

FIGURE 19.5 Growing organic food onsite at, Dalin Tzu Chi Hospital. Physicians and other health professionals participate in planting rice. (Photo courtesy of Chin-Lon Lin, M.D.)

the typical brown rice is chosen. It is used as a "transition food" to encourage replacing white rice with brown rice, providing a practical strategy to help patients adopt a healthier diet by increasing fiber intake that was discussed in Chapter 15.

During planting and harvesting seasons, the hospital regularly organizes recreational agricultural activities on the farm (Figure 19.5). This not only provides unique learning opportunities for health professionals and their families, but it also instills a sense of pride in our community while hospital employees reinforce the concepts of the "farm-to-table" model. It also creates a greater sense of appreciation for foods altogether. For example, Chia-Yi is a farming county and most patients are older farmers. The hospital's recreational agricultural events provide an opportunity for doctors and other health professionals to experience the daily-life activities of farmers, creating a greater understanding of the patient by the health provider. While the food grown at the hospital farm cannot supply the entire hospital's needs, most other foods are purchased locally to reduce the number of miles the food has traveled to reach the plate.

19.3.15 UPSTREAM FOOD SYSTEMS ISSUES

The upstream issues of food systems include the production of food and the overall impact of the food system. Raising cattle and other animals for food creates large amount of greenhouse gases such as methane as discussed in Chapter 3 (Steinfeld et al. 2006). The manure and other waste products contaminates rivers and lands while impacting microbial communities, resulting in devastating ecological consequences (Steinfeld et al. 2006). In order to raise cattle and other animals, large areas of rainforest such as the Amazonian rainforests have been degraded either to grow pasture or soy to feed animals, which drastically harms the natural ecology and the local biodiversity (Grosso 2009). Therefore, implementing a plant-based diet by reducing meat and choosing local organically grown whole plant foods is a key factor to prevent the loss of biodiversity while promoting environmental sustainability.

As mentioned, all of the six Tzu Chi hospitals in Taiwan and another, the Taiwan Adventist Hospital, provide complete vegetarian meals to patients, staffs, and visitors. Each hospital has its own unique way of serving a vegetarian diet according to its local cultural preferences. The Taipei Tzu Chi Hospital has a vegetarian food court that serves vegetarian meals from different cuisines, cultures, and traditions including a vegetarian buffet that serves more than 100 dishes per meal. Other units in the food court offer cuisine from around the globe. It also has the first and perhaps the only vegetarian Starbucks Café in the world. The Taiwan Adventist Hospital has a vegan buffet and a bakery that feature whole foods made without processed oil or sugar. In all of these vegetarian hospitals in Taiwan, meals for patients are planned by Registered Dietitian Nutritionists according to the guidelines for medical nutrition therapy while using whole plant-based foods.

19.4   STRATEGIES TO INCREASE ORGANIC FOODS

Impressively, 60%–90% of the foods served at The Gentofte and Herlev Hospitals in Copenhagen, Denmark are organically grown (Hernàndez 2016). In order to do so without increasing their budget, they have implemented several strategies: (1) reduced meat and increased beans and lentils procurement (2) use of seasonal fresh produce rather than semi-finished products (3) replace more expensive products with good quality but less expensive alternatives, such as replacing olive oil with local cold pressed canola oil or replacing white wine in sauces with local apple juice (4) bake their own bread instead of purchasing finished products and (5) reducing food waste. Some renovations were needed when using fresh local produce such as purchasing vegetable peeling machines.

As government policies have an important influence on food choices and food procurement, the governments in Denmark and locally in Copenhagen support organic farming. As of 2017, 89% of ingredients served in public canteens in Copenhagen are organic (IFOAM EU Group). In contrast, the government agricultural departments that subsidize land settlements, manipulate crop prices, and support the processing of cereals used to feed livestock rather than humans have been shown to have an independent and large deleterious effect on soil fertility, fresh water supplies, biodiversity, and atmospheric carbon (Williams 2017).

19.4.1   DOWNSTREAM FOOD SYSTEMS ISSUES

Downstream food system issues include the management of food waste, disposable food-serving containers and utensils, and packaging waste. Hospitals have a median plate waste of 30% (range: 6%–56%) (Williams and Walton 2011). Commonly used methods to reduce waste include carefully monitoring food waste, adhering to a strict inventory management system, improving meal quality, and serving appropriate portion sizes. Some hospitals implement composting to turn food waste into natural fertilizers that bolster the soil and biodiversity. Unserved and leftover foods could also be used creatively to make other dishes. Leftover food can be sold at a discounted price at the end of the day for employees—or it can be donated to local charities for immediate consumption.

19.4.2 EXAMPLES OF PREVENTING FOOD WASTE

The Freeman Hospital in Newcastle has an average waste of 6% of the foods it serves, which is lower than the 30% average hospital food plate waste (William and Wolton 2011). Two different choices of portion sizes are available for patients, which is associated with decreased food waste (Hernàndez 2016). Another example comes from The University Hospital Complex in Santiago de Compostela in Spain, where only 2.5% of its food is wasted. With its cook-chill system, the hospital is able to accommodate a patient's food request from 8am to 10pm, ensuring that food is ordered and provided when needed (Hernàndez 2016).

19.5 GREEN PURCHASING

"Green purchasing" is a practice where items considered safer and more sustainable are intentionally sourced and purchased. The City of Vienna Climate Protection Program, ÖkoKauf Wien, or "The Eco-Buy, Vienna" has created a database on the contents of commercial disinfectants, making the potentially toxic and harmful ingredient of disinfectants transparent to hospitals in order to encourage procurement of products that are safe and environmentally friendly.

Implementing green purchasing practices forces the institution to consider the environmental impact of all aspects of the product as discussed in Chapter 18. In addition to the primary factors traditionally considered in purchasing decisions such as cost, quality, efficacy, and availability, life-cycle assessments (a description of the environmental impacts of the product or service and its materials during manufacture, distribution, use, and end-of-life or disposal) are also considered. For instance, the Tzu Chi hospitals no longer buy mercury-laden thermometers or sphygmomanometers whenever feasible. The Tzu Chi hospitals purchase green products that carry the Taiwan Green Mark and Taiwan Carbon Label as certified by Taiwan's Environment Protection Bureau.

VIGNETTE 19.1   Khoo Teck Puat Hospital, Singapore

Stewart Tai

INTRODUCTION

Khoo Teck Puat Hospital (KTPH) is a 727-bed general and acute care hospital that opened in June 2010. Serving more than 700,000 people living in the northern sector of Singapore, KTPH combines skilled medical expertise with high standards for personalized care that is set within a visually beautiful healing environment. The building has garnered numerous awards for its green and energy efficient design. From natural ventilation to splendid views of Yishun

Pond, the entire facility connects patients to nature while substantially reducing impact on the natural environment. Yishun Pond supports biodiversity and creates a healing space for patients.

Set amid verdant landscape and soothing water features, KTPH is both "a hospital in a garden" and "a garden in a hospital." Sustainable development and the preservation of biodiversity are important components of KTPH's environmental philosophy. Vast areas of KTPH have been earmarked for landscaping and planting to encourage the creation of wildlife habitat and healthy ecosystems. Terrace and roof gardens along with therapeutic green spaces provide calming surroundings that soothe and rejuvenate. The citrus and edible gardens also provide an organic source of herbs and spices for the hospital.

The provisions offered are designed to promote health for employees, patients, and visitors. For example, the food court offers healthy yet delicious foods prepared with less oil, salt, and sugar that are priced lower to encourage the selection of healthier food choices. KTPH also provides a self-screening health kiosk where users can check their weight, Body Mass Index (BMI), and blood pressure. KTPH regularly conducts activities to educate and empower patients, staff, and community members on maintaining a healthy lifestyle.

KTPH is firmly grounded in its green and energy efficient design. A total savings of 34.6% from our Building Energy Baseline is achieved and verified by an external auditor for Green Mark certification. The Green Mark rating system awards points for low energy consumption, green building design, waste reduction, and reduced carbon emissions.

Conserving water is also a priority. Water from Yishun Pond is channeled to the hospital's irrigation system and is used for landscaping needs. When it rains, sensors are used to regulate this water source and prevent waste. KPTH reduced potable water consumption by 3% and new water use by 6% and was thereby awarded a Water Mark Award in 2016. This is the highest accolade given to an institution for excellent achievements in water efficiency and the conservation of water resources in Singapore.

HARNESSING TECHNOLOGY

Numerous energy conservation measures in the hospital reduce energy consumption such as demand-controlled ventilation, heat recovery systems, and efficient lighting design.

The air-conditioning system is provided by super-efficient chillers with an efficiency of 0.47 kW/refrigeration tons. This is 27% more efficient than the recent range of chillers available. Demand-controlled ventilation also ensures comfortable conditions of temperature and fresh air for patients. Heat pipe technology was adopted to reduce energy waste in operating theatres that use 100% outdoor fresh air. The heat pipe system serves to pre-cool the incoming fresh air using the coolness of the exhaust air from the operating theatres without cross contamination. To ensure the continuous operating efficiency of the chillers, auto tube-cleaning brushes are installed to keep the condenser tubes clean and minimize scaling.

Clean and renewable energy is harnessed through solar energy systems to help offset our carbon footprint. Solar panels or photovoltaic (PV) panels are used to convert solar energy directly into electricity, while a solar thermal system produces hot water for the hospital. The solar thermal system, together with the solar heat pumps, produces all the hospital requirements of approximately 21,000 liters of hot water per day. For the efforts supporting environmental sustainability, KTPH has been awarded the Building and Construction Authority (BCA) Green Mark Platinum Award in 2010, and again in 2016. Also in 2016, KTPH established and implemented an Energy Management System in line with International Organization for Standardization (ISO) 50001 Energy Management System, which ensures high levels of efficient energy performance and continuous improvement. KTPH obtained ISO 50001 certification in December 2016.

SHARING KNOWLEDGE

KTPH continuously engages customers and the public through interest groups and knowledge-sharing sessions. A new energy "dashboard" was built for employees and visitors. It offers a window into KTPH's conservation practices and encourages participation in conservation projects. Guided tours are conducted to visualize the efforts accomplished throughout the hospital.

CONCLUSION

Although hospitals and healthcare institutions are major contributors to environmental problems, they can be a solution by reducing their environmental footprints through their policies and operations. These strategies include but are not limited to: (1) reducing energy and water usage through implementing better architectural designs and technology (2) adopting a policy for green purchasing and creating low-impact food systems by replacing animal products with locally grown fresh whole plant-based foods, and reducing food system-associated waste (3) adopting new ways of eliminating, reducing, reusing, recycling, and upcycling medical and office-related materials and, finally, (4) continuously finding innovative ways to become greener and more sustainable (Healthcare Environmental Resource Center 2017).

REFERENCES

The Australian Healthcare and Hospital Association Policy Brief. 2012. Australian healthcare services and the climate change debate. http://ahha.asn.au/publication/issue-briefs/australian-healthcare-services-and-climate-change-debate

Bellarby, J., B. Foereid, A. Hastings, and P. Smith. January 7, 2008. *Cool Farming: Climate Impacts of Agriculture and Mitigation Potential*, p. 8. Amsterdam, Netherlands: Greenpeace International.

Bernstein, H.M. and M.A. Russo. 2009. Water Use in Buildings Smart Market Report. Bedford, MA: McGraw-Hill Construction.

Branegan, J. 1990. Island of greed: A wave of wild wealth washes over Taiwan. *Time* 135(12): 50–51.

Carraro, E., S. Bonetta, C. Bertino, E. Lorenzi, S. Bonetta, and G. Gilli. 2016. Hospital effluents management: Chemical, physical, microbiological risks and legislation in different countries. *Journal of Environmental Management* 168: 185–199.

Chen, K. May 17, 2016. Taiwan: The world's geniuses of garbage disposal. *Wall Street Journal.*

Chung, J.W., and D.O. Meltzer. 2009. Estimate of the carbon footprint of the US health care sector. JAMA 302(18): 1970–1972. City of Vienna, Austria. https://www.wien.gv.at/english/environment/protection/oekokauf/disinfectants/.

Davies, T., and A.I. Lowe. 1999. Environmental Implications of the Health Care Service Sector. Washington, DC: Resources for the Future.

Dziegielewski, B., J.C. Kiefer, E.M. Opitz, G.A. Porter, G.L. Lantz, W.B. DeOreo, P.W. Mayer, and J.O. Nelson. 2000. *Commercial and Institutional End Uses of Water.* Denver, CO: American Water Works Association Research Foundation.

Eckelman, M.J., and J. Sherman. 2016. Environmental impacts of the U.S. health care system and effects on public health. *PLoS One* 11(6): e0157014.

Fatta-Kassinos, D., S. Meric, and A. Nikolaou. 2011. Pharmaceuticals residues in environmental waters and wastewater: Current state of knowledge and future research. *Analytical and Bioanalytical Chemistry* 399: 251–275.

Grosso, M. 2009. *Amazon Cattle Foodprint.* Paulo: Greenpeace Brazil.

Healthcare Environmental Resource Center. 2017. Incinerators. https://www.greenpeace.org/usa/wp-content/uploads/legacy/Global/usa/report/2010/2/amazon-cattle-footprint.pdf Accessed June, 2017.

Hernàndez, P. 2016. Health care without harm Europe. *Food Waste in European Healthcare Settings.* https://noharm-uscanada.org/documents/food-waste-european-healthcare-settings.

IFOAM EU Group. 2018. Organic on every table leading by example. https://euorganic2030.bio/initiatives/organic-on-every-table/ Retrieved on February 20, 2018.

Interagency Workgroup on Industrial Ecology, Material and Energy Flows, Materials. August 1998. http://www.umich.edu/~indecol/materials.pdf

Kohn, L.T., J.M. Corrigan, and M.S. Donaldson. 2000. *To Err Is Human: Building a Safer Health System.* Washington, DC: National Academies Press.

Kosjek, T., E. Heath, and A. Krbavčič. 2005. Determination of non-steroidal anti-inflammatory drug (NSAIDs) residues in water samples. *Environmental International* 31: 679–685.

Kühling, J.G., and U. Pieper. 2012. Management of health care waste: Developments in Southeast Asia in the twenty-first century. *Waste Management and Research* 30(9 Suppl.): 100–104.

National Health Service (NHS). January 2009. England carbon emissions: Carbon Footprint modelling to 2020. https://www.sduhealth.org.uk/policy-strategy/reporting/nhs-carbon-footprint.aspx

Paut Kusturica, M., A. Tomas, and A. Sabo. 2017. Disposal of unused drugs: Knowledge and behavior among people around the world. *Reviews of Environmental Contamination and Toxicology* 240: 71–104.

Rafiee, A., K. Yaghmaeian, M. Hoseini, S. Parmy, A. Mahvi, M. Yunesian, M. Khaefi, and R. Nabizadeh. 2016. Assessment and selection of the best treatment alternative for infectious waste by modified sustainability assessment of technologies methodology. *Journal of Environmental Health Science and Engineering* 14: 10.

Steinfeld, H., P. Gerber, T.D. Wassenaar, V. Castel, M. Rosales, and C. de Haan. 2006. *Livestock's Long Shadow: Environmental Issues and Options.* Rome: Food and Agriculture Organization of the United Nations.

Taiwan News. 2017. Taiwan's garbage disposal system gets praise from foreign media because of the unique system, Taiwan's recycling rate stands at an impressive 55 percent. http://www.taiwannews.com.tw/en/news/3123172. Retrieved June14, 2017.

Tauxe-Wuersch, A., L.F.D. Alencastro, D. Grandjean, and J. Tarradellas. 2005. Occurrence of several acidic drugs in Environ Monit Assess sewage treatment plants in Switzerland and risk assessment. *Water Research* 39: 1761–1772.

Thornton, J., M. McCally, P. Orris, J. Weinberg. 1996. Hospitals and plastics. Dioxin preven-
     tion and medical waste incinerators. *Public Health Reports* 111(4): 298–313.
Tzu Chi Foundation. July 29, 2009. Implement environmental protection, purify the mind,
     and hold nature in Aw. http://tw.tzuchi.org/en/index.php?option=com_content&vie
     w=article&id=289%3Aimplement-environmental-protection-purify-the-mind-and-
     hold-nature-in-awe&catid=62%3Aenvironmentalprotection&Itemid=186&lang=en.
     Retrieved June 14, 2017.
Tzu Chi Foundation. April 30, 2016. Tzu Chi, 2015 Buddhist Tzu Chi foundation sustainabil-
     ity report, p. 75. http://www.tzuchi.org.tw/doc/2015CSR_complete_small(with_links).
     pdf
Tzu Chi USA. 2017. Ethical eating day – Tzu Chi USA. https://www.tzuchi.us/ethical-eating-
     day/. Retrieved June 14, 2017.
US Energy Information Administration. March 18, 2016. 2012 commercial buildings energy
     consumption survey. https://www.eia.gov/consumption/commercial/
US Environment Protection Agency. 1997. Mercury study report to congress, volume II, an
     inventory of anthropogenic mercury emission in the United States December, 1997.
     https://www.epa.gov/mercury/mercury-study-report-congress
US Environment Protection Agency. April 4, 2013. Hospital/medical/infectious waste incin-
     erators (HMIWI): Promulgated amendments to the federal plan to implement standards
     of performance for existing facilities and promulgated amendments to the new source
     performance standards (NSPS) fact sheet.
U.S. Environmental Protection Agency. 1994. *Medical Waste Incinerators – Background
     Information for Proposed Standards and Guidelines: Industry Profile Report for New
     and Existing Facilities*, EPA-453/R-94-042a. Research Triangle Park, NC: U.S. EPA,
     Office of Air Quality Planning and Standards.
US Environment Protection Agency. August, 2013. Revision: An inventory of sources and
     environmental releases of dioxin-like compounds in the United States for the years
     1987, 1995 and 2000. Washington, DC: National Center forEnvironmental Assessment.
     Office of Research and Development. https://www.nrc.gov/about-nrc/radiation/around-
     us/sources.html
US Nuclear Regulatory Commission. 2014. Sources of Radiation, Updated October 17, 2014.
United Nations Population Fund (UNFPA). June 13, 2013. World population to increase by
     one billion by 2025. http://www.unfpa.org/news/world-population-increase-one-bil-
     lion-2025. Retrieved June 14, 2017.
Wenzel, R.P., and M.B. Edmond. March–April, 2001. The impact of hospital-acquired blood-
     stream infections. *Emerging Infectious Diseases* 7(2): 174–177.
Weinstein, R.A. July–September, 1998. Special issue – Nosocomial infection update.
     Emerging Infectious Diseases 4(3): 416–420.
Williams, H. August 2017. Agricultural subsides and the environment. Oxford Research
     Encyclopedia of Environmental Science, doi: 10.1093/acrefore/9780199389414.013.310.
Williams, P., and K. Walton. 2011. Plate waste in hospitals and strategies for change. *The
     European e-Journal of Clinical Nutrition and Metabolism* 6: e235–e241.

20 The Smallest Sprouts
Engaging Children in Healthy Food Systems

Katrina Hoch

CONTENTS

20.1 INTRODUCTION

Parents and teachers learn the lesson that in any activity, kids will be more enthusiastic if they have participated in decisions and preparations. The soup bubbling on the stove is not so strange to a child if they have stirred it themselves. A child who has been a decision-maker, choosing the bell peppers over the carrots, knows what's in the soup and may feel a sense of pride in it. Food can be a contentious issue in families. Parents want their kids to eat foods that will help them grow and stay healthy, and kids want to maintain autonomy in an area of life that can feel imposed on them. Involving kids in preparing food can create a positive outlook on a meal and may lead to acceptance of new or unusual foods.

If we broaden our lens beyond the individual household, we can envision involving children in food preparation as part of involving them in a healthy food system. Helping in the kitchen is just one way kids can get involved—and accepting unfamiliar foods is just one of the positive outcomes that may result. We can trace the food system upstream from the kitchen to the farms where the food is grown; the process of growing the food; and more broadly to the ecosystem where the growing takes place and the goal of nurturing biodiversity. Schools and community centers are developing programs to get kids involved in each of the steps in this process, and individual households can also implement these activities. Involving children in healthy food systems also includes engaging them in spending time outdoors, gardening, purchasing food from local farms, and cooking.

20.2   SPENDING TIME OUTDOORS

Spending time in the natural world gives kids a context in which to understand the food system. The outdoors is part of the answer to both where food comes from and why they should care. The "biophilia hypothesis" posits that humans have an innate tendency to affiliate with living organisms, and some researchers understand this hypothesis to recognize an innate connection between children and nature (Hand et al. 2016; Soga et al. 2016). Many point out that this connection needs to be cultivated and preserved, as the modern world works against it. Children's exposure to nature is declining as a result of urban development, participation in structured activities, increased access to technology, and the prioritization of vehicles over pedestrians (Hand et al. 2016). We need to ensure we create time and space for kids to be outside.

The benefits of getting kids outside operate on multiple levels, from individual health to environmental consciousness. Mandy LeBlanc, a National Leadership Fellow for the School-Based Health Alliance, points out that walking in nature provides enjoyable physical activity, stress management, and a new perspective on the world. Time spent outside can provide a break from our gadgets, giving us time alone and time for in-person conversations (Turkle 2015). A walk in nature can also restore energy and improve concentration (Taylor and Kuo 2009; Berman et al. 2008). Research indicates that opportunities for outdoor play are associated with lower blood pressure, lower incidence of allergies, increased physical fitness, and increased attention span (Hand et al. 2016; Ohly et al. 2016).

In addition to providing individual and social benefits, building a connection to nature can be part of a framework for addressing environmental challenges. A 2016 cross-sectional study of 397 children living in Tokyo found that experiences with nature were positively associated with positive emotions and attitudes towards biodiversity and willingness to conserve biodiversity (Soga et al. 2016). Additional studies have found the same association (Soga et al. 2016). Research also indicates that the absence of childhood opportunities to experience nature is associated with a lower motivation to protect nature (Hand et al. 2016). This body of research suggests that spending time in nature helps build a conservation mindset that can be a foundation for thinking about food systems and biodiversity.

20.3   GARDENING

Moving one step closer to the realm of food, gardening is another way to get kids engaged with healthy food systems. Gardening, similarly to hikes and walks, provides time away from gadgets and it builds familiarity with fruits and vegetables. Participating in gardening projects can expose kids to a greater variety of produce than they are likely to see at the store (Guitart et al. 2014).

Programs that involve kids in gardening have sprung up all over the U.S. and in many countries (Gibbs et al. 2013; Berezowitz et al. 2015; Morgan et al. 2010; McAleese and Rankin 2007; Robinson-O'Brien et al. 2009; Guitart et al. 2014; Ohly et al. 2016). Gardening can be part of the school curriculum or can be offered as an after-school activity. It can be combined with cooking classes, science classes, or nutrition education. Alternatively, families can involve kids in growing food in the backyard—on an apartment balcony—or in a community garden. Kids love to get dirty; they love to feel competent and helpful—and they're fascinated by watching shoots emerge from the soil. Studies of gardening programs indicate that including a cooking and tasting component creates more robust impacts on kids' behaviors and attitudes (Gibbs et al. 2013).

A 2015 systematic review of 13 studies investigating the impact of school garden programs on health outcomes found that participation led to increased preference for vegetables (Davis 2015). The review also found that participation led to increased willingness to taste vegetables, ability to identify vegetables, and self-efficacy in preparing and cooking vegetables. The results connecting garden programs to actual increases in vegetable intake were inconclusive. This finding of clear effects on preferences and attitudes with unclear effects on concrete behaviors is a feature of other studies and reviews of school garden programs, and suggests that actual behavior change requires a longer and more multifaceted intervention (Davis 2015; Gibbs et al. 2013; Ohly et al. 2016; Berezowitz et al. 2015; Morgan et al. 2010; Robinson-O'Brien et al. 2009). Researchers who have produced similar results have reasoned that changes in intake are difficult to capture in a few months to two years and are more likely if an intervention encompasses not only school-based exposure, but also increased opportunities to eat vegetables at home (Davis 2015; Ohly et al. 2016; Berezowitz et al. 2015; Morgan et al. 2010; Robinson-O'Brien et al. 2009).

A 2016 systematic review of the impacts of school gardening in several countries found qualitative evidence for these programs' positive impacts on children's health, well-being, social development, educational attainment, and awareness of environmental issues (Ohlyet al. 2016). The primary health impacts observed were increased willingness to try new foods and preference for vegetables. Impacts on personal well-being included feelings of achievement, satisfaction and pride from nurturing plants, increased confidence and self-esteem, increased ability to manage emotions, decreased depression and stress, and empowerment in particular for kids who don't usually excel in an academic setting. Social well-being impacts included building relationships, increased teamwork and cooperation, and a sense of purpose and cultural exchange. Educational benefits included attainment of new skills, increased confidence in school attainment, and increased motivation and engagement in schoolwork. Impacts on environmental consciousness included greater awareness of water conservation, seasonality, composting, local wildlife, the food chain, sustainability, and recycling, all echoing previous research suggesting that garden programs increase kids' "ecoliteracy" (Gibbs et al. 2013; Ohly et al. 2016). This review found that quantitative evidence was often lacking due to reliance on study participants' self-report or because outcomes of interest were not measured quantitatively (Ohly et al. 2016).

Increasing kids' fruit and vegetable consumption is an important public health goal, but many plant foods contain bitter or sour flavors that are uncommon in popular children's snacks (Gibbs et al. 2013; Pitts et al. 2015). Accepting unfamiliar tastes requires recurring exposure to new foods (Gibbs et al. 2013). The more accustomed children become to the flavors of a variety of fruits and vegetables, the more likely they will be to accept them. This suggests that lifelong participation in gardening and tasting the harvest has a better chance of changing kids' intake than a one-year intervention.

The individual, interpersonal, and social benefits of school gardens are often intertwined, supporting the view that participation in everyday activities like gardening can engage kids in broader themes such as protecting biodiversity. Tending vegetables can make kids more interested in eating them, and at the same time, helps kids understand the challenges of food production and environmental stewardship.

20.4   BUYING PRODUCE FROM LOCAL FARMS

Learning about where food comes from encompasses not just gardening, but also following food up the chain to local producers and distributors such as Community Supported Agriculture (CSA) programs and farmers markets. As discussed in Chapter 13, a CSA is a type of alternative food network in which consumers join a program set up by a local farm and pay up-front for a weekly share of the farm's harvest for an entire season (Hayden and Buck 2012; Bougherara et al. 2009). The farmers sell directly to consumers, garnering funding at the start of the season for expenses and investments. Consumers get fresh local produce, and some enjoy the surprise and challenge of preparing whatever vegetables the farm harvested that week (Hayden and Buck 2012; Bougherara et al. 2009). They also get to participate in a sustainable food system. A survey conducted of 264 households in France found that CSA consumers are motivated by environmental considerations such as reducing "food miles" (Bougherara et al. 2009). In an ethnographic study of participants in a New York CSA, the researchers observed that participation in the CSA was an effective way to learn about the "where and how" of food production, and the environmental issues connected to it (Hayden and Buck 2012).

While studies investigating CSAs have generally focused on adults, receiving a weekly "box of surprises" can be fun for kids, and the inclusion of less common vegetables in the weekly share can help introduce these foods to children's palates. Additionally, by participating in the ritual of picking up their box of produce from a local farmer each week, kids can learn about the environmental considerations and values that motivated their families to join (Bougherara et al. 2009).

Farmers' markets have grown in popularity and abundance during the past two decades, drawing families with live music, food stalls, and local crafts as well as local farmers selling fruits, vegetables, and flowers (McCormack et al. 2010). Shopping at farmers' markets can also help kids learn about seasonality and local farms. Public agencies have developed programs to make produce from farmers' markets more affordable for low-income consumers (Pitts et al. 2015). A 2015 cross-sectional analysis of Supplemental Nutrition Assistance Program (SNAP) participants in Pitt County, North Carolina found that fruit and vegetable intake was positively associated with shopping at farmers' markets (Pitts et al. 2015). A 2010 review found that farmers' market programs for the Women, Infants and Children (WIC) program and seniors increased participants' intake of fruits and vegetables (McCormack et al. 2010).

20.5   COOKING AND TASTING

Involving kids in cooking can take many forms, from choosing recipes to measuring ingredients to stirring soup. Cooking can also be included in school nutrition or science curricula. One such program was implemented with fourth graders in Northern

Colorado. The study *Fuel for Fun: Cooking with Kids Plus Parents and Play* incorporated a cooking and tasting curriculum and a set of strategies to reinforce the classroom experience in the cafeteria, as well as a separate component to engage parents (Cunningham-Sabo et al. 2016). The researchers found that the intervention was associated with increased cooking self-efficacy for children with no previous cooking experience, particularly for male students, and increased preference for fruits and vegetables, though not increased intake. As with studies of gardening programs, the results showing positive impacts for attitudes about food suggest that behavior change may follow if interventions are continued.

Garden programs tend to have greater success if paired with a cooking program. In the Stephanie Alexander Kitchen Garden Program, 764 kids spent 45–60 minutes per week in garden class and 90 minutes per week in kitchen class. A two-year study of this program compared six program schools and six non-program schools (Gibbs et al. 2013). Both qualitative and quantitative results showed that kids reported an increased willingness to try new foods as a result of the study, yet only qualitative evidence showed an actual increase in healthy eating. The cooking component included learning knife safety, cooking three-course meals using fresh produce, and sharing meals at the end of each class. Kids made bread, pastries, pasta, salads, curries, and desserts from scratch (Gibbs et al. 2013). As with garden programs, this program did not change kids' dietary intake, but it did produce a more positive attitude towards dietary diversity—a first step that, if expanded for a longer duration and into the home environment—would be likely to produce more concrete effects (Gibbs et al. 2013).

20.6 CONCLUSION

The activities discussed above have documented benefits for attitudes about food, and many are likely to change behaviors in the long term. Gardening, shopping at farmers' markets, participating in CSAs, and cooking increase kids' willingness to try new foods, particularly fruits and vegetables. This willingness is important not only for individual health, but also for the food system. Sustainability researchers have pointed out that, if our goal is to ensure that sustainably grown foods are accessible, affordable, and available to all, it is not enough to work towards changing production and distribution systems. We must also ensure that consumers want to purchase, prepare, and consume these foods (James and Friel 2015). Consumer demand shapes the adoption and execution of sustainable diets (Jones et al. 2016). This in turn shapes the economic viability of biodiversity in the agricultural sector, which includes expanding the variety of available fruits and vegetables beyond the familiar supermarket staples (Davis 2015). Conserving biodiversity and promoting healthy food systems requires fitting sustainable foods into busy families' daily routines and making them appealing to kids. Involving kids in outdoor walks, gardening, buying from local producers, and cooking are enjoyable ways to realize those goals.

REFERENCES

Berezowitz, C.K., A.B. Bontrager, and D.A. Yoder. 2015. School gardens enhance academic performance and dietary outcomes in children. *Journal of School Health* 85(8): 508–518.

Berman, M.G., J. Jonides, and S. Kaplan. 2008. The cognitive benefits of interacting with nature. *Psychological Science* 19(12): 1207–1212.

Bougherara, D., G. Grolleau, and N. Mzoughi. 2009. Buy local, pollute less: What drives house holds to join a community supported farm? *Ecological Economics* 68: 1488–1495.

Cunningham-Sabo, L., B. Lohse, S. Smith, R. Browning, E. Strutz, C. Nigg, M. Balgopal, et al. 2016. Fuel for fun: A cluster-randomized controlled study of cooking skills, eating behaviors, and physical activity of 4th graders and their families. *BMC Public Health* 16: 444.

Davis, J.N. 2015. Sustenance and sustainability: Maximizing the impact of school gardens on health outcomes. *Public Health Nutrition* 18(13): 2358–2367.

Gibbs, L., P.K. Staiger, B. Johnson, K. Block, S. Macfarlane, L. Gold, O. Ukoumunne, et al. 2013. Expanding children's food experiences: The impact of a school-based kitchen garden program. *Journal of Nutrition Education and Behavior* 45(2): 137–146.

Guitart, D.A., C.M. Pickering, and J.A. Byrne. 2014. Color me healthy: Food diversity in school community gardens in two rapidly urbanizing Australian cities. *Health & Place* 26: 110–117.

Hand, K., C. Freeman, P.J. Seddon, A. Stein, and Y. van Heezik. 2016. The importance of urban gardens in supporting children's biophilia. *PNAS* 114(2): 274–279.

Hayden, J., and D. Buck. 2012. Doing community supported agriculture: Tactile space, affect, and effects of membership. *Geoforum* 43: 332–341.

James, S.W., and S. Friel. 2015. An integrated approach to identifying and characterizing resilient urban food systems to promote population health in a changing climate. *Public Health Nutrition* 18(13): 2498–2508.

Jones, A.D., L. Hoey, J. Blesh, L. Miller, A. Green, and L.F. Shapiro. 2016. A systematic review of the measurement of sustainable diets. *Advances in Nutrition* 7: 641–644.

McAleese, J.D., and L.L. Rankin. 2007. Garden-based nutrition education affects fruit and vegetable consumption in sixth-grade adolescents. *Journal of the American Dietetic Association* 107(4): 662.

McCormack, L.A., M.N. Laska, N.I. Larson, and M. Story. 2010. Review of the nutritional implications of farmers' markets and community gardens: A call for evaluation and research efforts. *Journal of the American Dietetic Association* 110(3): 399.

Morgan, P.J., J.M. Warren, D.R. Lubans, K. Saunders, G. Quick, and C.E. Collins. 2010. The impact of nutrition education with and without a school garden on knowledge, vegetable intake and preferences and quality of school life among primary-school students. *Public Health Nutrition* 13(11): 1931.

Niaki, S.F., C.E. Moore, T.A. Chen, and K. Weber Cullen. 2017. Younger elementary school students waste more school lunch foods than older elementary school students. *Journal of the Academy of Nutrition and Dietetics* 117(1): 95.

Ohly, H., S. Gentry, R. Wigglesworth, A. Bethel, R. Lovell, and R. Garside. 2016. A systematic review of the health and well-being impacts of school gardening: Synthesis of quantitative and qualitative evidence. *BMC Public Health* 16: 286.

Pitts, S.B.J ., A. Gustafson, Q. Wu, M. Leah Mayo, R.K. Ward, J.T. McGuirt, A.P. Rafferty, et al. 2015. Farmers' market shopping and dietary behaviours among supplemental nutrition assistance program participants. *Public Health Nutrition* 18(13): 2407–2414.

Robinson-O'Brien, R., M. Story, and S. Heim. 2009. Impact of garden-based youth nutrition intervention programs: A review. *Journal of the American Dietetic Association* 109(2): 273.

Soga, M., K. Gaston, Y. Yamaura, K. Kurisu, and K. Hanaki. 2016. Both direct and vicarious experiences of nature affect children's willingness to conserve biodiversity. *International Journal of Environmental Research and Public Health* 13: 529.

Taylor, A.F., and F.E. Kuo. 2009. Children with attention deficits concentrate better after walk in the park. *Journal of Attention Disorders* 12(5): 402–409.

Turkle, S. September 26, 2015. Stop Googling. Let's talk. *New York Times*. Sunday Review.

Index

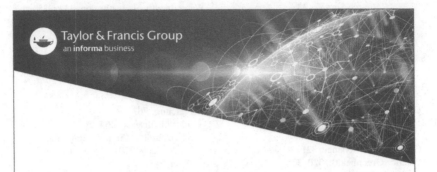

Printed in the United States
by Baker & Taylor Publisher Services